Ethics for Graduate Researchers

Ethics for Graduate Researchers
A Cross-disciplinary Approach

Edited by

Cathriona Russell
University of Dublin,
Trinity College,
Dublin, Ireland

Linda Hogan
University of Dublin,
Trinity College,
Dublin, Ireland

Maureen Junker-Kenny
University of Dublin,
Trinity College,
Dublin, Ireland

ELSEVIER

AMSTERDAM • BOSTON • HEIDELBERG • LONDON • NEW YORK • OXFORD
PARIS • SAN DIEGO • SAN FRANCISCO • SINGAPORE • SYDNEY • TOKYO

Elsevier
32 Jamestown Road, London NW1 7BY
225 Wyman Street, Waltham, MA 02451, USA

First edition 2013

Notices
Knowledge and best practice in this field are constantly changing. As new research and experience broaden our understanding, changes in research methods, professional practices, or medical treatment may become necessary.

Practitioners and researchers must always rely on their own experience and knowledge in evaluating and using any information, methods, compounds, or experiments described herein. In using such information or methods they should be mindful of their own safety and the safety of others, including parties for whom they have a professional responsibility.

To the fullest extent of the law, neither the Publisher nor the authors, contributors, or editors, assume any liability for any injury and/or damage to persons or property as a matter of products liability, negligence or otherwise, or from any use or operation of any methods, products, instructions, or ideas contained in the material herein.

British Library Cataloguing-in-Publication Data
A catalogue record for this book is available from the British Library

Library of Congress Cataloging-in-Publication Data
A catalog record for this book is available from the Library of Congress

ISBN: 978-0-12-416049-1

For information on all Elsevier publications
visit our website at store.elsevier.com

This book has been manufactured using Print On Demand technology. Each copy is produced to order and is limited to black ink. The online version of this book will show color figures where appropriate.

Working together to grow libraries in developing countries

www.elsevier.com | www.bookaid.org | www.sabre.org

ELSEVIER   BOOK AID International   Sabre Foundation

Contents

About the authors

Amy Daughton is Tutor in theology and the Director of studies at the Margaret Beaufort Institute of Theology at Cambridge. She primarily teaches systematics, but co-teaches public theology and is Module Leader for the core course of Narrative and Identity on the Masters in Christian Theology. She gained her PhD in theological ethics from Trinity College Dublin. While at TCD, she supported and co-taught several years of a National fourth level Generic Skills Module for graduate researchers in ethics. She built on this by developing a new seminar series for arts, humanities and social science post-graduates through her Postgraduate Fellowship with Trinity Long Room Hub. These modules focused on shared themes across disciplines and used inter-disciplinary discussions between post-graduates to enable them to identify ethical concerns. Her current research involves the publication of her work on the ethics of inter-cultural hermeneutics. Website: http://www.margaretbeaufort.cam.ac.uk/about-us/staff/dr-amy-daughton/

Gladys Ganiel is Assistant Professor in conflict resolution and reconciliation at the Irish School of Ecumenics (Belfast campus). She serves on the editorial board of the Africa Peace and Conflict Network and has been a Visiting Scholar at the universities of Cape Town and Zimbabwe. Her primary research interests are religion and conflict, Northern Ireland politics, evangelicalism, congregational studies, qualitative research methods, and religion and transition in South Africa and Zimbabwe. She is an investigator on the 3-year IRCHSS funded research project Visioning 21st Century Ecumenism. Previously funded research projects include *Religion, Reconstruction and Reconciliation in Zimbabwe* (the Association for the Sociology of Religion Fichter Grant) and her doctoral research on *Evangelicalism and Conflict in Northern Ireland* (Royal Irish Academy). She received her BA in political science from Providence College, USA in 1999, and an MA (2001) and PhD (2005) in politics from University College Dublin. Website: http://www.gladysganiel.com/my-cv/

Frank Gannon is the Director of The Queensland Institute of Medical Research in Brisbane, Australia since January 2011, and was formerly Director General of Science Foundation Ireland from 2007. Professor Gannon was Executive Director of the European Molecular Biology Organisation and Senior Scientist at the European Molecular Biology Laboratory, based in Heidelberg, Germany (1994–2007). He was also during this time director of the National Diagnostic Centre (1981–2007) and Professor at the Department of Microbiology at University College Galway, Ireland. He has served on a range of high-level scientific advisory boards at institutes throughout the world and was co-founder of the European Life Sciences Forum and the Initiative for Science Europe (ISE). The ISE played a significant role in the establishment of the European Research Council. His major research interest is the regulation of gene expression by the estrogen receptor, in particular related to its role in breast cancer and osteoporosis. He has published over 200 research articles. He holds a BSc from NUI Galway, a PhD from the University of Leicester and was a post-doctoral fellow at the University of Madison, WI. Website: http://www.imb.uq.edu.au/index.html?page=12244.

Sigrid Graumann is Professor for Ethics at the University of Applied Sciences in Bochum, Germany. She studied biology and philosophy at the University of Tübingen and received her PhD in human genetics there in 2000 and a second PhD in philosophy from the University of Utrecht in 2009. From 1994 to 2002, she was Researcher at the Interfaculty Centre for Ethics in the Sciences and Humanities at the University of Tübingen. From 2002 to 2008, she was Senior Researcher at the Institute Mensch, Ethik, Wissenschaft, Berlin, which was founded by nine disability organizations, and taught ethics at the Medical School of the Charité, Berlin. From 2009 to 2011, she was Senior Researcher at the Institute of Social Sciences, University of Oldenburg. Her research interests are in biomedical ethics, human rights and disability. She is a member of the Central Ethics Commission of the German Medical Association, a board member of the Academy of Ethics in Medicine (Germany), a member in the Commission for Genetic Diagnosis of the German Government and a member of the Expert Commission on the Rights of Persons with Disabilities, Family and Bioethics of the Federal Ministry of Social Affairs (since 2011). She has edited and co-edited books and published articles on bioethics, disability and human rights. Website: http://www.efh-bochum.de/homepages/graumann/.

Hille Haker holds the Richard A. McCormick Chair of Ethics at Loyola University, Chicago, having been Professor of Moral Theology and Social Ethics at the Johann Wolfgang Goethe University, Frankfurt, Germany. She received degrees in catholic theology, German literature and philosophy (1989–1991) from the University of Tübingen where she completed her PhD in 1997 and her Habilitation in theological ethics in 2001. At Tübingen's Interfaculty Centre for Ethics in the Sciences and the Humanities, she also served as Scientific Coordinator of the European Network for Bioethical Research. From 2003 to 2005, she was Associate Professor of Christian ethics at Harvard Divinity School, Harvard University, Cambridge, MA. She has served on the board of several international journals. Her research areas in which she has published three monographs include fundamental ethics, narrative ethics, biomedical ethics, and political and social ethics. She is a member of the European Group on Ethics in the Sciences and New Technologies at the European Commission. Website: http://www.luc.edu/theology/facultystaff/haker.shtml.

Linda Hogan is Vice-Provost and Chief Academic Officer at Trinity College Dublin, where she also holds the Chair in Ecumenics. Previously, she held the post of Lecturer in gender, ethics and religion in the Department of Theology and Religious Studies, University of Leeds. She is a theological ethicist with research and teaching interests in the field of social and political ethics. She has published widely on the ethics of human rights, on inter-cultural ethics, and on the ethics of gender. She has been a member of the Irish Council for Bioethics and has worked on a consultancy basis for NGOs and other national and international organisations. She has also published essays and journal articles in the fields of social and political ethics, feminist theological ethics and inter-cultural ethics. She has a BA from the Pontifical University Maynooth and a PhD from Trinity College Dublin. Website: http://www.tcd.ie/vpcao/office/bio.php.

Maureen Junker-Kenny is Associate Professor of Theology in the Department of Religions and Theology, Trinity College Dublin. She studied English literature, catholic theology and philosophy at the universities of Tübingen, Münster, and Trinity College. In 1989, she completed a PhD on F. Schleiermacher's Christology and theory of religion at the University of Münster and in 1996 her Habilitation on J. Habermas's discourse ethics in Tübingen where she was a Lecturer before coming to Trinity College Dublin in 1993. She has been a Fellow of Trinity College Dublin since 1998 and is currently Head of the School of Religions, Theology and Ecumenics (Aspirant). From 1996 to 2008, she was a member of the board of directors of the international theological journal *Concilium*. Her research interests are in religion and public reason, philosophical and theological theories of action, discourse ethics, P. Ricoeur, F. Schleiermacher, and biomedical ethics. Website: http://www.tcd.ie/Religions_Theology/staff/junker-kenny_maureen.php.

Alan Kelly is a Professor and Dean of Graduate Studies at University College Cork (UCC), Ireland with responsibility for institutional graduate education strategy. He has been a Lecturer in UCC since 1996 and is currently Associate Professor in the School of Food and Nutritional Sciences. He is also Director of Training of the Food Graduate Development Programme, funded by the Department of Agriculture and Food, in partnership with UCD and Teagasc. He has been an editor of the International Dairy Journal since 2005, and serves on several international agricultural and dairy research committees, including the Danish Agency for Science, Technology and Innovation. He leads an active research group on the chemistry and processing of milk and dairy products and has published over 150 research papers, review articles and book chapters, with recent research relating to innovative food technologies. He has also, in his capacity as a Dean of Graduate Studies, been at the forefront of reform of post-graduate academic policies in Ireland. He is a graduate of Dublin City University (BSc Biotechnology, 1990) and UCC (PhD Food Technology, 1995). In 2003, he received the Award for Innovative Forms of Teaching and Learning, and in 2005 the President's Award for Excellence in Teaching, UCC. Website: http://publish.ucc.ie/researchprofiles/D018/akelly.

Dietmar Mieth, who since 2009 is longtime fellow of the Max Weber Centre for Advanced Studies at the University of Erfurt, Germany, held the Chair of

Theological Ethics/Social Ethics at the universities of Fribourg, Switzerland (1974–1981) and of Tübingen, Germany (1981–2008). He was a member of the board of directors of the international theological journal *Concilium*, Founder and Chairman of the Centre for Ethics in the Sciences and the Humanities at the University of Tübingen, a member of the European Group on Ethics in the Sciences and New Technologies at the EU-Commission in Brussels (1994–2001), and Ethics Advisor at the Council of Europe and at the German Parliament. He received the Federal Cross of Merit of Germany in 2007. He has written 30 books in the areas of Christian mysticism, narrative ethics, social ethics and bioethics, as well as articles on gene therapy, cloning, embryo research, genetic diagnosis, predictive medicine, enhancement and doping. Website: http://www.uni-tuebingen.de/fakultaeten/katholisch-theologische   fakultaet/lehrstuehle/theologische-ethik-sozialethik/emeritus.html

Elizabeth Nixon is a lecturer in developmental psychology in the School of Psychology and a Senior Research Fellow at the Children's Research Centre, Trinity College Dublin. She received a PhD in developmental psychology from TCD. Before taking up her lectureship in the School of Psychology in October 2006, she worked as a Research Fellow at the Children's Research Centre, where she was involved in the first national study of international adoption in Ireland, funded by the Adoption Board (published in 2007). She has received funding from the Department of Children and Youth Affairs to conduct research into parenting practices and styles of discipline in Ireland (published in 2010). She was principal investigator of an Irish Research Council-funded study of parenting of newborn infants among immigrants in Ireland and she is currently a co-investigator of Growing Up in Ireland, the first national longitudinal study of children in Ireland. Her research interests include children's agency, parenting processes and the influence of family transitions on children's development. Website: http://www.tcd.ie/childrensresearchcentre/people/personnel/liznixon.php.

Desmond O'Neill is a Professor of medical gerontology at Trinity College Dublin. He was appointed as Lecturer in geriatric medicine in the University of Bristol (1990–1992) and as Consultant Physician in geriatric and stroke medicine since 1992. A member of both the Trinity College Institute of Neurosciences and the Trinity Consortium on Ageing, he has been Medical Director of the Alzheimer Society of Ireland (1993–2004), Chair of the Government Working Group on Elder Abuse and subsequent policy implementation body (1999–2010), Founder Chair of the Council on Stroke of the Irish Heart Foundation (1997–2009), and President of the Irish Gerontological (2003–2008) and European Union Geriatric Medicine Societies (2009–2011). He teaches medical ethics at the under-graduate and post-graduate level. His areas of interest include biomedical ethics, ageing, memory and other cognitive processes. He has over 250 peer-reviewed publications, has edited one book and three further books are in progress. He received his BA, MB, BCh, BAO and MD from TCD and is a Fellow of the American Geriatrics Society and of the Royal Colleges of Physicians in Dublin, Glasgow and

London. In March 2010, he received the All-Ireland Inspirational Life Award for his advocacy for older people and is a regular contributor on health issues in the Irish media, including a monthly column in the Irish Times. Website: http://www. tcd.ie/Neuroscience/partners/PI%20Profiles/Desmond_ONeill2.php.

Cathriona Russell is Adjunct Assistant Professor in the School of Religions and Theology at Trinity College Dublin and Director of the Masters in Ecology and Religion at All Hallows College, Dublin City University. Before her work in theology, she studied horticulture at University College Dublin and was employed in nursery management. She undertook her doctoral work at TCD with Professor Maureen Junker-Kenny and published her PhD in 2009 under the title *Autonomy and Food Biotechnology in Theological Ethics*. She administered and co-taught the fourth level Generic Skills Module at TCD. She currently teaches at the undergraduate and post-graduate level in environmental ethics, cosmology and anthropology, and in hermeneutics at TCD and All Hallows, and post-graduate cosmology and anthropology on the Masters in Theology for Ordinands at the Church of Ireland Theological Institute. She has taught ethics to medical students at TCD in collaboration with Professor Desmond O'Neill and has been a Tutor and Lecturer at the Dominican Priory Institute, Tallaght. She has published on food biotechnology and environmental and medical ethics and served on the Research Ethics Committee of St. James' and Tallaght Hospitals for several years. She has been a volunteer tour guide at the Chester Beatty Library, Dublin Castle since 2000. Website: http://www.tcd.ie/Religions_Theology/staff/Cathriona%20Russell.php.

Deirdre Stritch is a Project Officer with the National Qualifications Authority of Ireland (NQAI), where she plays a key role in the maintenance and enabling of the implementation of the National Framework of Qualifications and related policies and in enabling and promoting the recognition of international qualifications. Before joining the NQAI, she worked in the Policy and Planning Section of the Higher Education Authority, where she contributed to policy development and the management and delivery of projects informing the higher education agenda. Previously, she was the Researcher to the Royal Irish Academy's policy report *Advancing Humanities and Social Science Research in Ireland* (2007) and lectured in Greek archaeology at Trinity College Dublin. Areas of work in which she is currently involved include developing the qualifications recognition service of the NQAI and the establishment and co-ordination of a university sector Framework Implementation Network. She gained her BA and PhD in archaeology at Trinity College Dublin. She undertook her doctorate in archaeological heritage-management policy in Israel and the Republic of Cyprus with the Programme for Mediterranean and Near Eastern Studies at Trinity College Dublin in 2006. Website: http://www.nqai.ie/about_staff.html.

List of Contributors

Amy Daughton Director of Studies, Margaret Beaufort Institute of Theology, Cambridge, UK

Gladys Ganiel Irish School of Ecumenics (Belfast), Trinity College, Dublin, Ireland

Frank Gannon The Queensland Institute of Medical Research, Herston, Brisbane, QLD, Australia

Sigrid Graumann University of Applied Sciences, Bochum, Germany

Hille Haker Theology Department, Loyola University Chicago, Chicago, IL, USA

Maureen Junker-Kenny Department of Religions & Theology, Trinity College, Dublin, Ireland

Alan L. Kelly University College Cork, Cork, Ireland

Dietmar Mieth Max Weber Center for Advanced Cultural and Social Studies, University of Erfurt, Germany

Elizabeth Nixon School of Psychology and Children's Research Centre, Trinity College, Dublin, Ireland

Desmond O'Neill Centre for Ageing, Neuroscience and the Humanities, Trinity College, Dublin, Ireland

Cathriona Russell Department of Religions & Theology, Trinity College, Dublin, and All Hallows College, Dublin City University, Dublin, Ireland

Deirdre Stritch National Qualifications Authority of Ireland, Ireland

Introduction

Linda Hogan
University of Dublin, Trinity College, Dublin, Ireland

There are four key fields of research ethics mapped in this book: core concepts in ethics; ethics governance in Europe and internationally; the contextualisation of ethical principles in practice; and finally, the emerging debates in research ethics and indeed in ethics research. Readers can engage with this material at different levels; the introductions to the key principles link to the podcasts of the discipline-specific lectures, and then to the texts of the complete papers. The uniqueness of the collection is that it combines an analysis of complex ethical debates about the nature of research and its governance, with case-based and discipline-specific approaches. As such, it is intended to be a relevant and accessible resource for graduate students in all disciplines.

In Section 1, Linda Hogan introduces ethics as a core competency in research excellence. Ethical reflection and evaluation are central to the manner in which research programmes are articulated and developed. It is recognised that researchers need to be encouraged to develop their own skills of ethical reflection and evaluation, and that research training for graduates ought to incorporate skills development in this field. The teaching programme from which this collection derives drew on graduate researchers from across many fields: science and engineering; the health sciences, including medicine; and from the humanities and social sciences. In this way, early researchers were able to interrogate the objectives and progress of their specific research projects, not only in terms of the contribution to knowledge, but most especially in relation to the ethical questions raised by the research and in the company of peers from very different disciplines.

In Section 2, international documents — from the United Nations, the Council of Europe and the European Union — are examined as frameworks for research. Maureen Junker-Kenny introduces this section with reflections on the role of ethics committees, on the principle of precaution and on the goal of transparency in research.

In Section 3, Cathriona Russell introduces the contextualisation of ethical principles in practice. In the ancient world, this was part of what was referred to as 'practical wisdom' and is an aspect of ethics that now sometimes falls under the general category of 'applied ethics'. Ethics in this light is not first and foremost prescriptive but is better characterised as integrative, inter-disciplinary and interpretive.

In Section 4, Linda Hogan returns to that adage that *the more things change, the more things stay the same*. Research is an inherently dynamic activity, and its successes are critical to the economic, social and political well-being of individuals and communities worldwide. Yet, even as major innovations in research continue to be announced, especially in science and technology, many of the fundamental ethical issues persist. Historically, the major issues of concern have revolved around three main themes: the nature and purpose of research; the status and treatment of research subjects; and the conduct of research. More recently, two further themes have emerged in research ethics: first, the issue of social justice and the distribution of the benefits of research; and second, the role of research in a globalised society, and specifically whether and how social responsibility and accountability can be achieved.

We are grateful for the generous funding we received for this initiative and for the collegial hospitality from our hosts at TCD, UCC and NUIG. We particularly wish to thank all the specialists in Audio Visual and Media Services at TCD, who worked with us in filming the input of speakers and processing the podcasts. We are most particularly thankful for the meticulous and thoughtful input of the Chief Technical Officer Martin Murphy and for the patience and kindness of Jimmy Cumiskey. We are equally in debt to the students who took time from their busy schedules and took a risk, too, in joining us on the programme. They offered insights and well-thought out comments and also drove the development of the programme to become a collaborative and project-specific feedback process tailored to the specific needs and demands of the disciplines in which they worked.

Introduction to Section 1

Developing Ethics as a Core Competency: Integrity in Scientific Research

Linda Hogan

University of Dublin, Trinity College, Dublin, Ireland

Abstract

This section introduces ethics as a core competency in the research process. It suggests an approach that both builds on the ethical integrity of the researcher and that develops research practices to ensure that the institutional context in which research is pursued supports, reinforces and mandates responsible research.

Key Words

Ethical integrity, core competence, compliance, traditions of argumentation, ethical abuses

It is difficult to overstate the importance of ethical reflection in the context of research. Ethical reflection and evaluation is central to the manner in which research programmes are articulated and developed. It plays an important role in the determination of the fundamental objectives of research programmes and has a continuing role in the assessment of the methods and means by which such research objectives are pursued. Within this context, moreover, it is recognised that researchers need to be encouraged to develop their own skills of ethical reflection and evaluation, and furthermore, that research training for graduates ought to incorporate skills development in this field. With its focus on developing skills and competencies in research ethics, this collection proposes that training in research ethics ought to be available to graduate researchers in all fields, ideally in cross-disciplinary fora, and that it ought to form an integral part of all graduate education. However, while there is now a broad recognition that research in science and technology must proceed according to the highest ethics standards and researchers in this field need training in ethics, there is still a failure to appreciate fully that

Ethics for Graduate Researchers. DOI: http://dx.doi.org/10.1016/B978-0-12-416049-1.00030-1

researchers in the humanities and social sciences may also face significant ethical dilemmas as they pursue their research. In order to mitigate this, the teaching programme from which this collection derives drew on graduate researchers from across many disciplinary fields, in science and engineering, in the health sciences including medicine and in the humanities and social sciences. In this way, early researchers were able to interrogate the objectives and progress of their specific research projects, not only in terms of the contribution to knowledge, but also, most especially, in relation to the ethical questions raised by the research, in the company of peers from very different disciplines.1

In 2006, the Irish government, through the Higher Education Authority, announced a series of initiatives that were designed to support innovation in higher education. Under the umbrella of the Strategic Innovation Fund, over €510 million has been invested in the sector, with a significant portion of this multi-annual fund focused on developing graduate education and training. In the context of this initiative, Trinity College Dublin entered into a strategic alliance with University College Cork (UCC) and NUI Galway to add value to the already substantive provision of individual institutions. The aim has been to enhance the quality and effectiveness of training for graduate researchers, particularly through the development of new generic skills training at the highest level. There is no doubt that graduate researchers benefit from generic skills training in a number of important areas. The programme within which this research ethics training has been situated incorporates a host of other skills-based modules, including commercialisation of research and technology transfer, communications skills and statistics and data analysis. Indeed, this programme of graduate education has been tremendously successful and has been a catalyst for further innovations in the sector. The commitment to inter-institutional collaboration in particular has garnered significant support, as students and academics alike have benefited greatly from such interactions. Indeed, the 'Research Ethics for Graduate Researchers' programme actively pursued this inter-institutional model, both in the development of the curriculum and the delivery of the modules.

The central premise of this collection, and of the teaching programme on which it is based, is that the graduate researcher him/herself must think through the ethical issues that he/she encounters as the research proceeds. It is important, therefore, that research ethics is not simply associated with compliance, but rather that it is understood to be integral to good research. Of course, if graduate researchers are to develop the skills of ethical reflection, then they need to be introduced to key aspects of the history, philosophy and sociology of ethics, because it is through such exposure that the researcher can think critically about his or her core values and the values of the disciplines and institutions in which they work. Indeed, this focus on the individual graduate researcher provides the major focus for this first section, as it is from this platform that all ethical reflection ultimately proceeds. In support of this approach, the collection aims both to introduce researchers to the core concepts and principles in research ethics and to provide specialist in-depth explorations of these principles as they are contextualised in practice across key disciplines. The material is presented so that readers can engage with it at different levels, thus the introductions to the key principles link to the podcasts of the discipline-specific lectures, and then to the texts of the complete papers. The uniqueness of the collection, therefore, is that it combines an analysis of complex ethical debates about the nature of research and its governance, with the best of case-based and discipline-specific approaches. As such, it is intended to be a relevant and accessible resource for graduate students in all disciplines.

The collection opens with a discussion of the different traditions of argumentation in philosophical ethics. Through this consideration of the different ways in which ethical argumentation has traditionally proceeded, graduate researchers are enabled to recognise the fundamental frameworks that are at play in ethical reflection, and to identify the approaches that most resonate with their own values and principles. Maureen Junker-Kenny's chapter opens with the reminder that, at its most basic level, ethical reflection invokes the shared human capacity to generate value judgements based on our ability to be self-reflective, and that, historically, such reflection has generated a host of different articulations of these values and principles. In Chapter 1, Junker-Kenny analyses the different traditions of argumentation that are embedded particularly in Western philosophical discourse, and highlights the manner in which these traditions allow for different values to be foregrounded and promoted. Her discussion highlights the strengths and weaknesses of five major ethical traditions, namely virtue ethics, utilitarianism/consequentialism, deontology, contract ethics and discourse ethics. There is no doubt that each approach highlights an important dimension of ethical reflection. Virtue ethics, for example, stresses that ethics ought not to be focused only on acts, or rules or quandaries, but rather ought to be concerned with character formation, with the development of certain basic attitudes and with enabling the individual to make prudential decisions. Utilitarianism, by contrast, is concerned with the consequences of particular actions and assesses the merits of decisions on the basis that it contributes to 'the greatest happiness of the greatest possible number'. Utilitarian ethics has nuanced its original conception of 'happiness', which ought not to be equated simply with pleasure, but rather with a more rounded account of human well-being. Deontology fundamentally disputes the utilitarian approach and holds that some choices can never be justified according to their consequences, no matter how good such consequences appear to be. Thus, an individual may never make certain choices, because certain fundamental principles may never be compromised. Classically, deontology insists that human beings may never be instrumentalised and may never be used only as a means to a particular good — no matter how admirable that good may be. Contract ethics views morality in terms of a contract entered into out of self-interest, whereas discourse ethics tries to identify conditions for reaching a moral consensus in a public sphere in which citizens participate in their function both as authors and as addressees of laws. Junker-Kenny compares the different approaches in terms of their understandings of self, agency and inter-subjectivity that contribute to how they treat the ethical issues associated with the protection of vulnerable subjects. She concludes by drawing out the consequences for graduate researchers as they become able to contribute to the professional and public deliberation on such issues, aware of major variations in regulation between countries and of the argumentations conducted in the public realm of different political cultures.

Alan L. Kelly, Dean of Graduate Studies at UCC, continues this reflection on developing ethics as a core competency in Chapter 2 that focuses directly on the practical questions that researchers encounter as they design and develop their research methods. Kelly focuses in particular on scientific research, although his concerns certainly transcend these disciplines. Kelly notes that there is an increasingly well-defined set of principles which establish the parameters of responsible conduct in research, and he insists that these ought to be clearly articulated and frequently communicated. In terms of the practice of research, such principles recognise the importance of operating honestly when handling and reporting on data, and he highlights the serious hazards associated with dishonesty in the treatment of the results of research. Kelly also discusses the norms that ought to guide the designation of authorship, reminding researchers that the attribution of authorship is indeed an ethical issue and warning that the inequalities in the relationship between supervisor and graduate student should not be exploited in this context. Kelly discusses a number of the high-profile cases of scientific misconduct that have emerged over the past 20 years. In doing so, he highlights the manner in which the ever-increasing pressure for success can, and often does, corrupt the research process. As a result, he argues, graduate researchers must be attuned, not only to the norms of ethical scientific conduct, but also to the traditions of reflection and evaluation that will enable them to recognise and to respond to the ethical challenges embedded in their own research programmes.

The final chapter in this section (Chapter 3) is by Professor Frank Gannon, who is currently the Director of The Queensland Institute of Medical Research in Brisbane, Australia, but who, when he contributed to the module on research ethics, was the Director General of Science Foundation Ireland. Gannon's chapter speaks directly to the issue of ethical integrity, arguing that this is at the core of all ethical behaviour in research. Gannon begins by insisting that because research is a public and social good, it must be governed by sound ethical principles. Research, especially in science and technology, gives rise to a host of fundamental ethical questions, and the significance of these issues (e.g. stem-cell research or human enhancement) confirms the importance of maintaining the highest of ethics standards in science and technology. Quite simply, he argues, the behaviour of scientists must match the challenges that they face. His chapter focuses on the laboratory, and therein he outlines the multiplicity of challenges that the researcher faces in the pursuit of sound scientific research. He argues that the potential for misconduct lurks everywhere, notwithstanding the noble intentions of most researchers. Gannon structures his chapter around the key roles of researcher and research supervisor and analyses the pressures associated with the research process in the natural sciences and the hazards that are associated with the desire for success and for results. His chapter provides a salutary warning for idealistic early researchers who may not yet be attentive to the rationalisation and self-deception in which researchers can engage. Gannon's conclusion, however, is that within the laboratory each individual has an important role to play in ensuring that ethical standards are adhered to and in establishing a context in which individuals are habituated in the norms of ethical research. High ethical standards are essential in the research context, both in terms of the integrity of the research process, and ultimately in terms of the quality of the research itself.

The three chapters in this section share a common concern, namely to further the development of programmes that will improve the ethical articulacy and competence of graduate researchers. They share the conviction that good practice in research ethics begins with a commitment to self-critical reflection and with a determination to pursue each research programme with integrity and honesty. The chapters also recognise that education in research ethics requires ongoing engagement throughout a researcher's career. It requires researchers to develop a degree of fluency in ethical argumentation, as well as an understanding of the manner in which certain values and principles are embedded, for better or worse, in the various moral frameworks that are operative in different research settings. Ultimately, they make the case that ethical reflection and critical thinking will flourish only in a culture that prizes such skills and regards them as integral to the excellence of the research process itself.

Captions and links for PODCAST files for this section.

Linda Hogan

1. Introducing a module in Ethics for Graduate Researchers.

Maureen Junker-Kenny

1. Communicative reason and the Frankfurt School.

Alan Kelly

1. Encountering ethical concerns as a graduate researcher.
2. Scientific misconduct in ethical perspective.

Frank Gannon

1. Responsibilities throughout a scientific researcher's career: doing a PhD.
2. Moving on to post-doctoral research.
3. The pressure to publish.
4. Running a research foundation.
5. Sharing results with peers.
6. Ethical questions in the funding of research.

These can be found at http://booksite.elsevier.com/9780124160491

1 Recognising Traditions of Argumentation in Philosophical Ethics

Maureen Junker-Kenny

Department of Religions & Theology, Trinity College, Dublin, Ireland

Abstract

In this chapter, I take the human capacity for ethical evaluation as the shared basis for the different articulations of values that have been worked out in the history of ethical thinking. One influential method of operationalising ethics in research settings has been principlism. Beginning from an analysis of the effect of a technological culture on conceiving human agency, I compare five classical approaches to ethics from antiquity to modernity in relation to their frameworks and their criteria of protection for vulnerable subjects. I conclude by drawing the consequences for graduate researchers and illustrating these using a study that compares how the political cultures in three Western countries shape their responses to new biotechnologies.

Key Words

Agency, technological age, virtue, Utilitarianism, deontology, contract, discourse ethics, law, political culture

The term "ethics" will appear in many different understandings throughout this book. To avoid misunderstandings, and to be able to recognise at which level claims are, and are not, disputed, it may be helpful to distinguish three dimensions. At its origin, ethics is the human capacity to generate judgments of value, based on the ability of a self-reflective being to take a stance towards his or her thoughts and actions. All the diverse approaches to ethics presuppose this foundational faculty, although they explicate it in different terms. As the human capacity for evaluation, this faculty unites the plural worlds into which individuals are born and into which they shape from within their own cultures and in their encounter

Ethics for Graduate Researchers. DOI: http://dx.doi.org/10.1016/B978-0-12-416049-1.00001-5

with others.[1] Arising from this primary capacity for judgment come, secondly, the distinctive theories of ethics that are chosen and elaborated, repudiated, differentiated and specified; they will be characterised and compared in the second part of this chapter. A third form in which ethics appears is in the methods adopted in professional settings and in international consensus documents, making it operational by identifying guiding principles and values. The principlism that has shaped institutional decision-making in medical settings by providing the four cornerstones of autonomy, non-maleficence, beneficence and justice has provided a model for ethics assessments also in other areas.[2] Respect for autonomy and avoidance of maleficence were translated into a requirement for informed consent performed by signing a document. How ethical principles can be made operational within different disciplines will be discussed further in Section 3 of this book.

The reasons to establish ethics governance and to specify oversight procedures were several: they included the realisation that, even in democratic states after 1945, human rights abuses had been committed by researchers; that the pluralism of worldviews and values within Western societies called for renewed reflection on the principles shared by citizens for living together in one state and in one world; and that ethical, civic and political opinion formation and decision-making were needed to catch up with the unprecedented pace of acceleration that the new scientific and technological possibilities presented for existing lifeworlds and self-understandings.

Thus, before turning to ancient and modern traditions of conceptualising the basic human experience of ethical and moral evaluations, it is necessary to analyse the

---

[1] Greisch, J., "Ethics and Lifeworlds", in Kearney, R. and Dooley, M., (eds), *Questioning Ethics. Contemporary Debates in Philosophy* (London/New York: Routledge, 1999), 44–61, 56–59.

[2] Beauchamp, T. and Childress, J. F., *Principles of Bioethics* (New York/Oxford: OUP, 1989). In a critique that would merit further unpacking, Charles Bosk points out how the main problem he sees with this method, its universalism, is mitigated by the plurality of principles which in their different possible combinations allow for culturally sensitive applications. From a different angle of critique, the core principle of 'autonomy' would have to be investigated for its provenance from either I. Kant or J.S. Mill. Cf. Bosk, C.I. "Professional Ethicist Available: Logical, Secular, Friendly" in *Daedalus* 128 (1999) 47–68, 62: 'Here, I want simply to call attention to leading assumptions of principlism: namely, that the individual is the proper measure of all things ethical, that tools for measurement transcend culture, and that there is a single, correct solution for each ethical problem, which is largely independent of person, place, or time. At the time that this ethical universalism is gaining ascendance in the world of medicine, it is being rejected in virtually every other sphere of society. In academia, cultural relativism had made the assertion of a single ethical standard applied across cultures highly problematic. In the public arena of political culture, the spirit of cultural pluralism made the assertion of such a single standard not only unfashionable but also a badge of great insensitivity. The fact that bioethics embraced principlism, and that this embrace took root in such a complex community as is the modern medical center, is peculiar, to say the least. Of course, the very nature of principlism gave it a curious dual aspect. On the one hand, the four principles seemed to provide something like a moral methodology for public discussion of ethical issues. John Evans has even suggested that principlism functions in ethics much as double-entry bookkeeping does in accounting: it makes commensurable what was formerly incommensurable. On the other hand, despite the seemingly privileged place of autonomy, the fact that principlism allows the four principles to be combined and deployed in any configuration allows a wide range of cultural preferences legitimation under its aegis. Principlism has then the seeming advantage of being both authoritative and sensitive to cultural difference.'

cultural situation in which the need for ethics governance in research has also become so pronounced. Beginning with hermeneutical and ethical reflections on the technological age (Section 'Agency and Ethics in a Technological Culture'), I compare five schools of ethical thinking that are informing such assessments in the contemporary international debate (Section 'Traditions of Ethical Argumentation'). I conclude by drawing some consequences for research ethics from a recent comparison of how the forces of law, ethics and the market sphere, with producers and consumers, are organised in different political cultures, each of them marked by their own historical memories and civic aspirations (Section 'Cultural Memory and Political Institutions as Decisive Contexts for Research Parameters and for Public Debate').

Agency and Ethics in a Technological Culture

At least as implicit components, approaches to ethics contain assumptions about human agency. A minimal presupposition shared by them is that actions are not completely determined but are sufficiently free so as to be able to come under reflective judgement. Yet, before such evaluation is the more basic question of how initial views of the world, structured symbolically by language and culture, shape a person's desires and self-understanding. The capacity for moral reflection, although universally human, only exists as embedded in symbolic worlds that are prior to individual initiative and that both enable and limit it. In relation to modern societies, how do current reflections decipher what they call the technological condition? Unlike sociological or political power analyses of empirical factors, interests and decision-making processes which equally need to be carried out, a hermeneutical enquiry is directed towards elucidating how humans relate to the worlds in which they find themselves. From this perspective, framing the debate in terms of technology being either a tool for free human agents, or a force of domination, does not do justice to the inevitable shaping of human agency by all cultural conditions; it is too simple, it is a 'stale dichotomy'[3] :

> We are not victims of a technological fate, any more than we are masters of a technological destiny. This gives some indication of the problems with identifying human capability in the absolute terms that force us to take sides on the question of technological neutrality or determinism.

So, rather than assess specific developments as either liberating or as alienating and destructive, it is more accurate to identify modern technology as a deci-

---

[3] Lewin, D. "Ricoeur and the Capability of Modern Technology", in Mei, T. S. and Lewin, D. (eds.), *From Ricoeur to Action. The Socio-Political Significance of Ricoeur's Thinking* (New York/London: Continuum, 2012), 54–71, 54.

sive 'context in which the question of human freedom arises'.[4] In Lewin's analysis, the hermeneutical philosopher Paul Ricoeur identifies two dangers in this. First, that the imaginative pole of resources of narrative, myths of origin, conflict and utopias could be depleted by an experience of world that is reduced to the mere functionality of technological devices. The vital tension between the symbolic stocks of a culture and the rationality from which its productivity emerges is impoverished when rationality is only available as instrumental reason. There is no risk of otherness in such predictable, pre-programmed utilities. Thus, and this is the second danger, that the gain in function through a new technology could be a loss in other ways of coping with the world and affect the ability to encounter a genuine other. Ricoeur's critique of the homogenising effects of consumer culture already in the 1960s complements the analysis of indirect incapacitating implications of the technological advances produced by humans in their creative agency.[5] Thus, rather than specific devices − which may increase ease of communication and facilitate encounters with others − it is the technological condition that deserves attention as a new mode of relating to objects and to the world we can shape. It is a view that does not demonise technology but analyses it as the product of human action in its effect on human initiative and receptivity.

Similarly, a perspective from human agency is at work when technology is presented not as a given, but as something socially constructed and supported by societal systems, and therefore answerable to socially desired goals. In her two articles, Hille Haker proposes to turn around the burden of proof and to regard 'science and technologies as social practices that need to be justified in light of the normative framework'. There are deontological dimensions to this framework, such as the Millennium Development Goals, to which technological advances need to contribute, and teleological ones concerning 'social imagination and social visions, but also norms of social interaction, practices of solidarity or group identities'.[6]

---

[4] Ibid., 58. However, Lewin points out that its destructive force does put into question the power of human agency to contain the consequences: 'With the catastrophes at Hiroshima and Nagasaki, the assumption that technology could simply be the servant of human will came to an end. Such was the destructive power that the notion that any technology was simply a neutral tool became a moot point, even though the potential benefits of nuclear power were given due consideration. Ethical questions were important in coming to terms with this destructive potential, but equally important were questions of agency and responsibility.' (55−56) For an analysis of how much also the peaceful use of nuclear energy is connected to national identity, business and government interests and requiring more effective safety control by global agencies such as the IAEA, see Pfotenhauer, S. M., Jones, C. F., Saha, K., and Jasanoff, S., "Learning from Fukushima", in *Issues in Science & Technology* 28 (2012) 79−84, 79: 'Technologies such as reactors, risk models, and safety mechanisms are embedded in social values and practices; similarly, national identity, risk regulation, and corporate culture are materialized in the production and operation of nuclear power plants...a sociotechnical approach... uncovers a different set of lessons and points to novel responses that include participatory technology policy, global nuclear governance, and a more reflexive approach to modeling.'

[5] Ricoeur, P., "Universal Civilisation and National Cultures" (1961), in *History and Truth*, trans. and introd. by Ch. A. Kelbley (Evanston: Northwestern University Press, 1965), 271−284.

[6] Haker, H., "Synthetic Biology: an Emerging Debate in European Ethics", in this volume, 213−224.

To elucidate the various ways in which the human capacity for ethical evaluation has been conceived, I shall now compare different traditions of argumentation in their use of key terms and in their disputes with opposite schools. The criterion I shall use to assess their strengths and weaknesses will be a core requirement of ethics, namely the 'protection of the vulnerable'. Other aspects will be their understandings of self and human agency, motivation and inter-subjectivity.

Traditions of Ethical Argumentation

The five approaches to philosophical ethics that are to be introduced in this section each offer aspects that are relevant for coming to decisions on which courses of action in research can be justified ethically. Some of their options overlap, evidently, for example, in the fact that each of them is oriented towards the goal of justice. Conceptions that diverge from this goal or that offer profound critiques of the values developed in Western ethics because Plato and in biblical monotheism will not be considered here. The alternative value system they offer is based on advocating the 'will to power'. The legacies of Hobbes and Nietzsche would be relevant because they influence the political philosophies that frame policy proposals but are not always analysed and they would have to be discussed if current bioethical debates such as transhumanism were treated.

Because all five schools assume that humans are capable of ethical reflection, it may appear that the overlaps outweigh the differences. Yet, the extent to which they offer alternative reconstructions of this ability becomes clear when one takes each of them as a coherent set of philosophical claims. Even if at times they may come to the same practical conclusion, they will do so for different reasons and objectives. To researchers in other disciplines, it may seem as if the variations between them may well give a lifetime of satisfying intellectual quarrels to theorists inclined towards conceptual hair-splitting, though without much yield for practical decision-making in the decisive fields of applied ethics. However, the different starting points and emphases of virtue ethics, Utilitarianism/consequentialism, deontology, contract ethics and discourse ethics become evident in the points they consider to be relevant for coming to decisions across different fields of research. I shall summarise each of them in their basic framework, outline the distinction and advantages they claim over other ethical systems and conclude with an evaluation of what others find lacking in them.

Virtue Ethics

In its basic framework, virtue ethics is oriented towards the development of certain attitudes, stable dispositions and long-term orientations; it seeks to enable the individual to make context-sensitive, prudential decisions in a concrete socio-historical community. It is interested in the conditions under which stable identities can be developed that put values into practice in a reliable way marked by continuity, rather than turns, or once-off decisions. What makes it attractive in complex societies marked by system imperatives — such as economic rationality, that get into tension with the communicative values people want to follow in their lifeworlds — is its emphasis on personal authenticity. It conceives of the moral subject not in terms of a deliberating individual but as a participant in and a contributor to a shared cultural enterprise. With its interest in formation, socialisation and ethical growth in commitment to a community, it offers a hermeneutical starting point from shared self-understandings to the realisation of ethical values. The corrective features offered by virtue ethics are: it begins with the human orientation towards a flourishing life, trusting in the evidence of good moral characters; it opts for prevention rather than damage limitation after disasters; and it invests in the building of long-term basic attitudes over against individual decision-testing and in steady personal responsibility over against the anonymous forces of unrelated systems. Examples of this mode of ethics for different fields of research include the Hippocratic Oath from around 400 BCE that formulated the ideal attitude of the physician just before Aristotle (384–322 BCE) developed his concept of virtues. The emphasis given, in many chapters of this book for graduate researchers, to the values of integrity, precaution and sustainability can be seen as belonging to a virtue ethical model. In their ability to fill institutions with life, virtues are unrivalled.

The distinction from and advantage over other approaches has been worked out especially since its renaissance in the late 1970s. Some of the key authors on virtue have pitched this antique understanding against modern foundations of ethics, preeminently against Immanuel Kant's. In *After Virtue*, Alasdair MacIntyre sets out to undo what he sees as the devastating effects of the Enlightenment by advocating a return from its subjectivism to the supportive contexts of communities.[7] Other authors have followed suit in their opposition to features which they attribute to a Kantian concept of ethics that they see as focused on acts, rules or quandaries, rather than on character formation and on being and the basic attitudes behind individual acts. Ethics in modernity is seen as dissecting the moral life into a series of isolated acts, as a method of application of a universal set of rules or rational principles. The deficiencies virtue ethics wants to overcome thus include individualism, an understanding of ethics as legislation centred on acts, and abstract and universal criteria, i.e. standards of evaluation that are independent of the context and situatedness of agents and communities. Such contexts are to be recognised as being before legislation, supplying decisive conditions for the training of character, in which the models of concrete lives can be seen and imitated as formative examples. These late twentieth century forms of virtue ethics take up once again Hegel's critique of Kant insofar as the existing ethos of living communities is invoked over against the foundation of Kant's ethics. In contrast to virtue ethics, Kant's ethics is founded not on the good habits formed in lived community but rather on the experience of morality as an irrepressible part of the autonomous individual's self-understanding. For Kant, we owe recognition to others on account of their equally original freedom as humans, not because they are members of the same particular

---

[7] MacIntyre, A., *After Virtue* (London: Duckworth, 1981).

community. The obligation to others expressed as self-government (autonomy) by the moral law is the standard by which actions are to be judged. The fact that it can never be fully realised is seen by Hegel and his followers as denying moral quality to existing relationships and social bonds. While the contemporary form of virtue ethics does not share the Hegelian justification of the state,[8] it supports the shift from an ethics of individual obligation to one of confidence in the community's resources of goodness.

From the perspective of the main alternative position, as identified by current key supporters of virtue ethics, namely Kant's ethics of autonomy, I see three areas that need evaluation: the understanding of self, the scope of protection for vulnerable subjects and the status of ethics.

Self and Conscience, or Character?

While the Aristotelian orientation towards the goal of a flourishing life implies a teleological concept of motivated agency, and while the inter-subjective setting of the training in virtues is one of its distinctive features, questions arise with regard to the concept of self.

The emphasis on character and on being as before action is meant to underline steadfastness and continuity over against a focus on disjointed acts. Yet, in line with Hegel's critique of conscience in its subjectivity, it risks downplaying the role of individual conscience over against dispositions acquired within a supportive ethos; it minimises the possible divergence from the community, as well as differences within it. And the lack of a more encompassing horizon than the particular group of origin makes it unable to recognise and critique in-group ideologies.

Compared with other analyses of the self, which are equally critical of a Cartesian foundationalism, such as Ricoeur's, the key function given to character in virtue ethics presents it as a unitary concept, rather than as a relationship between the *idem* pole of continuity, and the *ipse* as the centre of spontaneous agency and reflection. Ethical selfhood needs to take account of both, i.e. to give equal consideration to the pole of human reflexivity which is not captured in the term character.

The Scope of Protection for Vulnerable Subjects

A strong point of virtue ethics is its appreciation that education, cultural self-expression, political participation and religious practice need a community that is valued not just as a conduit to a next higher (individualistic) stage. Yet, by

---

[8] This critique also comes from a nuanced position on the roles of Kant and Hegel for ethics in modernity, Paul Ricoeur's: 'What, finally, is inadmissible in Hegel is... the thesis of the state erected as a superior agency endowed with self-knowledge... For us, who have crossed through the monstrous events of the twentieth century tied to the phenomenon of totalitarianism, we have reason to listen to the opposite verdict [on moral consciousness], devastating in another way, pronounced by history itself through the mouth of its victims. When the spirit of a people is perverted to the point of feeding a deadly *Sittlichkeit*, it is finally in the moral consciousness of a small number of individuals, inaccessible to fear and to corruption, that the spirit takes refuge, once it has fled the now-criminal institutions.' *Oneself as Another*, trans. K. Blamey (Chicago: University of Chicago Press, 1992), 256.

conceiving all social relations in terms of community, there is not only a danger of promoting social conformity but also a danger of excluding fellow-humans from view who are not members of one's own circle or culture of origin. If one takes the communitarian background of this school seriously, responsibility for the vulnerable is shrunk to the home territory of virtuous agents.

A further missing factor is a concept that can express relations to anonymous others, first, within one's own society. It may also be possibly extended to the cosmopolitan horizon in which Kant situates his ethics of peaceful coexistence and collaboration of republics. This is the concept of legality, the 'most important non-Aristotelian element in our modern ethos', as the German philosopher Herbert Schnädelbach points out in his critique of Neo-Aristotelianism.[9] It expresses the level of formal legal relationships that autonomous subjects will honour but that do not presuppose a shared communal background.

The Status of Ethics

A final objection against conceiving virtue as an alternative to autonomy, that is, not as a matter of *complementing* but of *challenging* the modern foundation of ethics on the autonomy of the subject, relates to the ensuing status of ethics. The question arising from a uniquely hermeneutical understanding of ethics is whether ethics can only explore the internal logic of a given ethos. Are moral judgments always situated elucidations of the self-understanding of a community and its agents? Or are context-independent principles possible? Schnädelbach criticises the first position as a '*phronesis* ideology' which is in danger of emphasising the contingent, singular and contextualised nature of human action so much that no general evaluation according to recognised criteria is possible. He also points out the intellectual neighbourhood in which the renunciation to 'strong normative claims' sits:

> *If it is no longer possible to attach strong normative claims to an idea, a radical critique can also no longer be founded. Theoretical skepticism always favours the power of what is established... The historically enlightened Neo-Aristotelian can in fact only be a skeptic..., leaving praxis – in equal distance both to a Kantian ethics of obligation and to platonising ethics of value – to practical cleverness and unburdening himself and us from normative challenges as far as possible.*[10]

How far virtue ethics, with its orientation towards continuity of character and a shared framework of communal values, can cope with either radical breaks in self-understanding or a pluralism in which previously taken-for-granted standards

---

[9] Schnädelbach, H., "Was ist Neoaristotelismus?" in *Zur Rehabilitierung des animal rationale* (Frankfurt: Suhrkamp,1992), 205–230, 228.

[10] Ibid., 214.

are challenged, is an open question. It depends on how far this tradition wants to distance itself from typically modern insights and problems.[11]

Utilitarian/Consequentialist Ethics

The basic tenets of Utilitarianism are reconstructed systematically in their sequence by the political philosopher Otfried Höffe. It proposes to evaluate actions and rules on the basis of four principles, beginning with the theory decision that gives it one of its names, to judge by the consequences, rather than by the original intention or the inherent quality of an act. The criterion by which consequences are to be judged is their utility in regard to the good. This second principle explains its other name, Utilitarianism. The third principle defines what this good consists in through the criteria of experiencing pleasure and avoiding pain, of positive and negative utility or happiness, therefore, of an initial hedonism that was developed into a more nuanced account of human well-being, taking its starting point in satisfying basic needs. The question of how to determine utility leads to the fourth principle through the criterion of maximising the good for those affected, the social principle. It concludes the steps of evaluation by judging an act/rule to be good when following it contributes to 'the greatest happiness of the greatest possible number'.[12] For the time of its origin, the year of the French Revolution,[13] this was a socially progressive proposal that recognises the empirical needs of the human person and offers an understanding of justice that begins with these needs. Examples for fields of research in which its criteria of maximising the number of those who will benefit are relevant could be ecology, because the happiness of the greatest possible number depends on sustaining living conditions for future generations; or public health in the name of which individual interests (e.g. smoking) or corporate lobbying (e.g. for advertising alcohol or against food labelling) can be overridden.

It is distinct from ancient approaches because unlike the original Greek setting of virtue ethics, Utilitarianism is concerned with how the happiness of a majority of persons is affected by decision-making. Bentham's concept of pleasure is differentiated by John Stuart (1806—1873) into higher and lower pleasures, while still retaining the goal of maximum happiness in both quantitative and qualitative terms. By offering a substantial definition of the goodness of actions as those that result in the greatest happiness of the greatest possible number, it provides a user-friendly formula that does not impose the pain of overly demanding moral standards, such as an unconditional and one-sided realisation of the moral imperative to recognise

---

[11] I have discussed philosophical critiques and theological receptions of virtue ethics in greater detail in "Virtues and the God Who Makes Everything New", in Mayes, A. and Jeanrond, W. (eds.), *Recognising the Margins: Essays in Honour of Sean Freyne* (Dublin: Columba Press, 2006), 298—320.

[12] Höffe O., (ed.), *Einführung in die utilitaristische Ethik. Klassische und zeitgenössische Texte* (München: Beck, 1975), 7—11, quoted in Anzenbacher, A., *Einführung in die Ethik* (Düsseldorf: Patmos, 1992), 32.

[13] J. Bentham (1748—1832) published *An Introduction to the Principles of Morals and Legislation* in 1789.

the other. With its empirical brand of rationalism, it can attract support from different schools of social thought, as its social principle — that requires the basic needs of majorities to be met — would be agreeable without the need to resolve differences on more controversial anthropological assumptions. Its empirical view of the human person as those who have interests and can justify them may not be shared by other approaches, but can remain open for the time that the demand to ensure conditions for survival is being satisfied, as is required, for example, by the Millennium Development Goals.

In relation to its concepts of agency, self and inter-subjectivity, a more in-depth discussion of current utilitarian thinking would have to differentiate and take account of its ability to take on board many critiques, as Mill did by refining its underlying anthropology. The following objections would have to be tested in view of its more recent proposals. Yet, already in comparison with virtue ethics, the motivation that drives agency invites further questions. How direct and unmediated is the way towards achieving happiness? For Aristotle, it was connected to a rationality that included virtue, existence in a well-governed *polis* and time for *theoria* (contemplative reflection), thus indicating that it could not be an end on a par with others that could be made happen by straightforward action. While the self can evaluate and choose the type of pleasure it pursues, the possibility for such reflection is not explained. As to inter-subjectivity, Mill's empirical view of autonomy as independence from external influence seems to take the presence of others as a negative factor for self-determination and cast the exercise of one's freedom in an unnecessarily competitive mode. The social principle which offers some common ground with other traditions is defined by average utility and lacks precisely the factor that is central for a theory of justice, namely a principle of distribution — be it happiness, basic goods or life chances. The calculus of consequences that Utilitarianism proposes denies that human reflection can identify a moral quality that is imminent in actions and that agents can stand over in their conscience, even if they were unsuccessful in achieving the intended outcome. Consequences other than the satisfaction of basic needs are difficult to assess for reasons of principle, namely, because the effect of actions on other persons is as unpredictable as their free responses are.

Regarding its scope of protection for vulnerable subjects, the lack of a principle of distribution already indicates that it is not the individual in her basic rights who is the measure for the justice of a system. No theoretical argument is available that establishes the just treatment of each individual as the standard by which consequences need to be judged. How is it possible, on the basis of which criteria, to distinguish between mere wishes, preferences or private interests which can be sacrificed (such as smoking), and basic individual rights, which cannot? The average and additive calculation of happiness with its implicit sacrificial principle leaves Utilitarianism open to the charge that the terms in which it has been developed at least originally do not allow for a categorical prohibition, itself an achievement of cultural insights and historical struggles, to instrumentalise or violate fellow-humans in the interests of a majority. Additional assumptions borrowed from other traditions of thinking are necessary.

Deontological Ethics of Human Dignity

The central insight that gives deontology its name is that in moral reflection, the self discovers that an act ought to be done; it owes it to itself to do justice to this obligation. Agency is not only a straightforward drive, a movement of expansion, but also governed by a reflection that links it back to the self as its author. The ability to turn back on itself and to halt an action that is not in keeping with the agent's view of himself needs to be explained in its possibility. This is what Kant (1724–1804) does in a transcendental analysis that seeks to uncover the condition of the possibility of knowing and acting within the self. In this metatheoretical move, one goes behind what is experienced – for instance, that there are actions that are done out of respect for the moral law – to understand the condition of its possibility. This condition that one has to assume, but cannot prove empirically, is freedom. While Kant admits that it is equally thinkable that human beings are completely determined by nature, he takes the experience of obligation or sensitivity to moral concerns as a reason against a purely naturalistic explanation of human consciousness and action. A deontological account of ethics thus sees the human person as capable of perceiving duties and rights, of understanding that the other person in her equally original freedom is a limit to one's action if this action means that I instrumentalise her for my own plans. The humanistic formulation of Kant's 'Categorical Imperative' is: 'Act in such a way that you always treat humanity, whether in your own person or in the person of any other, never simply as a means but always at the same time as an end.[14] ' How demanding this account of morality is can be seen in the fact that this obligation holds regardless of whether the other person returns the recognition offered. Even if the relationship is not mutual, thus, also in cases of silence or of enmity, morality demands of the self to continue to extend respect even if it remains one-sided. We owe it to our dignity not to act in certain ways. As the capability for morality, dignity is the foundation of autonomy, which means self-government by the moral law. Not to do justice to this dimension is heteronomy.

In distinction from virtue ethics, the autonomy approach puts forward a formal rule of judgment, left to the agent's conscience to decide, instead of substantive and concrete contents, such as courage or compassion. Intentions or maxims of actions are judged by the principle of universalisability of whether every one could do so. Thus, its measure is not the social expectation of a specific cultural context. On the contrary, it submits these contexts to moral evaluation, transcending their historical values and judging them by principles based on moral self-reflection, discerning whether a maxim or intention respects or violates the other or humanity in oneself. Its horizon is not communitarian but cosmopolitan. With such an extensive scope of ethics, namely all humanity, the question arises where such an encompassing perspective can be anchored. For Kant, it is in the 'good will' that is a human disposition.[15] Ricoeur sees a parallel in it to Aristotle's most comprehensive and

---

[14] Kant, I., *Groundwork of the Metaphysic of Morals*, trans. H.J. Paton (New York: Harper, 1964), 96.

[15] The opening sentence of Kant's *Groundwork of the Metaphysic of Morals*, 61, is: 'It is impossible to conceive anything at all in the world, or even out of it, which can be taken as good without qualification, except a *good will*.' (BA 1)

leading virtue, the capacity for justice.[16] Good action is not, however, anchored in the striving for a happy or flourishing life congruent with the typical features of human nature. The quest for meaning or happiness is recognised in Kant's concept of the highest good that comprises both moral goodness and happiness, but the second has to be proportionate to the first. Morality is an order of its own, the two have to be distinguished, and their conflict leads to the antinomy of practical reason. The harmonious view of human striving as coinciding with what is good is not shared by Kant; the painful experience that good intentions can fail to reach their goal or be counteracted is acknowledged as a problem so serious that it puts into question the foundations of ethics.

The decisive difference to Utilitarianism is that it excludes the sacrificial principle. Deontology insists that individuals may never be instrumentalised and fundamentally disputes that moral choices can be justified by their consequences. The only feature that can make an act good is the intention that guides it, the good will. This is what distinguishes it both from antique ethics and from Utilitarianism: the shift from ends towards which we strive naturally (as in virtue ethics) to an emphasis on the will. One can see the influence of the heritage of biblical monotheism in Kant's repositioning of the good from the *cognitive* sphere of insight to which it was linked in Greek philosophy to the quality of the *will*. Kant's insistence that acts need to be judged imminently, rather than by their external results, recognises the decisive role of conscience and self-reflection that modern Neo-Hegelian virtue ethics and Utilitarianism downplay for different reasons. What is crucial for an adequate analysis of Kant's theory of practical reason is that it is not based on rationality as such, as in the *Critique of Pure Reason* but on the will that realises the human capability to be moral, which is the foundation of human dignity.

Evaluating this approach in terms of its concepts of self, agency and inter-subjectivity, its historical achievement is that it provides a definition of human dignity that is the source of human rights and the uniting foundation of respect for pluralistic self-understandings.[17] Several chapters in this book refer to how it operates as a guiding principle in constitutions, United Nations declarations and documents both of the Council of Europe and of the European Union. Its decisive quality is the argument and the scope it gives for the protection of vulnerable subjects. Human freedom and its actualisation in the good will is not of an order that can be demonstrated and proved empirically, as some current definitions of personhood by empirically verifiable features – consciousness, or ability to voice one's interests – assume. The capability for morality has to be assumed as belonging to every human being, regardless of their actual cognitive or other capacities.

---

[16] Ricoeur, "Ethics and Human Capability: A Response," in J. Wall, W. Schweiker and D. Hall (eds.), *Paul Ricoeur and Contemporary Moral Thought* (London/New York: Routledge, 2002), 279–290, 285–289.

[17] For treatments of this principle from different disciplines, cf. *Cambridge Handbook of Human Dignity. Historical Traditions, Philosophical Interpretations, Legal Implementation and Contemporary Challenges*, ed. by M. Düwell, J. Braarvig, R. Brownsword, D. Mieth (Cambridge: CUP, forthcoming 2012).

It has, however, in its emphasis on morality as distinct from self-interest and from striving for a flourishing life, reduced the sphere of practical reason to an analysis of its deontological dimension. The rationality in determining priorities of values that Aristotelian ethics excelled in has been outside of its purview. Its major deficits are seen in the failure to provide a link to what motivates agency, such as the hope for a flourishing life in keeping with the virtues, and the gap between justification and application. It needs middle axioms or intermediary principles to specify what dignity means in concrete cases, such as of children's rights. Kant provides categories for differentiated proposals, such as the distinction between perfect and imperfect duties, and designates decision-making on concrete cases to the faculty of judgment (*Urteilskraft*) which mediates between principles (e.g. to tell the truth) and concrete situations. However, the uniqueness that is discussed in relation to artists and their standard-setting works in the *Critique of Judgment*, urgently needs to be extended to persons in their singularity, as Ricoeur has shown convincingly in his critique of the contradiction between the 'universal law' and the pluralist ('persons as ends in themselves') formulations of the Categorical Imperative.[18]

The final two schools are Neo-Kantian in that their social and political ethics proposals start out from 'free and equal' citizens. They agree to the difference between the 'right' and the 'good' that has arisen from Kant's distinction between duties of law and duties of virtue. Much of the debate between and about them is on how they reinterpret their Kantian heritage.[19]

Contract Ethics

Contract ethics seeks to reconcile the freedom and the equality of citizens by presupposing an agreement on sharing benefits and burdens concluded in a fictional contract situation. The most famous recent version of this foundation proposed in 1762 by Jean-Jacques Rousseau (1723–1790) is John Rawls's *Theory of Justice* (1971).[20] It develops its two principles of justice with the help of the device of an 'original position' in which participants choose behind a 'veil of ignorance' regarding their position and assets the game-setting rules for society. For Rawls, the outcome of this thought experiment is an agreement on justice as fairness.

The first foundation of *Theory of Justice* is a contract which is entered into out of self-interest. It has been much discussed whether Rawls's use of rational choice theory for this part of his argumentation undermines the ethical foundations of justice in the 'sense of justice' he equally assumes to be shared by humans. A second foundation can be discovered in his reference to the 'considered convictions' of citizens that point to historically achieved standards.

---

[18] Ricoeur, *Oneself as Another*, 262–273.

[19] Cf. in relation to medical ethics, the chapter on "Autonomy, Individuality and Consent" in O'Neill, O., *Autonomy and Trust in Bioethics* (Cambridge: CUP, 2002), 28–48.

[20] Rawls, J., *A Theory of Justice* (Cambridge/MA: Belknap Press, 1971).

In the cultural situation after the civil rights movements of the 1960s and 1970s, the contract approach with its regard for equal autonomy found much resonance. It also supported the move from a medical ethics based on the virtue of physicians with its latent paternalism to an autonomy-centered patient ethics in which informed consent became key. The strength of this approach in research settings is that it is based on reciprocity, with the researcher or the physician as a technical expert and the informed citizen as their counterpart.

Rawls understood his *Theory of Justice* with its insistence on individual rights as setting out an alternative to the prevalent Utilitarianism in English-speaking social ethics. His second book, *Political Liberalism*, written in realisation of the 'fact of pluralism', argues for the need of a different level than any of the 'comprehensive' traditions of thinking, such as virtue ethics, Kantianism or Utilitarianism, a neutral level he calls 'public reason'.[21] For him, also Kant's analysis of morality as a universal feature of humans, as well as the Preamble and Article 1 of the UN Declaration of Human Rights with its principle of human dignity are such particular proposals,[22] what he calls comprehensive doctrines that cannot constitute a basis for consensus. Instead, all that can be achieved is an 'overlapping consensus' in which different worldviews and values systems coincide for contingent reasons.

In the evaluation of this approach, casting agency in terms of rational choice has been controversial. Separately, his recourse to the contract tradition has been critiqued for cutting out the pre-political foundations of democracy in cultural and intellectual traditions to which citizens belong and which they reinterpret in their 'co-foundation' of the public sphere.[23] The second foundation in 'considered convictions', and *Political Liberalism's* understanding of pluralism in terms of comprehensive doctrines which need to be translated into 'public reason' leave this pure contract foundation behind. Yet, its individualism is retained in that no interaction between citizens and their traditions is required for translation into public reason.

Protection for vulnerable subjects can be seen as the core motif of *Theory of Justice* in its rejection of the sacrificial principle implied in Utilitarianism. However, its scope is affected by several theory decisions: With no shared moral consensus, only contingently overlapping ones, and no principle of human dignity as the source of human rights, it depends completely on the convictions of the comprehensive doctrines as to whether this rejection of sacrificing a minority will be upheld. In addition, the horizon is not cosmopolitan but that of a 'bounded society' so that, for instance, despite the 'just savings principle' for a country's future generations, questions of climate justice and of transnational justice of resources will

---

[21] Rawls, *Political Liberalism* (New York: Columbia University Press, 1993).

[22] Rawls, *The Law of Peoples, With 'The Idea of Public Reason Revisited'* (Cambridge/MA: Harvard University Press, 1999), 80, Fn. 23: 'some seem more aptly described as liberal aspirations, such as Article 1...: 'all human beings are born free and equal in dignity and rights. They are endowed with reason and conscience and should act towards one another in a spirit of brotherhood.' Articles 3-18 count as 'human rights proper.'

[23] Ricoeur, *Reflections on the Just*, trans. D. Pellauer (Chicago: University of Chicago Press, 2007), 105.

find a limited reception.[24] Moreover, the idea expressed in *Theory of Justice* that more effective measures might be taken if justice could commence at the level of genetics, rather than in already entrenched social structures[25] (with its admittedly dangerous neighbourhood to eugenic ideas), has attracted the critiques of authors on disability. Its view of nature just in terms of individual assets in an unquestioned competitive society asks for a response that offers a different view of human embodiment.

Discourse Ethics

Discourse ethics interprets its Kantian foundations by replacing the categorical imperative, seen as monological, with a consensus to be reached in domination-free inter-subjective discourse. It tries to identify conditions for reaching a moral consensus in a public sphere in which citizens participate in their function both as authors and as addressees of laws. It thus goes beyond the negative rights prevalent in liberalism to a participative understanding of the project of democracy. Judgments in concrete cases have to be deliberated and pass the test of a discursive procedure according to universalisable criteria. Climate conferences or citizens' fora on scientific and technological developments that will impact on their lifeworlds would be examples relevant for research settings.

Discourse ethics distinguishes itself especially from liberalism by insisting on the possibility of an impartial moral point of view, rather than a merely overlapping consensus. With its origin in the critical theory developed by Max Horkheimer, Theodor W. Adorno, Erich Fromm and others in the 1930s in the Frankfurt Institute of Social Research, it is keen to keep the difference between a factual consensus and a true consensus as a task for ongoing self-critical reflection. The author who has shaped it in the last half century, Jürgen Habermas, has defended this model especially against the renaissance of Nietzschean and neo-conservative thinking. In relation to his fellow Neo-Kantians, he has pointed to the typically liberal neglect to consider the effects of individual citizens' decisions on third parties. His diagnosis of the pathologies of a society that pitches 'individual liberties exclusively against one another like weapons'[26] is aimed at reinvigorating a

---

[24] O'Neill, O., *Bounds of Justice* (Cambridge: CUP, 2000), 133, on *The Law of Peoples*: 'When Rawls finally relaxes the assumption that justice is internal to states, he argues only for selected principles of transnational justice. He repeats the thought experiment of the original position... but claims to establish only those principles of international justice which are the analogues of his first principle of justice: non-intervention, self-determination, *pacta sunt servanda*, principles of self-defence and of just war. There is no international analogue of the difference principle, and hence no account of transnational economic justice.'

[25] Rawls, *Theory of Justice*, 107–108. Buchanan, A., Daniels, N., Wikler, D. and Brock, D., *From Chance to Choice* (Cambridge: CUP, 2001).

[26] Habermas, J., *Between Naturalism and Religion*, trans. Ciaran Cronin (Cambridge: Polity Press, 2008), 107: An 'uncontrolled modernization of society could certainly corrode the democratic bonds and undermine the form of solidarity on which the democratic state depends even though it cannot enforce it. Then the very constellation that Böckenförde has in mind would transpire, namely, the transformation of the citizens of prosperous and peaceful liberal societies into isolated, self-interested monads who use their individual liberties exclusively against one another like weapons.'

participative public sphere inspired by the original Kantian understanding of the public use of reason oriented towards arguing out what can be considered to be in the interests of all.

There have been long-standing debates with German- and English-speaking colleagues in philosophy and theology, the individual social sciences and law, on the core concepts of this theory. Beginning from inter-subjectivity, it does not consider the reflexivity of the self which it attributes to a philosophy of consciousness that it sees as superseded by the paradigm change to language theory. In the last decade, however, in Habermas's critique of proposals for the genetic enhancement of children, Kierkegaard's concept of self has been the key argument in conjunction with Kant's idea of autonomy and relations of equality applied to parents and children.[27] It has developed a comprehensive and detailed theory of action in dialogue with different individual sciences, as initiated by the interdisciplinary research project of the first generation of the Frankfurt School. Yet, the idea of the flourishing life, or, as Ricoeur specifies, of 'living well with and for others in just institutions',[28] remains foreign to this approach which therefore cannot account for the motivation needed to sustain the high expectations to citizens as moral subjects and their discourse.

Its scope of protection for vulnerable subjects is cosmopolitan, and its idea of embedding moral discourse on the enormous new challenges posed by new technologies, such as cloning, in a 'species ethics', offers interesting perspectives. It also asks for wide-ranging debates and mutual 'translations' between citizens with and without religion as part of their self-understanding in view of the social pathologies that pressures of commercialisation and system imperatives have inflicted on communicative lifeworlds. The vitality of all cultural resources and their mutual exchange are needed to come up with equitable and inventive proposals for parliaments to process further. With its explication of rationality as communicative, the trust of this school of thinking is in the public sphere and includes proposals for the European project as a peaceful and diverse political experiment between constitutional democracies. In the third part of my overview, I can now explore how the contexts of different political cultures shape the perception of the potential and of the ethical challenges of science and new technologies and of research therein.

Cultural Memory and Political Institutions as Decisive Contexts for Research Parameters and for Public Debate

The embedded nature of concrete moral judgment is made evident in studies of how states differ regarding their permissiveness or restrictiveness in new biotechnologies. These patterns can be reconstructed from what the Harvard theorist

---

[27] Habermas, *The Future of Human Nature*, trans. Hella Beister and Wiliam Rehg (Cambridge: Polity Press, 2003).

[28] Ricoeur, *Oneself as Another*, 172.

of technology studies Sheila Jasanoff calls their 'political culture'.[29] This includes the way in which a society structures the connection between law and ethics as the legal and the moral normative orders, and how it regulates private companies, consumer demand and state support in health care institutions for citizens' options.

Jasanoff concludes that 'public responses to biotechnology are embedded within robust and coherent political cultures and are not ad hoc expressions of concern that vary unpredictably from issue to issue'. In the United States, the market takes the place of the expert committees and institutions that regulate bioethical innovations in the United Kingdom. In Germany, regulation is entrusted to the law. It should be added that this law is tied to the opening principle of the German Constitution that 'human dignity is inviolable' which 'to respect and protect... is the duty of all state authority'.[30] Jasanoff summarises:

> In the United States, where the market is the dominant form of social ordering, it is no accident that biotechnology has been construed as a stream of products, the goods that the market is best positioned to deliver and regulate. In Britain, where the state regulates innovation by creating a shared empirical culture of taken-for-grantedness, it again seems natural to focus on, and be seen to master, a process that visibly remakes life in forms not yet well understood by experts or publics. And German attentiveness to possibly dangerous programmatic alliances between technological innovation and the state is coupled to a postwar legal and political order that is exceptionally resistant to the idea of ungoverned or ungovernable spaces and to categories that defy the controlling capacity of the law.[31]

The form of regulation has consequences for the public sphere:

> In particular, regulatory choices invariably affect the degree to which publics can unpack and deliberate on the underlying purposes of innovation. Which of the brave new worlds opened up by biotechnology are worth our collective investment? Which, perhaps, will produce lives we will regret living with, or living at all?... Not surprisingly, opportunities for deliberating on the aims of innovation

---

[29] S. Jasanoff, 'In the democracies of DNA: ontological uncertainty and political order in three states,' in New Genetics and Society 24 (2005) 139–155, 154, Fn. 2. She defines this concept of political culture without naming the role of cultural memory and of philosophical traditions, although they are referred to in her comparison of factors contributing to each country's outlook: Political culture is the 'systematic means by which a political community makes binding collective choices. The term encompasses structured modes of action, such as litigiousness in the United States, but also the myriad unwritten codes and practices with which a polity supplements its formal methods of assuring accountability and legitimacy in political decision-making. Political culture in contemporary knowledge societies includes the tacit, but nonetheless powerful, routines by which collective knowledge is produced and validated. It embraces institutionalized approaches to reasoning and deliberation. But equally,...political culture includes the moves by which a polity, almost by default, takes some issues or questions out of the domain of politics as usual.' The quote is taken from S. Jasanoff, Designs on Nature: Science and Democracy in Europe and the United States (Princeton: Princeton University Press, 2005), 21.

[30] German Basic Law, Art. 1, paragraph 1.

[31] Jasanoff, "In the Democracies of DNA", 151–152.

have been most conspicuously absent in the United States, the country most hospitable to the fact of innovation. Farmed out to public intellectuals and, lately, to presidential ethics commissions of uncertain legitimacy and purpose, the task of reflecting on the directions of biotechnological advancement has largely been excluded from the public sphere. In Britain, the shock of the 'mad cow' crisis, coupled with turn-of-the-century pressures for political reform, converted expert ignorance and uncertainty into a more political issue than ever before... But questions of what is have to date occupied the British political imagination more than questions of what ought to be... Only in Germany has the temptation to privatize ethical deliberation been successfully resisted and the normative and political questions surrounding biotechnology have been extensively debated in the public sphere. But the response has been to erect high, some would say unacceptably high, barriers against social and technological creativity.[32]

Table 1.1 neatly spells out the distinctive orders of priority and accountability between state government, parliament, courts, civil society and the market, showing profoundly different attitudes towards risk, unforeseeable consequences and threats to human dignity.[33]

Table 1.1 National Strategies of Normalisation

United States	United Kingdom	Germany
Monsters encouraged	Monsters permitted	Monsters forbidden
Market-regulated innovation	Expert-regulated innovation	Law-regulated innovation
Decentralized norms	Centralized norms	Centralized norms
Winner-take-all settlement of controversy	Consensual settlement of controversy	Reasoned (principled) settlement of controversy
Judicial accountability	Parliamentary and administrative accountability	Legislative accountability

What can be seen as encouraging in Sheila Jasanoff's analysis of legislation in four bioethical areas (abortion, assisted reproduction, embryonic stem cells and genetically modified (GM) crops and foods) is that states are still able to be guided in their decision-making by what Rawls has called 'considered convictions': insights and judgments drawn from historical experience and from processes of consensus formation, some of them painful. It speaks against the impression that biotechnological advances are beyond the control of democratic processes as if they were a force of nature.

The consequence of an analysis that advocates the resource of political deliberation is that the individual graduate researcher is released from the burden to have to assess and stand up for the moral probity of their research all by themselves. Such an exclusive delegation to experts would disempower the public. Conditions

---

[32] Ibid., 153.
[33] Ibid., 151.

conducive to public opinion formation can be identified and supported, a vibrant public sphere is the best ally for researchers keen to explore the potential of new applications of science for defensible social goals; the role of assessing on behalf of society their potential for disrupting standards achieved in historical struggles for equality is not only theirs. By helping to create a research culture that discharges its obligation to be transparent and educate both ordinary and expert lay people who have specialised in other areas, they give back to the public realm what it needs to discuss and to move on to the legislative level of parliament. While the strenuous task of sifting the evidence belongs to researchers, assessing the societal and global impacts of new technologies is a matter for their interdisciplinary translation and collaboration. Encouraging the capacity for moral judgment in fellow citizens, multiple circles of belonging, communities, universities and churches offer sounding boards in coherently developed traditions of thinking. As co-founders of the public space, such 'heterogeneous traditions' provide the foundation of democratic authority in an awareness of their own historical shortcomings: they provide 'a multiple foundation, a diversity of religious and secular, rational and Romantic traditions, that mutually recognize one another as cofoundational... themselves... reinvigorated and driven by their unkept promises'.[34]

Graduate researchers know that their ethical responsibility is not exhausted by having consent forms signed. Their moral reflection is advanced by trying to understand different heritages of 'collective sense-making'. These give rise to convictions rooted in reflections on successful and on flawed courses of action, resulting in changed self-understandings in response to historical experiences, in striving for wisdom in judgment under conditions of finitude.

Bibliography

Anzenbacher A. *Einführung in die Ethik*. Düsseldorf: Patmos; 1992, 32.

Beauchamp T, Childress JF. *Principles of Bioethics*. New York/Oxford: Oxford University Press; 1989.

Bosk CL. "Professional Ethicist Available: Logical, Secular, Friendly". *Daedalus* 1999;128:47−68.

Buchanan A, Daniels N, Wikler D, Brock D. *From Chance to Choice*. Cambridge: Cambridge University Press; 2001.

Düwell M, Braarvig J, Brownsword R, Mieth D, editors. *Cambridge Handbook of Human Dignity. Historical Traditions, Philosophical Interpretations, Legal Implementation and Contemporary Challenges*. Cambridge: Cambridge University Press; 2012, forthcoming.

Greisch J. "Ethics and Lifeworlds". In: Kearney R, Dooley M, editors. *Questioning Ethics. Contemporary Debates in Philosophy*. London/New York: Routledge; 1999. p. 44−61. 56−59.

Habermas J. [Beister H, Rehg W, Trans.] *The Future of Human Nature*. Cambridge: Polity Press; 2003.

---

[34] Ricoeur, *Reflections on the Just*, 105.

Habermas J. [Cronin C, Trans.] *Between Naturalism and Religion.* Cambridge: Polity Press; 2008.

Haker H. "Synthetic Biology: an Emerging Debate in European Ethics," in this volume.

Höffe O, editor. *Einführung in die utilitaristische Ethik. Klassische und zeitgenössische Texte.* München: Beck; 1975.

Jasanoff S. "In the Democracies of DNA: Ontological Uncertainty and Political Order in Three States". *New Genet Soc* 2005;24:139−55.

Junker-Kenny M. "Virtues and the God Who Makes Everything New". In: Mayes A, Jeanrond W, editors. *Recognising the Margins: Essays in Honour of Sean Freyne.* Dublin: Columba Press; 2006. p. 298−320.

Kant I. [Paton HJ, Trans.] *Groundwork of the Metaphysic of Morals.* New York, NY: Harper; 1964.

MacIntyre A. *After Virtue.* London: Duckworth; 1981.

Mei TS, Lewin D, editors. *From Ricoeur to Action. The Socio-Political Significance of Ricoeur's Thinking.* (Continuum Studies in Continental Philosophy) New York/London: Continuum; 2012.

O'Neill O. *Autonomy and Trust in Bioethics.* Cambridge: Cambridge University Press; 2002.

O'Neill O. *Bounds of Justice.* Cambridge: Cambridge University Press; 2000.

Pfotenhauer SM, Jones CF, Saha K, Jasanoff S. "Learning from Fukushima". *Issues Sci Technol* 2012;28:79−84.

Rawls J. *A Theory of Justice.* Cambridge/MA: Belknap Press; 1971, 107−108.

Rawls J. *Political Liberalism.* New York, NY: Columbia University Press; 1993.

Rawls J. *The Law of Peoples, With 'The Idea of Public Reason Revisited'.* Cambridge/MA: Harvard University Press; 1999.

Ricoeur P. "Universal Civilisation and National Cultures (1961)". In: Kelbley ChA, editor. *History and Truth.* Evanston: Northwestern University Press; 1965. p. 271−84 [trans. and introd].

Ricoeur P. [Blamey K, Trans.] *Oneself as Another.* Chicago: University of Chicago Press; 1992.

Ricoeur P. "Ethics and Human Capability: A Response". In: Wall J, Schweiker W, Hall D, editors. *Paul Ricoeur and Contemporary Moral Thought.* London/New York: Routledge; 2002. p. 279−90. 285−289.

Ricoeur P. [Pellauer D, Trans.] *Reflections on the Just.* Chicago, IL: University of Chicago Press; 2007, 105.

Schnädelbach H. *"Was ist Neoaristotelismus?" Zur Rehabilitierung des animal rationale.* Frankfurt: Suhrkamp; 1992, 205−230, 228.

2 Navigating the Minefields: Ethics and Misconduct in Scientific Research

Alan L. Kelly

University College Cork, Cork, Ireland

Abstract

Scientific research today involves an increasingly well-defined set of principles of what constitutes good responsible conduct, and conversely what constitutes misconduct. These principles cover areas such as honesty in handling and reporting data and results, authorship of scientific principles and the manner in which scientists interact with other researchers. These developments have been catalysed by a number of high-profile cases of scientific misconduct in the last 20 years or so, and awareness of the norms of scientific conduct are today recognised as priorities for the training of future researchers. This chapter summarises some of the key aspects of scientific research conduct and ethics, in the context of an introduction to the area for graduate students.

Key Words

Ethics, publication, scientific misconduct, plagiarism, fabrication, falsification

Introduction

Scientific research may be described as an idealistic quest for truth, particularly knowledge about the natural world. In a simplistic description of 'how science works', scientists have ideas which inspire them to undertake experiments or studies, trials or measurements; if they succeed, they communicate their research in a written format, principally through publication of articles in the scientific literature, if deemed to be interesting and reliable following review by peers in the field. By the outputs of their research, scientists are then judged, in terms of their success as professional researchers, and this has subsequent implications for their career and funding opportunities.

Ethics for Graduate Researchers. DOI: http://dx.doi.org/10.1016/B978-0-12-416049-1.00002-7

Of course, in this idealised scenario, a key underlying assumption and expectation is that scientists are honest at all stages of the scientific endeavour. In other words, they must be honest when they propose to do research, in the manner in which they acquire their ideas, in the way in which they undertake their research and interact with others and, in particular, in the manner in which they report the outcomes of their research.

In recent years, however, a number of high-profile cases where researchers have failed to adhere to these accepted norms of scientific conduct have occurred. Such cases of research misconduct, including what may be termed ethical breaches, have gained attention from the media, policy-makers and funding agencies; possibly the most infamous recent example would be the wide range of ethical breaches involved in the stem cell work led by the Korean scientist Hwang Woo-Suk.[1] As a result, there has been an increasing focus on the importance of a high level of awareness of ethics and good research conduct among researchers at all levels.

It is recognised that a key opportunity to create responsible researchers with a good understanding of ethical principles lies in graduate education, where students should be, as part of their training in research, introduced to principles of good research conduct and learn about appropriate ethical principles alongside their studies towards a doctoral degree.

The objective of this chapter is to summarise some key implications of research ethics in a manner which is accessible and suitable for postgraduate research students. I will first outline what is meant by research ethics, and then consider the factors that influence misbehaviour, what constitutes misconduct, and issues of authorship and peer review, plagiarism, treatment of colleagues and dealing with error.

What Is Meant by Research Ethics?

A dictionary definition of research ethics will typically refer to the principles of conduct governing an individual or group, a set of moral principles or values, or the moral uprightness of an action or judgment. Thus, ethics fundamentally concerns issues of right or wrong in the area under discussion. The interpretations of this in the specific context of scientific research will be the primary focus of this chapter.

Ethical considerations in scientific research typically fall into two principal areas:

1. Ethical considerations associated with particular types of research, such as that involving human subjects, confidential information, interview data or animal experimentation.

---

[1] For one account of this case, see Cyranoski, D. "Verdict: Hwang's human stem cells were all fakes." *Nature*, 439 (2006), 122–133.

2. Ethical issues involved in the conduct of research itself, and in particular with the reporting of the results thereof, e.g. fabrication or falsification of data, or plagiarism (all of which will be discussed later in this chapter).

While it is acknowledged that not all research students will be working in the fields which entail specific ethical concerns, as in the first category above, it must equally be recognised that all students must have an awareness or the expectations of good research conduct (i.e. the second category), and the importance of avoidance of fabrication, falsification, plagiarism and other incidences of misconduct which apply to *all* disciplines. This is critical so that young researchers begin their careers in research with a strong set of appropriate values and principles.

Why Might Scientists Misbehave?

For many years, perhaps until the 1980s, it was taken for granted that scientific researchers were honest in their dealings at all stages of the research process, but a number of unfortunate and high-profile cases since that time have drawn attention to the possibility that this may not have been the case; a number of cases of this type will be discussed later in this chapter.

A key question which may be asked concerns why would scientists be dishonest. To try and unravel the reasons why a researcher would behave in a way which could be considered as misconduct, it must first be acknowledged that reputation is key to scientists. A researcher's reputation depends heavily on publications (today, more and more this is measured in terms of quality, e.g. by citations for their articles and impact factors of the journals in which they publish, rather than just quantity), and their career prospects (and therefore personal earnings) depend on this productivity. Thus, as in many spheres of human activity in which advantages can be acquired by certain questionable or prohibited actions, there may be individuals who try to take short cuts, for reasons of personal gain, advancement or other reward. Other drivers for misconduct may include insecurity, a wish to impress or a reluctance to admit failure.

Working from the principle that one of the most important assets of a researcher is the list of their publications, it follows that a critical area of potential ethical challenge is credit and authorship, and indeed it is quite probable that the most likely ethical dilemmas to be encountered by a graduate students concern authorship of their papers. Today, there is great focus, among authors and editors alike, on unacceptable practices such as honorary or ghost authorship; these will be discussed in more detail later in this chapter.

Another area of potential ethical concern for scientists involves the need for openness regarding conflicts of interest. This includes declaration of all information relating to a piece of research (especially regarding the source of funding) which may influence the conclusions which a reader might take from that research, and their subsequent actions.

Thus, the research environment today is somewhat of a minefield, with a wide range of areas where there is an increasing need to define understanding of what constitutes acceptable behaviour, and increasing scrutiny for transgressions thereof.

The Nature of Scientific Misconduct

The nature of scientific misconduct has been the subject of discussion and consideration for many years. Perhaps the first systemic study of the topic was undertaken by the early computer scientist Charles Babbage (1791–1871), who referred to practices such as:

- hoaxing (e.g. faking results perhaps in a humorous manner, where it is generally expected that the hoax will be eventually discovered);
- forging (where results are faked, i.e. data are generated by the researcher and not their measurements or instruments, and not expected to be discovered; this is now generally referred to as fabrication);
- trimming ('clipping' off bits of observations to make patterns look neater and more accurate); and
- cooking (omission or concealment of less desirable results, generally to make patterns and trends look clearer or more in line with the researcher's bias as to what the result should be; this is now generally referred to as falsification).[2]

Over the intervening years, many famous scientists have had their work scrutinised for evidence that they could be said to have engaged in any such practices. To take but two examples, questions have been raised about the suspicious 'goodness' of the data yielded by Mendel in his famous experiments on pea genetics, while the famous physicist Robert Millikan has been frequently criticised for the manner in which he reported the results of his famous 'oil-droplet' experiments, from which he measured the charge of the electron, which has been criticised by a number of historians of science as being less than transparent.[3]

Thus, it is recognised today that there are key areas where awareness of good research conduct is acute. Following on from Babbage, the three key areas which today are most frequently regarded as the main types of unethical misconduct are fabrication (the creation of data or results to not reflect experimental reality), falsification (the manipulation of existing data to give an outcome other than that which they would otherwise show) and plagiarism (the copying of data, ideas or text from other sources). In addition, of course, there are grey areas, involving questionable research conduct, some of which will be mentioned later.

While it has been stated earlier that principles of good research conduct and avoidance of fabrication, falsification and plagiarism are common to all disciplines, an interesting question arises as to whether the severity of the implication of

---

[2] For a good discussion of this classification, see Judson, H.F. *The Great Betrayal; Fraud in Science* (Harcourt, Inc., Orlando, FL, 2004).

[3] Holton, G. (1978) "Subelectrons, Presuppositions and the Millikan–Ehrenhaft Dispute" in *The Scientific Imagination: Case Studies* (Cambridge University Press, Cambridge, 1978), pp. 25–83.

misconduct is the same in all disciplines. For example, should a researcher who is found guilty of falsification or fabrication of data in the field of astrophysics be subject to the same moral code or ethical expectations (and subsequent penalties for misconduct) as a researcher working in the field where the outputs of the research impact directly on the lives of others, such as cancer research? Such questions, while undoubtedly of great interest within the field of ethical considerations in scientific research situations, are beyond the scope of this chapter.

A key question in any consideration of research ethics and research conduct in modern science is the extent to which principles of good conduct in research are adhered to by researchers, and conversely the level of misconduct which is found in reality. The answer will be very different depending on who is asked, with the view of those in media or regulatory agencies likely being very different to that of scientists themselves. There is no doubt that cases of misconduct which have been discovered and identified do not represent all the cases of misconduct which have occurred, and that many papers lie today in the scientific literature which, unbeknownst to the reader, contain false and fabricated data and should not be trusted. However, the important subsequent question is whether we are only seeing the tip of the iceberg of scientific fraud or whether we can see the bulk of the iceberg at this point.

An interesting study published in *Nature*[4] involved a confidential questionnaire to over 3000 scientists in the United States, which asked whether they had engaged in certain forms of conduct that would be regarded as inappropriate. For more serious transgressions, levels of responses, while not zero, were very low, i.e. < 5%; this included falsifying or 'cooking' data, ignoring major aspects of human subject requirements, or not disclosing commercial vested interest. Almost 1.5% of respondents indicated using ideas of others without permission or credit in their work, and a relatively high level (15%) indicated that they had changed the design, results or methods of study due to pressure from a funding source; 10% of respondents indicated that they had inappropriately assigned authorship or withheld details of methodologies from papers, and 15% indicated that they had dropped data based on the gut feeling that the data were inadequate, which is the charge usually levelled at Robert Millikan in the context of his oil-drop experiments.

Nonetheless, there has to be an assumption of trust in the scientific process. If researchers were deemed guilty until proven innocent, and every submitted or published manuscript regarded as potentially dishonest or falsified, then the only solution would be for every paper to be submitted to a journal to be accompanied by a deluge of raw data, copies of laboratory notebooks, instrument printouts and other raw material from which the case was built and eventually summarised in the neat tables and figures of the paper. While this may allow editors and reviewers to ascertain with a much higher degree of confidence if the results presented were honestly obtained, the time required to process each paper would increase vastly and the scientific publishing process would grind to a halt. Honesty must be

[4] Martinson, B.C., Anderson, M.S. and de Vries, R. "Scientists Behaving Badly." *Nature* 435 (2005), 737–738.

assumed, but researchers must live up to that trust and earn it (and not lose it by dishonest dealings), while editors and referees do what they can to try and verify the veracity and reliability of submitted claims.

In any area of scientific ethics, the question of what penalties the authors guilty of misconduct should face is a matter of current debate. In the United States, those found guilty of serious misconduct have been barred from seeking federal funds for their research for significant periods of time[5] ; this, together with the reputational damage which will arise from any high-profile case where a researcher is 'caught' (and ambitious scientists love to gossip as much as anyone) can effectively mean the end of a researcher's career. Suggested penalties which journals could impose for authors guilty of publishing dishonest material could include a prohibition on further publication in that journal, informing other editors of the authors' behaviour, or even notifying the authors' institutions or funding agencies. Overall, the stakes are unquestionably, and rightly, very high indeed, when scientists choose to wander off the path of proper behaviour.

Ethics and Authorship

A particular area where ethical issues come to light that can often impact directly on postgraduate students concerns authorship of scientific publications. One of the most difficult considerations or discussions which may sometimes be encountered concerns the assignment of authorship for a student's paper. Today, it is recognised that there are two categories of authorship which are of particular concern:

1. 'ghost authors', i.e. researchers who have contributed to the work reported in a paper but for some reason (e.g. a personal disagreement with the senior author) have failed to be included as authors;
2. 'honorary authors', i.e. researchers who have not contributed sufficiently to the work described in a paper to deserve authorship, but whose names nonetheless appear as co-authors of the paper in question.

Incidences of practices such as honorary authorships were more common in decades past where, for example the head of department or research centre could demand to have their name on a paper coming out of that unit irrespective of whether they had been directly involved in the research. Such behaviour is now widely acknowledged to be wholly inappropriate.

Some areas of scientific literature, in particular the biomedical literature, have now developed highly defined guidelines for criteria on determining authorship of scientific papers. These were most explicitly elucidated in a set of principles laid down by a group of editors of medical journals at a meeting in Vancouver, Canada

---

[5] Good case studies of the penalties for misconduct in the US would include Kevles, D. *The Baltimore Case: a Trial of Politics, Science and Character* (W.W. Norton and Company, New York, NY, 1988) and Reich, E.S. *Plastic Fantastic: How the Biggest Fraud in Physics Shook the Scientific World* (Palgrave Macmillan, Basingstoke, UK, 2009).

(later the International Committee of Medical Journal Editors), and first published in 1979.[6] These principles indicate very clearly what must be done to warrant authorship, including involvement in undertaking the work, writing the manuscript in question and final approval of the version being submitted. The protocols also explicitly state that some activities, such as management or directorship of the research group or acquisition of funding alone, do not warrant authorship of the manuscript. In other fields of research, these principles are less explicitly developed, but there is no doubt that young researchers must be well aware of the criteria governing authorship.

Ethics and Peer Review

One of the critical pillars supporting the scientific process is peer review, the process by which any paper submitted for publication to a journal is subjected to scrutiny by experts who recommend to the editor whether the paper is worthy to be published in that journal. However, this review process itself is also potentially fraught with ethical considerations. The semi-open system of refereeing applied by most scientific journals, where the names and identities of authors are known to reviewers, but the names of the reviewers are not known to authors, arguably allows for the possible problems. This might involve, on the one hand, bias (positive or negative), from a reviewer towards an author which may allow them to assert influence without fear of discovery, or, on the other hand, plagiarism or theft of ideas from submitted manuscripts by reviewers hiding under the cloak of anonymity.

There have been many debates in recent years about the nature of the peer-review process and the attendant dangers as mentioned here. Some steps have been taken, on the one hand the introduction of 'open refereeing' where referees are required to sign their review, or, on the other hand totally 'blind' reviewing, where authors see manuscripts without any indication of who the authors are. However, most journals today still use the semi-open system, as it seems to suit their purposes best.

A final comment on the ethical aspects of refereeing concerns the obligation of researchers to act as a referee when invited. There is no doubt that a special day in any researcher's career is the one when they are first invited to review a manuscript, by an editor who seems to be interested in their views. The novelty rapidly wears off, however, particularly when several invitations, sometimes from journals one has never heard of and on topics only vaguely related to one's field of expertise, appear in the email inbox. However, if every researcher was too busy to review papers, it is clear what would happen; the peer-review process, and hence any semblance of reliability in the scientific literature, would grind to a halt. It could be proposed (perhaps simplistically) that, if in most scientific fields the norm

[6] International Committee of Medical Journal Editors "Ethical Consideration in the Conduct and Reporting of Research" http://www.icmje.org/ethical_1author.html.

would be for two reviewers to scrutinise each submitted paper, a researcher should review two papers for every one they publish, to repay the courtesy shown to their work by others and thereby 'balance the books'. Thus, researchers should think carefully before declining an invitation to review a paper which they would consider within their area of expertise.

Plagiarism in Scientific Writing: A Plague on All Our Houses

Arguably, the biggest and the most widespread ethical problems faced by the editors and publishers of scientific journals today is plagiarism. Ready access to the majority of the scientific literature online places in the hands of researchers an easy opportunity to cut and paste text and claim it as their own. However, in parallel, there have emerged advanced and sophisticated tools for comparison of text in submitted articles to those already published. This has placed powerful tools for the detection of plagiarism in the hands of those responsible for safeguarding the literature (e.g. editors and university authorities), and the results have been broadly very disappointing.

When journal editors have started to use software to analyse the text of papers submitted to their journals for similarity to previously published work, they have often been shocked at the extent to which authors have seemed content to engage in plagiarism, particularly of their own work. Cases of what might be considered the typical meaning of plagiarism, i.e. the theft of the ideas or words of others, are somewhat less frequent than those of authors recycling text from their own prior publications. The second type of plagiarism can be regarded as laziness or dishonesty in presenting previously generated text as a new creation, while the first type is much more serious, as it constitutes intellectual theft.

Arguably, the most controversial aspect of plagiarism is in the 'Materials and Methods' section of an experimental paper, where there can literally be only so many ways to say that a certain test or piece of scientific research practice has been performed, but authors must always strive to present a minimalist account of their methodology, using references to direct the reader who wishes to find out more to the original sources. The cardinal rule concerning the description of methodology used in the text is that it has to be detailed enough to allow anyone wishing to repeat the experiment or study exactly to be able to do so.

Ethics and the Treatment of Colleagues (and Rivals)

There can be no doubt that scientific research is competitive, and tough, and requires a high degree of persistence and determination for success. Every research student, to complete their project, needs to be able to work with a whole range of others and be able to have them do what they need for their project to keep moving forward; a key 'survival skill' for research students could thus be defined as diplomacy. Obviously, the student–supervisor (apprentice–master) relationship is the primary relationship which a graduate student must cultivate and work to keep harmonious, and most students can identify others in their immediate circle who they can call on for advice and support, such as other students, post-doctoral researchers and perhaps technical staff. However, beyond these immediate circles, in other laboratories, or even other institutions, there may be apparently uninvolved staff or students, sometimes in different areas, who may not immediately strike a student as critical, but who one day may have the helping hand the student urgently needs. Thus, while every research student is in a class of one, working on his/her own project towards their unique thesis and examination thereon, he/she must learn to work in an often ill-defined and fluid team. Graduate students must, in their own way, quietly lead that team to their own goals, often at times when the student has far more to ask then they ever could return.

Beyond graduation, a researcher will grow in confidence and stature, and perhaps become less dependent on the kindness of relative strangers. However, the culture of science has certain expectations for what might naively be called 'fair play', in terms of dealings with others. Many a scientist will encounter situations where interactions with colleagues and competitors will strain civility and cooperation to the limit, but nonetheless, professionalism remains the expected standard of behaviour.

One of the most frequently discussed case studies of the manner in which a scientist should, or should not, deal with their colleagues and competitors concerns the discovery of the structure of DNA by James Watson and Francis Crick in the early 1950s in Cambridge.[7] Watson's classic account of the discovery, *The Double Helix*, published a decade or so after the event, painted in no uncertain terms a picture of two very ambitious scientists who suffered fools badly and were single-minded in the pursuit of their goals. Rivals in the race to unlock a key aspect of life's most fundamental workings were dismissed, even if they had the stature of Linus Pauling, undoubtedly the giant of biological science in the first half of the twentieth century, but it was their interactions with a team far closer to home, in King's College in London, which has drawn most comment. In brief, the key data that led to their model (they did no experimental work themselves) were generated by an X-ray crystallographer at King's College, Rosalind Franklin, whose relationship with Watson and Crick was icy at best. The specific data which provided the last piece of the structural puzzle were provided to Watson by Franklin's colleague Maurice Wilkins, in frustration at his own inability to forge a good working relationship with Franklin. It is said that Franklin never knew the manner in which Watson had acquired the intuition to develop the correct model, and she died in 1958, before both the publication of Watson's frank account of the matter, and the award of the Nobel Prize to Watson, Crick and Wilkins (Nobel Prizes may not be

---

[7] An excellent account of this discovery is by Judson, H.F. (1996) "The eighth day of creation: makers of the revolution in biology." Cold Spring Harbour Press, while Watson's own account (Watson, J.D. "The Double Helix," reprinted many times) is rightly acclaimed as a seminal account of scientific discovery.

awarded posthumously). Franklin was unquestionably not the easiest person to work with but was an outstanding scientist, and many feel that the manner in which her work was built on by others, before publication and without her consent, represents a striking example of the behaviour which researchers are supposed to avoid.

More recently, in April 2011, a case emerged of a post-doctoral researcher in the University of Michigan who admitted to sabotaging the work of a PhD student whom he was trying to 'slow down'. They admitted spraying alcohol on her cultured cells when no one was around, bar the unsleeping eye of a hidden camera placed in the laboratory when the student reported many inexplicable problems with her research.

Researchers, alas, are human, and perhaps the type of personality which leads one into research all too often comes encumbered by parallel foibles such as independence, ambition and determination. This can result in behaviour towards others which is not the idealistic picture of normative behaviour; nonetheless, science must involve a degree of trust in others to treat each other with fairness, just as we hope we can trust scientists that what they say and write is honest and not false.

Dealing with Error

Of course, sometimes (rarely, one might hope) a researcher might publish a paper which they later discover to be unreliable due to errors in its preparation, which is not picked up during review, where readers of the paper who do not know of these errors may waste time or effort or both trying to reproduce or build on this wrong information. In such cases, as difficult as it may be, it is the responsibility of the author to correct the mistake and avoid any such future scenario, perhaps by submitting to the same journal a correction or erratum. A superb example of how to manage this kind of situation arose when an English astronomer, Andrew Lyne, realised that his 'discovery' of a planet orbiting a pulsar, the first such reported planet outside our solar system, was in fact an artefact due to a calculation error.[8] Lyne thought he had checked all such alternative explanations before publication, as a scientist is supposed to do; indeed a researcher should be their own most sceptical critic. Not only had he thought he had made a career-defining discovery and published the resulting paper in *Nature*, but he was about to go to talk about it at the largest international gathering of astronomers in the world, as a scientific celebrity. What did he do? While perhaps others might have, or have, decided to keep their heads down and let the lie lie, as it were, a booby trap for the unwary in the literature, he stood up at the conference, admitted his mistake and concluded with these words: 'Our embarrassment is unbounded and we are truly sorry'. For this astonishing display of integrity and guts, he received a standing ovation and duly set the standard for expectations of admission of error thereafter.

[8] For an excellent account of this, see Ken Crosswell's *Planet Quest: the Epic Discovery of Alien Solar Systems* (Free Press, New York, NY, 1997).

Conclusions

Scientific research today is governed by an increasingly explicitly articulated set of ethical codes, setting down the standards of integrity that are expected of a modern researcher. Case studies of unacceptable behaviour unfortunately abound and do not need to be invented. While some are summarised above, limitations of space preclude discussion of perhaps the most extravagant case study of all, which shows transgression of so many ethical principles as to make it hard to believe it was not created as a textbook case for students of biomedical research to be forced to study; this is the Korean stem cell scandal led by Woo-Suk Hwang and his colleagues in the 1990s, as mentioned earlier, and those readers who wish to learn more are advised to consult the numerous summaries and articles on this case available online. For the graduate student today, the ethical problems encountered are likely to be less dramatic, but will exist in every field; most likely, the first will emerge once a graduate student starts to ask who belongs on their first scientific paper. The stakes involved increase every year as codes of conduct and attendant penalties become more stringent; an early question or scandal can blight a career before it even starts.

Acknowledgement

The author would like to thank Professor Paul Jelen, University of Edmonton, Canada, for insightful comments on the draft manuscript.

Bibliography

Crosswell K. *Planet Quest: the Epic Discovery of Alien Solar Systems*. New York, NY: Free Press; 1997.

Cyranoski D. "Verdict: Hwang's human stem cells were all fakes". *Nature* 2006;439:122−33.

Holton G. *"Subelectrons, presuppositions and the Millikan−Ehrenhaft dispute"*. The *Scientific Imagination: Case Studies*. Cambridge: Cambridge University Press; 1978. pp. 25−83.

Judson HF. *The Great Betrayal: Fraud in Science*. Orlando, FL: Harcourt, Inc.; 2004 [An excellent if somewhat pessimistic overview of the classification and famous cases of scientific misconduct.].

Judson HF. *The Eighth Day of Creation: Makers of the Revolution in Biology*. Cold Spring, NY: Cold Spring Harbour Press; 1996.

Kevles D. *The Baltimore Case: a Trial of Politics, Science and Character*. New York, NY: W.W. Norton and Company; 1988 [A great case study of the famous case where a researcher in the laboratory of David Baltimore, one of the pre-eminent biologists of the twentieth century, was accused of dishonesty in presentation of data in a paper in

Cell, and the years of enquiries, involving literally forensic analysis of notebooks and character alike, that followed.].

Martinson BC, Anderson MS, de Vries R. "Scientists Behaving Badly". *Nature* 2005;435:737−8.

Reich ES. *Plastic Fantastic: How the Biggest Fraud in Physics Shook the Scientific World.* Basingstoke, UK: Palgrave Macmillan; 2009.

3 Ethics and the Researcher

Frank Gannon

The Queensland Institute of Medical Research, Herston, Brisbane, QLD, Australia

Abstract

Research is an essential component of advanced society. Underpinned by an effort to understand life and nature, the consequences for health care, industry and lives of the general population are immense. Without research, it is unlikely that better treatments for illness would be available, technologies improved, nature's bounties harvested effectively or the ever-expanding world population provided with adequate amounts of food. The behaviour of scientists therefore has to match the challenges they face. In this chapter, I focus on the laboratory, the scientists who work there and the environment that is created by the heads of laboratories. The potential for misconduct lurks everywhere, but the structure of the laboratory society works to ensure that high standards are adhered to. Each person in the laboratory has serious individual responsibilities, and in most cases, the trust placed in them individually and collectively is not betrayed.

Key Words

PhD students, post-doctoral fellow, laboratory head, falsification, ethical standards

Introduction

A recent paper noted that of 27,000 articles submitted per week, 200 will have to have some correction or alteration and approximately 5 will have to be retracted.[1] This is a small number, but it is growing annually. So it is important to consider how this comes about. In doing so, we should see that the need to retract is just the extreme end point of a gradient of less visible misdemeanours, all of which come under the rubric of ethics in the laboratory. In life, there are minor, almost insignificant misdemeanours, such as crossing the road when there is no traffic but there is a red sign telling you not to cross. The societal environment in which you live will have a big influence on whether you cross. The same is true in the research world;

[1] van Noorden, R. "The Trouble with Retractions" *Nature* 478 (2011), 26−28.

Ethics for Graduate Researchers. DOI: http://dx.doi.org/10.1016/B978-0-12-416049-1.00003-9

the environment has a large impact on your behaviour. And just as crossing the
road illegally can, with extreme extrapolation, lead to tolerating driving with more
alcohol in your system than is legal (and that can do serious damage), a lax ethical
aspect in the laboratory can also lead to very serious escalations. In this chapter,
I examine some of these contexts and in doing so hope to increase the awareness of
all in the research environment of their responsibilities and perhaps encourage
some who were reluctant to act to do so.

The motivation for embarking on a scientific career is almost always noble, to
add to the understanding of the universe or to provide a solution to some big problem. But it is also the first step on a career that will allow the pursuit of such goals to
continue and hence the drive to succeed, to be better than some others at the same
delicate stage, can have an influence on behaviour. The apprenticeship of a
researcher is carried out in the laboratory of somebody who has worked their way to
a position of having the resources to be able to take on a PhD student. It follows that
the moral tone will be set by that person, and experience shows that all flavours of
individuals reach the position in which they control the laboratory in which the
research will be performed. So nobility of intention cannot be taken for granted, and
it is not always the head of the laboratory who causes the problem. An early-stage
researcher who has had repeated 'failures' with some experiment that should give a
predicted result may be tempted to provide that result at the next laboratory meeting
rather than admit that he/she was not capable of doing what seemed easy. Deception
can be too easy at that stage. If the result is the expected next step on a research
road, the data may not be challenged in a robust way. But a researcher's ethical
behaviour is not restricted to avoidance of falsification or fabrication. They are part
of a team and, in all such circumstances, the way in which the dignity and rights of
each member of the team is a personal responsibility for all in the group. Equally, a
supervisor may abuse his/her position of power in many subtle ways that I address
later. This includes bullying, lax approaches to health and safety and lack of consideration of the rights to researchers when deciding on publication authorship. Each of
these examples will be examined later from the perspective of the responsibilities of
the researcher and of the research supervisor. I am instructed by experience in the
life sciences, but believe that the general messages apply to all research.

The Researcher

The biggest challenge for a researcher is to generate data. The increased frequency
of reports highlighting the fact that not all published data are reliable, gives rise for
concern for all those in research.[2] However, inventing or falsifying data is clearly
an extreme situation and probably very rare. Not all data that are presented at laboratory meetings get included in a research paper. If there is a flaw in the anticipated
path of the research, then building on false data will, usually, lead to increasingly

---

[2] Begley, CG and Ellis, L.M. Drug Development: Raise standards for preclinical cancer research. *Nature*
483 (2012), 531–533.

incompatible results and the project dies. If it gets pushed far enough to be submitted for publication, then the peer-review system with three independent referees will have a good probability of identifying the data that are weak and demand more information before publication. But there are situations where more minor misdemeanours can cloud judgement and the truth of the situation can remain uncovered. In an earlier article that considered fraudulent activities in the laboratory,[3] I pointed to the questions that arise when a data point does not fit on the line that is anticipated; was the sample mislabelled, were the lanes mixed up, is it an outlier that can be ignored? Or if a cell gives a strange result, is it the growth conditions or the media that explain it and allow it to be ignored? Or if an animal experiment does not fit into a series of experiments, is it due to some small change in the feed, or an undetected infection and hence could be ignored. Presented in a stark manner like that, there is no shadow of doubt that the experiments should be repeated, and I anticipate that this is what happens in 99.x% of cases. But in some cases, the inconvenient result is not revisited and that usually points to some flaw in the individual or the laboratory environment. Clearly, in each of those examples, there is a need to have more than one set of eyes analysing the original data and doing so with an aggressive demand for accuracy. Some laboratories have internal systems that ensure that this happens. But not all do so, and in situations where massive amounts of data are produced, it may not be realistic to have a forensic analysis of every point. This is why the laboratory group environment is a very important factor. If there is an intolerance of any short cut, even if it delays an important publication, then it will become the norm for the individual, when analysing the data they generate, to exercise the same standard of behaviour.

Research today is very frequently a team effort. There are some areas where a team implies working together. Increasingly, research requires the input from different perspectives and methodological approaches from members of a team that work individually. This collective input to a publication or a research presentation often means that each component of the input is only examined for its consistency with the overall outcome that is being presented. It is possible, therefore, that a detailed examination of the primary data does not take place if the result that is presented fits with the direction of the data of others. There is an obvious danger in this situation. Presented with a research protocol and an anticipation of the outcome, it could be tempting for the over-pressurised, technically inadequate or overambitious researcher to fudge the results and that this does not happen frequently comes predominantly from the inherent moral quality of the individuals who are researchers. Such qualities are, of course, found in every other walk of life; scientists cannot claim to be more morally secure than others. And it is true that there are some who fail to maintain, at all times, the level of performance that is expected. With research, however, there are some extra safeguards that probably ensure that it is rare for falsification to occur. The word research itself sends the message that the quest for knowledge is an attempt to discover more than had been known heretofore. At the frontiers of knowledge, the road map is uncertain.

---

[3] Gannon, F. "Fraud in our Laboratories?" *EMBO Reports* 8 (2007), 1.

Repeatedly, there are surprises and what had been taken for granted is overturned. This may be less true for more applied sciences, but there also the limits of performance may not be defined with certainty. Under such circumstances, it is always a risk to invent a result. Although this is not an endorsement of the scientific community's moral fibre, it is a very practical deterrent to taking short cuts.

But the step of fabrication is an extreme on a gradient of less than totally ethical choices. Great accuracy is required when handling minute (micro-litre or less) volumes. A drop is a large volume by comparison. It follows that those with less than excellent technique can have some variability between samples. For this reason, many experiments are performed in triplicate. When a point on a curve does not fall correctly onto the line indicated by other samples, there is a moment of judgement when the experimentalist decides whether the deviant point is telling something real or whether it is within the scope of error of manipulation. Usually, this is a clear-cut decision and the canvas of experimental results are built by layering new information onto old and in this way, the deviation is revisited and either confirmed or shown to be a real variation on what seemed like a predictable stream of data points. The deviating data may affect the interpretation of the experiment or may be simply an error. The context of the other related results can usually guide which is the real situation. Repeating an experiment is never an error. When the context of the data point is a less sure guide, then a repeat experiment is the obligatory next step. In most laboratories, this is a decision made by the individual researcher. Whether she/he discusses it with others often depends on the structure and the degree to which the climate in the laboratory is supportive. But in that moment of decision, the researcher is probably revealing their own personality and the consequences of their family and academic upbringing. He/she also might be responding to external pressures; holidays are booked and there is no time to regenerate all the reagents, the next career move has been planned and the repeat will require that the move is postponed, others with alternative data may be moved to a more prestigious place on a publication or simply repeat an experiment might mean getting home late (again) with very negative consequences from a waiting partner or family. The moment when the researcher takes a short cut, does not repeat an experiment over which there is an inherent doubt, ignores and does not highlight in discussions with others the large error bars on a triplicate sample point, is the moment when the road is crossed even though there is a flashing red light saying that it is not the right thing to do. It may be the start of a lower degree of exigency when future and ambiguous data of potentially greater consequence show up in an experimental series. And, of course, if there are no consequences and the cut corners do not lead to results that are challenged – and may be right even if not correctly obtained – then that researcher will set a bad ethical tone and standard when they move up the career ladder and are themselves the supervisors of the group.

It should never be forgotten that a scientific research career is one that is built by being successful in competition for grants, fellowships and positions. Being careful and avoiding confrontation, either intellectual or personal, is not sufficient. Incremental advances are not sufficient to distinguish a competent researcher from one who has an added insight and skill. At every stage, the scope of the proposed research is very important and if it has a spark of inventiveness underpinned by some preliminary data, it can distinguish itself from other more predictable projects. The spark can come from either an intellectual analysis or an unexpected result. Investing excessive belief in that result could lead to a temptation to avoid challenging it adequately. Success also depends on the track record of the researcher, and the easiest surrogate to analyse this is the publication output of the applicant. The number of publications, the quality of the journal and the place the applicant has been allocated on a multi-author publication are all integrated into the opinion the selection committee form of the applicant. Obviously, these decisions have a comparative aspect so the profile of another applicant can define the ranking. Under those circumstances, it is clear that getting research published, in journals of the highest impact and being placed first on a multi-author publication, is a very powerful driver that demands high-quality research results and a clear ownership of the project, under the overall supervision of the senior (last) author. And as all research builds on the available knowledge gleaned from the literature and scientific presentations, it is obvious that in some other laboratory somewhere in the world another group is addressing the same problem with similar research tools. It does not require expansion of this concept to highlight the extreme pressure under which researchers work. Their highest ideals to contribute to a cure of some disease are dependent on their ability to get a job as a research scientist. Their own salary depends on it in many cases. It may not be a great exaggeration that the decision to lower ethical standards when faced with a result that will delay a paper is one that is a consequence of these immense life-defining pressures. It follows that all in a research group, and the supervisor in particular, have to be very attentive and challenging to any data that are presented as a result that is definitive and worthy of inclusion in a publication.

The Research Supervisor

There are different ways of describing the research environment, but one that is telling is to view it as a master—apprentice relationship. The novice researcher seeks out a laboratory in which they can learn how to do research. The expertise of the research supervisor has been recognised by the position to which she/he was appointed and by their success in attracting money required for the research to be performed. When a grant has been awarded, it is in the interest of the laboratory head to attract to their team a hardworking, skilled and intelligent student who will spend the next 3—4 years working on the problem defined by the laboratory head (usually). In doing so, the pre-doctoral student will take the first step on the ladder of their own career. So, there is a mutual interest in the research being successful and the PhD student being productive. Many laboratories have a second, intermediate layer between the PhD student and the laboratory head; the post-doctoral fellow. Having completed a PhD, she/he has moved to (or stayed on in) the laboratory because he/she believes that this is the best location for promoting their career. Sometimes the post-doctoral fellow has already great experience and skills related to the specific research problem, but sometimes the move to the laboratory is decided by an interest to learn something new or to enter a new field that best matches the long-term plans of the researcher. In laboratories where the principal investigator is very busy with diverse duties, or if the laboratory is particularly large, then the post-doctoral fellow may be the *de facto* supervisor of the work of others. Although more advanced, the post-doctoral fellow is also at a delicate stage in their career. They need the papers and they need to be well placed on them, as the senior author is usually the head of the laboratory who had developed the hypothesis and envisaged the next steps and got the funding for the work to be performed. The laboratory head is also under immense pressure. One's standing in the scientific community has a short half-life and failure to have dazzling new results, or to show that your understanding has advanced since the last expert meeting is noted and when promotion is considered, there can be a tellingly negative assessment of 'he has peaked and his output is modest since that great paper 5 years ago'.

Ego is a powerful driver for all in the research world. Often masqueraded or interchanged as a wish to cure some disease (in the area of the life sciences), it is also the element that makes researchers work long and hard, making real sacrifices in doing so. This is true for all stages of the career that has not reached an irreversible plateau. The laboratory culture therefore is not likely to be one that comforts the meek or tolerates the ineffectual. To be competitive, the output of the group has to be very high. Getting things wrong in the design or the execution of an experiment has impacts on the entire group and, indeed, on its financial resources. This is where the ethical question becomes a reality. If a delayed result stands in the way of the submission of a paper, or an important presentation at a meeting, then the person responsible for the failure will inevitably feel the pressure. It follows that there is a very major responsibility on the laboratory head to strike the right balance between demanding high-quality data in a time-efficient manner and breaking an individual in the process. Not all in a laboratory are equally skilled and some are at a stage of learning new techniques, so some patience has to be a part of the make-up of the supervisor. A long-term view is also important. The old adage that 'all work and no play make Johnny a dull boy' applies to those in a research group also and a supervisor must have an awareness of the work–life balance that is necessary for all to perform and deliver. Knowledge of the full life picture of the individual can be a help as matters outside the laboratory (an illness in the family, for instance) can be a damaging distraction that should be factored in when applying pressure to produce a result.

But the reality is that some, perhaps even many, of those who are laboratory heads have little time for any human frailties. They send macho messages about the need to work 24/7, as many of them do themselves. They can see an engagement with family and children as a distraction for their research group. They do not mind if they humiliate or harass if it ensures that the results are delivered. They are powerful and use the power when influencing the next stages of the career of those that work with them. They are bullies and they have no ethical compass to guide them.[4] Success, for this cohort, is the only output to be judged.

While this picture is a caricature that exaggerates for effect, there is some element of all of these traits in most research group leaders. Aspects of the depiction are to be found in researchers at earlier stages of their careers when they have more to prove and when their sense of their superior intelligence may not have been challenged by others with equal or greater brainpower. This is a very dangerous environment as all elements are present for output-driven behaviour, and data that are hard to obtain can be the barrier to that and thus to the development of a career. It is obvious that it is the responsibility of the laboratory head to ensure that ethical standards, even if they impinge on progress, are maintained at a high level. He/she should engage in discussions that challenge every result. When there is a difficult experiment that should be performed to confirm a result, she/he should insist that it is performed and examine the results from it very carefully. Expedience and an urge to show that progress is being made should not trump a meticulous commitment to finding the truth that resides in the system under study. An environment of openness that welcomes alternative views, draws out the reflections of the more timid, understands the difficulties with complex experiments, is one in which the behaviour of the group will ensure that output from the group is of the highest ethical and scientific standards.

In addition to setting the moral tone of the group, the supervisor has other practical tasks that must be delivered without deviation from the highest standards. Today, there is a great awareness of the potential dangers to health and safety for those working in laboratories. Adhering to these can be time consuming or even a barrier to some experiments. If the laboratory head does not reinforce the need to pay full attention to these aspects, then the laboratory culture will reflect that and can harm the result. Similarly, the need to follow all guidelines when working with animals can be rigorous, if the head of the laboratory supports all the ethical and practical directives, but can be slip-shod if not. For those working with humans, in research studies or clinical trials, the obligation to adhere to agreed protocols must be absolute and cannot be approximate and again the tone set by the laboratory head by his or her actions or even by side comments will tell those working in the group what is really tolerated, rather than what is written and required.

When it comes to publications, the laboratory head faces a new set of actions that require high ethical standards. Who should be on the paper? This may seem like a simple question, but sometimes an individual can be omitted because their contribution did not catch the attention of the person who decides the list of authors. In which order should the authors be listed? Again, the decision by the lead author has to be based on fairness and a balanced analysis of the input to the story by different approaches. This can be very difficult to do as it falls into the realm of subjectivity in many cases − but the author should ensure that they are well informed when making the decision. Unfortunately, as the position is often pre-decided by the circumstances that permitted the research to be performed, the

[4] Gannon, F. "Bullies" *EMBO Reports* 10 (2008) 937.

senior author may not pay sufficient attention to the fate of others. The need to give credit for ideas and insights is almost as important as identifying the source of the experimental data. Discussions in the laboratory and over coffee are often the start of a new experiment that opens the way to a fresh view on a problem. As this often happens in interplay of different perspectives, it is sometimes hard to say who really asked an unexpected question that was the source of the idea. Nonetheless, it is important not to exclude those that made the work possible through a contribution to the spark that resulted in a new insight, by an acknowledgement or by inclusion as an author depending on the significance of the input. Giving credit correctly is another aspect of the ethics of a laboratory and one that is sometimes ignored.

Senior researchers have another important role to play as the expert analysts of manuscripts submitted for publication in scientific journals. This is an onerous task that is an inherent part of the research communities system of checks and balances. It is also one where a scientist has privileged anonymous access to the most recent discoveries of others. The reviewer has the opportunity to examine every detail of the submitted material and most are courageous, meticulous and conscientious when they do so. Many papers are much improved by this process of peer review with the comments of the expert feeding into the research that is performed by the laboratory that submitted the paper. But a referee has also a position of trust that is betrayed occasionally. Peer experts are often in fact in competition with the group that submitted the paper. Delaying the paper by requesting difficult extra experiments, or blocking the paper by recommending that it is not published, are temptations to which it seems from anecdotal evidence that some succumb. But an even graver demeanour is when the insight in the manuscript is used by the reviewer to give his laboratory an unfair advantage. This can include rushing through a less complete paper in a journal that might not have the same quality requirements. Even if this happens rarely, there is no doubt that the opportunity to misbehave is present and again the need for high moral standards of behaviour must be re-iterated.

All of the above contexts (authorship, reviewing the work of others and health/safety/animal and human welfare), show the need for an environment where transparent discussions can take place on any aspect of how the laboratory functions and where deviations from the highest standards can be seen as such and can be highlighted without fear or negative consequences.

There is a final aspect of the role of the research supervisor that broaches a completely different aspect of ethical standards. Scientists are under increasing pressure to present their work as an answer to some need of society. It is wrong to promise a cure from a research project, if there is no realistic chance of it happening. It is hypocritical to suggest that work is unique, when it is known to experts that it is but one approach to a problem. It is unethical to be selective, when reporting on the outcome of a study that did not deliver what had been expected (or promised). All of these aspects are part of the scientific world today unfortunately,[5]

[5] Gannon, F. "Hope, Hype and Hypocrisy" *EMBO Reports* 12 (2007) 1087.

the combination of the rising costs to perform research and the increased linear and short-term linkage in funders' minds between the money provided and the outcome expected means that researchers are under pressure to promise a good return on investment. Much greater care should be exercised by the scientists when they are party to a press release and to those (same) scientists who sit on selection panels when presented with excessively optimistic promises of the consequences of the research. Hype should not be rewarded, not least because the hope it engenders in the community will in due course be replaced by mistrust. But we should also be aware that in this, as in other areas considered in this chapter, fear of practical negative consequences should not replace the application of sound ethical standards. Some aspects of the research world are to be judged by criteria that go beyond strategies and tactics.

When Things Go Wrong

It is obvious from the earlier discussion that there are very many opportunities for the behaviour of the researcher at every level to be less than ethics would demand. It would be trite to say that there are rare occasions when there is behaviour that falls short of the standards that should be expected. But the daily reality is that most people do not seem to see problems of behaviour that need correction. The early-stage PhD student needs to be sure that the system will protect and support them. In practice, this means that there must be opportunities where they are encouraged to speak up if there is something that seems incorrect. Some institutions have a thesis committee that examines the progress of a student. The committee often has a session where the student meets them in the absence of their boss. This can encourage some comments on anything that is troubling the student. Many institutes have protocols that ensure that complaints are handled in a manner that is supportive and protective of those that might, in the overall system, be vulnerable. But these do not exist everywhere and to be effective they have to have the moral support of the leaders of the institute. More can be done in this domain worldwide, and nobody should be immune to a well-founded criticism and take the appropriate consequences.

Although the correct social behaviour, where individuals are respected and credit for the outcome of research is fairly allocated, is indeed very important, there is little doubt that the most corrosive damage is done when data are falsified. As indicated in the introduction, this occurs in a very small percentage of cases, but the accurate statement is that this is detected in a very small number of cases. To avoid it happening, there has to be vigilance by all, an environment where data are shared and viewed by multiple members of the group, and where honest and challenging alternative interpretations can be considered and debated.

In the life sciences, when an unexpected new insight results from a series of experiments (rather than an incremental increase that is frequently the case), it is essential that the novel insight is challenged by a combination of different approaches where this new perception is the hypothesis that is being tested. One should ask why the result was not discovered previously. Often a new perspective will be part of the understanding of a problem within a research group for a year or more before it is presented in public. During that time, the published data will be re-examined from the new perspective and corroborating data will be generated; in some cases, it is appropriate to protect the resultant intellectual property. It is a best practice to ensure that different people in the group perform experiments that will allow the new understanding to be confirmed and extended. When the veil is lifted on the research, the external research community asks new questions and tests the solidity of the story that has been told. Researchers are trained to be sceptical and to challenge any departure from the well-established textbook version of events. This carries through overtly and covertly in the process by which the research is published. Scientific journals (as referred to above) typically will ask three independent experts to look very carefully at the data that are presented. Almost in all cases, the referees will suggest alternative and extra experiments that they require to satisfy themselves that there is not an alternative interpretation of the data. Usually, the results of these experiments are required by the editor and are re-examined by the referee. It is a demanding process that if followed perfectly should ensure that the published literature has passed through the most demanding filter. Unfortunately, the reality is that not all referees are adequate to the task, or they are too busy to delve deeply enough into the data or they are too tired when they do so and are under a time demand from the journal and its editor. So, things can slip through the net if those custodians are asleep on their watch. It points to another ethical demand, this time on those that are entrusted with the task of reviewing submitted papers. If they are correctly engaged and are well selected, then the inadequacies of the unethical researcher that generates the data will be exposed and their career will not progress.

While the problem of a pesky result that does not fit received wisdom has been presented as a major source of the lowering of ethical standards, experience shows that an equally challenging problem is that of the perfectionist researcher. Although working with imperfectly controlled material that is a characteristic of biological reagents (cells or animals), it is sometimes unacceptable to the perfectionist when this is reflected in the data that are produced. The temptation to improve may result in omission, and hence a potentially misleading result is presented. The data that are presented in a visual form might be cosmetically enriched on the computer to make the result more convincing. In this case, it is possible that the result is in no way altered by the presentation, but it is clear that any such practice is the first step towards greater misrepresentation up to the point of deception and falsification. Journals and referees are now well aware of the ease of enhancing figures, but as always the place for the controls to be imposed are at the laboratory level and not by the peer-review police.

A more challenging problem that may not be restricted to the perfectionist is the failure to report experiments that give a very unexpected result. Normally, this is a wonderful development, but if the head of the laboratory is particularly wedded to, and known for, a particular hypothesis, a researcher might feel threatened sufficiently to fail to share the result. For this to happen, it would seem that the laboratory environment is very defective; it is one thing to be slow to present the contrary result to a bullying boss, but it is another to keep it from others in the laboratory. Yet, one meets researchers that have moved from a laboratory rather than face the ire of proving that the edifice on which the laboratory is built is defective. The strength of the scientific endeavour however is that the cross-checking of the results of others is inevitable and as a field develops and places one stone of knowledge on another, the error or wrong interpretation will be exposed by a mismatch between the hypothesis and the result. In the long term, therefore, the failure to report a result in one forum will most likely be corrected by the results from elsewhere. It follows in all cases that all should feel and act freely and report what they find and not what was expected.

When any problem arises related to the data that are presented, the first imperative is to have access to the primary material – the experimental results. With the mobility of researchers and less than adequate storage systems for data that are increasingly converted into digital forms, it has to be acknowledged that this is not an aspect of laboratory life that functions well. Attempts to have signed laboratory notebooks are often seen as being too close to industry norms and hence rejected by those in research that chose not to go to industry. But in the absence of the primary data suspicions can only grow and in some cases an innocent career can be damaged by innuendo. And of course, a guilty researcher can escape for lack of proof. Both cases are undesirable and a collective effort should be made to improve on this situation.

Falsification is almost always the act of an individual. If performed with skill, it is difficult for those to whom the data are presented to know that they have been adjusted, or invented. Those working at the bench in the proximity of the culprit are sometimes well placed to know if a sudden wonderful result is to be expected from their neighbour. Even if the experiment is performed at night or the weekend, it is an unusual case that a scientist does not wish to share their excitement with a colleague or laboratory friend. But those that are sufficiently misguided, secretive and prone to working on their own could succeed. Detecting that devious and deliberate act performed with misused skill can be impossible to detect. It follows that, again, the group laboratory meeting is the critical crucible where new data are interrogated. When they are novel or of an unusual high quality (given the imperfections of the material that are used to generate them), then the heat applied to the analysis has to be commensurate. Perhaps, it is because of the social context that characterises most laboratories that cases of fabrication and falsification are rare. But even so, the need to be wary and critical remains essential aspects of the functioning of a laboratory where such problems do not arise.

Conclusion

The research laboratory is clearly an environment where much can go astray in terms of human behaviour. Lives can be broken, careers ruined, opportunities missed, even if everybody behaves ethically. Succeeding to imagine and deliver on an experiment is intrinsically difficult. Interpretation of the most clear-cut result requires a vast body of knowledge directly and indirectly related to the study that is ongoing. Intellectual flexibility is needed to see things in a new light and yet the knowledge that is required to understand a topic is not malleable, only hidden. In that environment, it is of prime importance that high ethical standards permeate the research adventure. Reflection on this has pointed to the importance of the individual and to the collective. The researcher alone, when faced with a new result, must be assured that it is saying something that will help unveil a mystery of life or nature. She/he must be un-waying in confirming, challenging and reporting that new perspective. Those who are his/her immediate and ultimate superiors have an equally unambiguous charge to adhere to the highest standards in all that they do and for which they are responsible. They have a secondary responsibility of ensuring that the environment in which the research is performed is open to internal criticism and unexpected results. Bullying and harassment are too often tolerated and must be seen for what they are rather than the prerogative of the supervisors. But if all behave correctly as individuals and as a collective the frontiers of knowledge are constantly re-defined and the benefits flow to society. As this is the track record of research for decades and shows no signs of abating, then one could conclude that the deviations from the norms of exemplary behaviour must be rare and the methods of detection and correction robust. By discussing the alternative unethical possibilities, it is hoped that the current positive assessment will remain the norm for all.

Acknowledgement

This chapter has benefitted from the critical reading by Susanne Mandrup, George Reid and Stephanie Denger.

Bibliography

Begley CG, Ellis LM. "Drug Development: Raise standards for preclinical cancer research". *Nature* 2012;483:531–3.
Gannon F. "Bullies". *EMBO Rep* 2008;10:937.
Gannon F. "Fraud in our Laboratories?" *EMBO Rep* 2007;8:1.
Gannon F. "Hope, Hype and Hypocrisy". *EMBO Rep* 2007;12:1087.
van Noorden R. "The Trouble with Retractions". *Nature* 2011;478:26–8.

Introduction to Section 2

Research Ethics Governance in the EU; the Role of Civic Debate, the Question of Limits in Research

Maureen Junker-Kenny

Department of Religions & Theology, University of Dublin, Trinity College, Dublin, Ireland

Abstract

This section treats international documents on research regulation, their processes of negotiation and ongoing differences at UN, Council of Europe and European Union levels. It concludes with current evaluations of the role of the scientist, of the media and of civic debate for determining the directions for new biotechnologies.

Key Words

Cloning, consensus, nanomedicine, political subsidiarity, precautionary principle, transparency, research ethics governance, civic debate, limits in research

Section 1 was dedicated to ethics as a core competency, both at the level of understanding the different background traditions that define the meaning of ethical principles and in terms of the individual researchers' capacity for moral reflection in the workplace. Section 2 will treat some of the existing international documents that designate the boundaries within which research has to be conducted. Concluding the section, the geneticist and philosopher Sigrid Graumann considers a case study which is concerned with determining a consensus on an absolute limit for research on the issue of cloning. While there is a shared conviction across the various cultures and member states of the United Nations (UN) that cloning needs to be proscribed, the differences that have arisen between countries on what should be covered by the prohibition of cloning cannot be bridged. For some, legislation ought to include a ban on embryo cloning. For others, prohibition is sought only on

Ethics for Graduate Researchers. DOI: http://dx.doi.org/10.1016/B978-0-12-416049-1.00031-3

the process that would lead to the birth of a human being who is genetically identical with its one parent. The failure to reach agreement on this limit in the form of a UN Convention in 2005 may yet be addressed by new moves beyond the UN Declaration that was achieved. This deliberation illustrates the dilemmas in the ongoing task of ethics committees trying to identify common moral ground in the face of new technological possibilities.

In his first chapter on bioethics and biolaw in the European Union, the former member of the European Group on Ethics in Science and New Technologies, Dietmar Mieth highlights how the bioethical controversy in Europe can be summarised under two core principles, self-determination and dignity. The first leans towards individual choice, and the second considers the inviolability and integrity of the person. While in some approaches these two aspects are internally connected, their current divergent use is such that they exemplify different traditions of philosophical argumentation. This divergence gives rise to the question of whether international consensus documents serve to bridge or to obfuscate ongoing differences in interpretation. In the case of the European Union, while 'directives' are European laws that have to be translated into national law, below that threshold the principle of political subsidiarity applies. It leaves the decisions about which practices are to be permitted to national jurisdictions. Rather than aiming for a uniform policy, the autonomy of member states is respected by making subsidiarity a procedural principle. Thus, policies on matters that affect research governance can differ. The judgments on cases taken to the European Court of Human Rights in Strasbourg (as an institution of the Council of Europe with currently 47 member states) and to the European Court of Justice in Luxembourg (an institution of the European Union called on to give definitive interpretations on the application of EU law in all its member states) can have implications for, or even directly affect, the limits drawn for research.

In the case of the 1997 Council of Europe Convention on Human Rights and Biomedicine, the divergence was obvious when countries opted not only out of ratifying, but even out of signing the Convention. Germany and the United Kingdom refused their signatures for very different reason and Mieth explains why. The chapter closes with an example of how the demand for transparency in research can be specified, in 10 points proposed in the Enquete Commission of the German Parliament.

In his second chapter, Mieth analyses the practice of ethics in such committees. With the requirement and self-understanding that they should remain independent, ethicists are situated between the expectations of the appointing institution; the different disciplines relevant to the issue; the constituencies, moral perspectives and traditions of thinking they have been chosen to represent in their task of interpreting new scientific possibilities in the light of the principles of the constitutions and of the values articulated in European treaties. Against the background of an analysis of dilemmas both within science and society, and between them, Mieth shows how divergent assessments call for renewed debate in civil society. For him, the inbuilt tendency of international agreements towards less restriction puts into question a view which sees tolerance and respect for pluralism as the ultimate European values; this would have the paradoxical effect of abolishing the need for arguing out ethical differences, both in committees and in civil society. Committed to a universalist framework that takes the human capability for moral evaluation as a basic experience, and good will as the endowment of every human being, Mieth establishes human dignity as the benchmark by which policies have to be judged. In his capacity as a theological ethicist, Mieth argues against pitting the concept of God as creator against patenting sequences of genes – which the Church of Scotland does in its response to European policies – for the reason that genes remain elements of creatures. He recommends instead the shared moral ground of human dignity as the decisive reason why body parts such as gene sequences should not be patented. Human dignity as the source of human rights is a principle on which different ethical sources can come to a moral consensus that is not merely 'overlapping' for contingent reasons, but rather is endorsed by practical reason as genuinely shared.

Hille Haker, from the same autonomy school in theological ethics, and a current member of the European Group on Ethics, focuses her analysis on the search for criteria and methods that are adequate to deal with the major change with which hitherto guiding cultural self-understandings are confronted by the new technologies of nanomedicine and synthetic biology. It is remarkable that the final point of the EGE Opinion on synthetic biology calls for fora in the public realm to discuss and assess the challenge that these emerging technologies will pose for the relationship of humans to machines, nature and intersubjectivity. 'The EGE recommends that an open intercultural forum is initiated in order to address the issues, and to include philosophical and religious input' (cf. Chapter 15). Thus, ethics committees are aware that they cannot resolve such questions at the round tables they organise with stakeholders; ultimately the self-understandings of citizens will be decisive in determining which courses of action should be taken, and which ones are to be avoided. What professional ethicists can do, however, is to analyse which methods have been tried so far, and to give an account of the different options that can be used and possibly combined in technology assessments. She raises questions about how comprehensive the conventional ethical, legal and social aspects (ELSA) evaluation of new technologies is. In addition, she analyses the different methodological options, and asks whether a technological risk assessment should be employed, or a biomedical one or whether a different approach entirely has to be found, i.e. one that is adequate for the new dimension of nanomedicine. She distinguishes four approaches: theoretical approaches in philosophical ethics, with the alternative between a Kantian or a Utilitarian perspective of analysis; a case-by-case approach; systems theory; and a power analysis, tracing the heuristics and management of what is made to count as an ethical issue. She also provides a further range of criteria of assessment: should nanomedicine be judged in light of the four principles of autonomy, non-maleficence, beneficence and justice, or should human dignity be constituted as the highest principle from which rights flow? All these considerations demonstrate the need to reflect on the presuppositions, methods and criteria of technology assessments, rather than assume the ELSA exercise to be sufficient and self-explanatory. Haker proposes to turn the starting point and direction of ethics assessments by 180°. She begins with the moral standards reached and articulated in human rights documents and then classifies new technologies according to how they deliver on these goals and not the other way around. Technologies are human practices that need analysis and ethical orientation just like other social practices. The two tasks of ethical advisory boards then become clear and can be summarised as first assisting political bodies in legal regulation, and second as communicating between science and society.

Haker's starting point is the consciousness of ethical standards as cultural achievements that constitute a platform from which new practices can be assessed, and not that of taking the new developments as a given and ethics as merely construed and dependent on various relative and incommunicable standpoints. If this was all ethical reflection could deliver, it would be unable to form a serious counterpart to the dynamics of change through biotechnology that affect the lifeworlds of current and future citizens.

Each of the contributors in this section has been connected with an institution that has pioneered ethical reflection within the sciences in interdisciplinary cooperation in Germany, the International[1] Centre for Ethics in the Sciences and the Humanities at the University of Tübingen (IZEW). One is its founder, the other two are previous coordinators. Before the three Continental ethicists get to develop their analyses, however, I would like to complement their reflections with some English-speaking authors who are concerned with some of the same issues: (1) the role of ethicists in committees that relate to a public realm in which the media can have a polarising effect on citizens' opinion formation; (2) the difference in the cultural and political relevance of the principle of precaution on the two sides of the Atlantic; and (3) the goal of transparency in research.

Questions by Ethicists to their Role in the Public Realm

Because the work of ethics committees includes the task of mediating between science and society, the ethics experts especially continue to interrogate themselves as to how they are doing justice to the participative goal of their discourse. The sociologist Charles Bosk quotes two observers on the fear of failing in one's service to the public:

> In Carl Elliott's (2001) colorful turn of phrase, bioethicists 'look like watchdogs and act like showdogs' (p. 20) or in Jon Imber's (1998) more trenchant observation, 'bioethics is the public relations division of modern medicine, whether physicians (or bioethicists) like it or not' (p. 30).[2]

The ethicist's function is made more difficult by a specific trait of the media, which could otherwise perform an indispensable role of communicating

---

[1] Previously Interfaculty.

[2] C.L. Bosk, "Bioethics, Raw and Cooked, Extraordinary conflict and everyday practice," in *Journal of Health and Social Behavior* 51 (2010) 133–146, 135.

developments in science, the tendency to polarise, which turns contested issues into a 'spectacle'. Bosk compares the way in which such conflicts are staged. He applies the analytical category proposed by the sociologist Marcel Mauss in his ethnomethodological studies of exchanges and conflicts in primitive societies. He calls these conflicts a 'total social phenomenon'; he captures them as 'essentially-contested total social conflicts' (ECTSCs). This helps explain why a small number of individual cases have been the cause for major changes in legislation.

> *Essentially-contested total social conflicts appear to be the contemporary version of those exchanges in primitive societies that Mauss ([1950] 1990) labeled 'total social phenomenon' (p. 3). In such transactions, 'all kinds of institutions are given expression at one and the same time – religious, juridical and moral, which relate to both politics and the family ...' (p. 3). The fact that the institutional development of bioethics has depended on celebrated cases that have become ECTSCs becomes clear when we understand how landmark cases have served as the foundation for massive changes in social practice. For example, a relatively few cases (e.g., Tuskegee, Willowbrook, Gelsinger, Quinlan, Cruzan, Schiavo) became 'total social spectacles' in which all kinds of institutions were drawn into conflict within and among each other at the same time.*[3]

As a sociological observer of the staging of these conflicts, he notes how 'bioethics is the instant case that acts as a lightning rod for our collective attention':

> *First, media coverage of ECTSCs requires 'one-handed' experts to fuel dramatic differences of opinion. Thus, the principle of balance in reporting favors spokespersons from both extremes of a conflict while muffling the voices of moderation and compromise (Gamson and Modiglianni 1989). Ginsburg (1989) provides a particularly vivid account of how the media practice of balance serves to fuel public controversy by privileging the most extreme voices in a public debate.*[4]

It seems clear that one conclusion to be drawn from this analysis by professional ethicists is that their role should consist in providing sober analyses, comparisons and considerations on possible long-term effects for future relationships, such as those between parents and children, fellow citizens when they are well and when they are ill or those who can provide and those who cannot in their responsibility for a shared planet. When, instead, individual tragedies with unique features in their life stories are taken as the basis on which future directions are decided after being appropriated militantly by different sides and submitted to predictable exchanges, many others who will remain anonymous may be affected and caused to suffer by legislative decisions taken in view of persons in different circumstances. The role of ethicists should be to identify guiding principles and values that conflict in such cases in order to foster more reasoned debate. One such principle which is contested in its relevance is that of precaution.

---

[3] Ibid., S 135.
[4] Bosk, "Bioethics, Raw and Cooked," S 136.

Recognition of the Precautionary Principle |

From her professional basis in science and technology studies, Sheila Jasanoff points to a case in the politics of trade which illustrates the difference between the European handling of this principle and the US approach. While in the European Union, it acts as a legal constraint, the United States favours a more risk-friendly attitude, and have even taken the matter to the World Trade Organisation as an issue of competition:

> One manifestation is the US decision in May 2003 to bring a case in the World Trade Organisation challenging the EU moratorium on imports of genetically modified foods. This case directly pits US 'risk based' regulatory approaches against the European precautionary approach.[5]

In her discussion of the lessons to be learnt from the 2011 power plant catastrophe of Fukushima, having analysed the role acquired by nuclear power in post-war national identities, Jasanoff suggests how the precautionary principle could be operationalised by including forms of international peer review for national modelling assumptions. When sensitive security information is at stake, less open mechanisms such as panel-based review could be employed. This would facilitate a self-critical process that includes healthy and robust discussion of models and is aimed at learning over time.[6]

She recommends a move from an isolated 'predictive' mode of science to a 'participative' one.[7] Responses of citizens should go into the analysis as much as the anticipated interactions between different natural elements and contexts in models which harbour large margins of error in the unavoidable remaining indeterminacies and their evaluation. A further manifestation of the European adoption of the precautionary principle should consist in spelling out possible military uses of a new technology. As Hille Haker comments in her analysis of the EGE Opinion on nanomedicine, the military aspects have not, to date, been identified.

Transparency of Research

The requirement for research to satisfy criteria of transparency presupposes the honesty of scientists regarding their results. This was spelt out by Alan Kelly and Frank Gannon in Section 1. It also involves the distinction and choice between different self-conceptions scientists can adopt. In Jasanoff's review of a book concerned with identifying typical roles, scientists can choose between some parallels

---

[5] S. Jasanoff, "(No?) Accounting for Expertise," in *Science and Public Policy* 30 (2003) 157−162, 162, Fn. 1.

[6] S. M. Pfotenhauer, C. F. Jones, K. Saha and S. Jasanoff, "Learning from Fukushima," in *Issues in Science and Technology* 28 (2012) 79−84, 83.

[7] Ibid., 80. 83.

in analysis emerge with Mieth's discussion of the role of prejudice, which is operative also in science.

> *In this vision, the expert uses specialized knowledge to clarify policy choices and to inform decision makers of the range of options open to them. Using his two-by-two matrix, Pielke differentiates four theoretically possible advisory roles: pure scientist, issue advocate, science arbiter and honest broker of policy alternatives. ...He believes that scientists have an obligation to behave as honest brokers much more frequently than they currently do; all too often, he complains, they operate instead as issue advocates, propelled by their beliefs in the linear model and in interest-group pluralism. Pielke's greatest scorn is reserved for those scientist-experts who take politically interested advocacy positions without admitting to themselves or others that this is what they are doing. Borrowing a metaphor from weapons manufacture, he calls these dishonest experts 'stealth issue advocates'.[8]*

Where Jasanoff diverges from Pielke's programmatic outline of the types of links between science and political decision-making is both in her nuanced defence of the knowledge orientation of science and also in calling attention to the implicit values that should be articulated and submitted to public debate. In her view, Pielke offers an

> *imperfect understanding of what is wrong with the linear model of science policy. Scholars in science and technology studies have not claimed that science should never constrain or compel policy; nor have they said that there is something intrinsically wrong with doing science independently of concerns for its use in policy. Rather, they see as problematic scientists' tendency to naturalize or take for granted values and social preferences that are often embedded in the internal workings of science. As a result, many scientific priorities and methodological choices that should be open to wider debate remain insulated from critical scrutiny. A 1996 report of the National Research Council, Understanding Risk, explicitly recognized this problem when it called for an analytic-deliberative approach to decision making on risk. What STS scholars have insisted on is that the very process of collecting and codifying information is value-laden and should not be insulated from democratic accountability. Nor should ambiguities in the available knowledge be concealed behind monolithic claims of scientific certainty.[9]*

One further circumspect point to be added to this discussion is the observation by Mieth of how science projects are classified at the outset, and how their definition already includes the anticipation of offering results that will benefit people who suffer:

> *The distinction between 'health purposes' and 'basic research' is not so sharp. 'Research' in a broader sense includes the motifs and the options — in a strict*

---

[8] Jasanoff, "Speaking Honestly to Power," in *American Scientist* 96 (2008) 240–243, 240–241, a book review of R. A. Pielke, *The Honest Broker: Making Sense of Science in Policy and Politics* (Cambridge: Cambridge University Press, 2007).

[9] Jasanoff, "Speaking Honestly," 242–243.

sense it is distinct from them, because they are not 'scientific' in themselves. There is an input of hope which transforms the scientific purpose into 'health purposes'.[10]

It belongs to the requirement of transparency not to overstate the value of hoped-for results. Finally, as Bosk points out, there is also the danger that 'ethics' could be used as a placebo, when the response to problematic conditions needs a different level than ethics advisory panels can provide: 'As sociologists, we might ask, does the ethicization of all institutional problems serve to deflect attention away from larger structural avenues for reform? These are the questions that remain to be answered as we look toward the future.'[11]

Bibliography

Bosk CL. "Bioethics, Raw and Cooked. Extraordinary conflict and everyday practice". *J Health Soc Behav* 2010;51:133—46 135.

Jasanoff S. "Speaking Honestly to Power". *Am Sci* 2008;96:240—3.

Jasanoff S. "(No?) Accounting for Expertise". *Sci Public Policy* 2003;30:157—62.

Mieth D. "Bioethics and Biolaw in the European Union — Bridging or Fudging Different Traditions of Moral and Legal Argumentation?" Chapter 4 in this volume.

Pfotenhauer SM, Jones CF, Saha K, Jasanoff S. "Learning from Fukushima". *Issues Sci Technol* 2012;28:79—84.

Captions and links for PODCAST files for this section.

Dietmar Mieth

1. Conventions and protocols on research in the European Union.
2. Autonomy and the dignity of persons.
3. Contingency and finitude in problem solving.
4. Pluralism and tolerance in consensus building.
5. Distinguishing practical compromise from ethical judgement.
6. Is there a minimum threshold for participation in consensus building?

Hille Haker

1. Steps in ethical decision-making: normative reasoning.
2. Nanomedicine and ethics in the sciences.
3. The necessary but not sufficient standard assessment of new technologies: ELSA.

These can be found at http://booksite.elsevier.com/9780124160491

---

[10] Mieth, "Bioethics and Biolaw in the European Union — Bridging or Fudging Different Traditions of Moral and Legal Argumentation?," Ch. 4 in this volume.

[11] Bosk, "Bioethics, Raw and Cooked," S 143.

4 Bioethics and Biolaw in the European Union: Bridging or Fudging Different Traditions of Moral and Legal Argumentation?

Dietmar Mieth

Max Weber Center for Advanced Cultural and Social Studies, University of Erfurt, Germany

Abstract

In this chapter on bioethics and biolaw in the European Union and as a former member of the European Group on Ethics in Science and New Technologies, I highlight an important aspect of bioethical controversy in Europe. This concerns the relationship between two core and related principles, self-determination and dignity. My analysis gives rise to the question of whether international consensus documents serve to bridge or to obfuscate ongoing differences in the interpretation of these two principles. The compromise solution between the different member states in the European Union has been to leave the decisions about which practices are to be permitted to national jurisdictions. I examine why some countries opted out of signing the Council of Europe's Convention on Human Rights and Biomedicine (1997) but for very different reasons. I finish with suggesting that the 10 points proposed in the Enquête Commission of the German Parliament outline how the demand for transparency in research can be specified.

Key Words

Self-determination, dignity, European Group on Ethics, Convention on Human Rights and Biomedicine, Enquête Commission, transparency in research

At the centre of bioethical controversies in Europe are two concepts, self-determination and dignity, which I analyse in Section 'Two Traditions of Thinking: Self-Determination and Dignity'. In Section 'Controversies Between Different Traditions of Interpretation of Moral and Legal Concepts', I will give an overview of 'crucial points' to exemplify the conflict between different traditions of moral

Ethics for Graduate Researchers. DOI: http://dx.doi.org/10.1016/B978-0-12-416049-1.00004-0

and legal thinking.[1] This overview begins with the controversy about the European Convention on Biomedicine (1997), which for very different reasons was not signed by the United Kingdom or Germany. These divergences can also be seen in applications of bioscience and biomedicine such as genetic testing, gene therapy, research on supernumerary embryos, on genetic doping and enhancement, and in the regulations of good clinical practice.[2] I shall conclude with reflections on transparency in research and with recommendations developed in the Enquête Committee of the German Bundestag for how this requirement can be realised in medical research.

Two Traditions of Thinking: Self-Determination and Dignity

At one time, in 2000, the predecessor to the current European Group on Ethics in Science and Technology (EGE), then called the European Advisory Group on Ethics, compiled a list of ethical criteria that were used in the practical work of preparing 'opinions' for the European Commission. There were a lot of principles which indicated a so-called 'overlapping consensus' such as informed consent, respect for the private sphere, confidentiality of personal data, non-discrimination, non-exploitation, non-commercialisation of the human body, proportionality of risks and benefits, special protection of vulnerable persons and the principle of precaution (to expect the unexpected), to name those most often invoked.

But there was also a clear difference between more 'continental' approaches to human dignity as the unique principle which is the source of these criteria, and a more Anglophone approach, deriving everything from the autonomy of the person, as well as the mutual recognition of persons. In this case, autonomy is the source of the person's dignity, and if we speak about dignity of all humans, we do not mean exactly the same thing, because some human beings are not recognised as persons. Therefore, they fall under the criteria of 'respect for human life', which is not the same as 'having personal rights'. This discussion is also happening on the Continent, mainly in France and Germany. The German Constitution, which is the source of the first sentence of the draft of the European Constitution states, '*Die Würde des Menschen ist unantastbar*', human dignity is inviolable.

In a different tradition of thinking, dignity is replaced by self-determination. The concept of self-determination is often used as an instrumental term for justifying the dominance of the joint forces of science, technology and the economy. However, this term and what it denotes can be seen as an absolute contradiction as

---

[1] Nearly all Recommendations on Ethics and Law in Europe and beyond can be found in the *Jahrbuch für Wissenschaft und Ethik* (Berlin: De Gruyter), vols. 1–15.

[2] For other important themes, see the papers of the EGE on Nanomedicine, Opinion 21, Brussels 2007 and on the "Ethics of Synthetic Biology," Opinion 25, Brussels 2009. The Issue 13 of the Secretariat of the EGE "Ethically Speaking" of December 2009 informs about the activities of the National Ethics Committees in the EU. For international aspects, see the Report of the 2nd Meeting of the European Commission's International Dialogue on Bioethics, Madrid, 4–5 March 2010, Luxemburg 2010.

it is based on an atomistic individualism. It puts information in the place of mutual advice and counselling and bureaucratically formulated lists of consent in the place of relationships. What is paradoxical about self-determination is that it is regulated from the outside. Decisions are not made by the self, but externally, for example, on whether a specific woman belongs to the percentage of those justified as exercising self-determination. The content of the offer of self-determination is decided upon externally as well: suggested reformulation which offer do we make to whom, for example, through our health systems?

In theory, the offer could be different; it could be an offer of other alternatives. But no one thinks seriously about alternatives in offers or in the needs of persons. The 'dictatorship of the genes' swallows up what could be large segments of potential medical progress in other fields. Will other alternatives in the therapy of Parkinson disease continue to be explored and financed if many countries choose the stem cell option? Countless other examples come to mind.

Self-determination is worthy as a criterion and in itself is not to be challenged. But the following questions must continue to be raised: which understanding of self-determination is in use, within which limits, to whose advantage? A self-determined self-determination in the tradition of thinking I referred to first is a self-committing self-determination. In Kant's understanding, true autonomy is exceedingly aware that one's own self is not at one's disposition and that 'the other' remains unavailable and not objectifiable. The term 'dignity' does not denote an addition or summation of values but establishes inviolability.

Self-determination is often coupled with the conception of not having to bear 'unnecessary' suffering (a formulation of the Council of Europe in 1977). But the question is how to decide what is 'unnecessary'. This question is no excuse for inactivity or for the failure to lend support to people who are in distress or who suffer. But does the current level of technology determine what a need is, and what solidarity there should be among citizens, demanding personal involvement? Especially in dealing with the experience of suffering, technology is taking on roles that would otherwise be questions to the willingness and resources of a culture to address human suffering. If one uses the terminology of rights, this point leads to the distinction between 'negative' rights and 'positive' rights. We have the right that no harm or suffering is forced upon us; yet, we do not have the right to make others the instrument for the fulfillment of needs, the non-fulfillment of which causes us to suffer. Nor can others be made instruments for the reduction of suffering.

My first proposal is to distinguish between two aspects of human dignity: the aspect of self-reliance and self-determination, for which we need all kinds of support (e.g. non-directive counselling) to make this possibility a capability of each person (in the sense the economist Amartya Sen gives to 'capability'), and an aspect of the dignity of humanity in every human being, in Kant's terms, 'respecting the humanity in every human being'. These two aspects are not in a hierarchy to each other, and they cannot be separated from each other. Distinction is not separation. Human beings and persons cannot be separated, but they are connected by potentiality, identity and continuity. The distinction is made to search for the best integration of these two aspects of one and the same dignity.

My second remark is about the contingency or finitude in human agency. Human beings cannot foresee all the new problems which will arise from their problem-solving. Our history gives us enough proof of mistakes which cannot be taken out of the world, even if we wanted to do so. Thus, we have to act in favour of the reversibility of our decisions on scientific, technical and economic progress.

Controversies Between Different Traditions of Interpretation of Moral and Legal Concepts

The European Convention of Human Rights and Biomedicine (1997) is a convention which is a Treaty of the Members of the Council of Europe (45 at the time of signing), signed by approximately two-thirds of the members, and ratified meanwhile by more than a third. Three protocols have been added since that time, starting with the protocol on cloning (1998), genetic testing and research on humans.

Germany has not signed the Convention. The main problems in the view of Germany are the distinction and the relationship between the concepts of the 'human being' and the 'person', which remains unclear; the question of embryo research and clinical trials on people not able to give consent. On the other hand, the United Kingdom has not signed it either and not accepted the norm supported by the convention not to create embryos for research (by nuclear transfer).

The European Union (EU) is not a signing partner, but the Convention is often used as a point of reference, especially in the making of directives, such as the directive on bio-patenting, the directive on good clinical practice or the directive on tissue banking. Such directives must then in turn be adopted by the EU member states. The EGE (an advisory group of the EU Commission since 1992) also quotes in their references the Convention on Human Rights and Biomedicine.

Genetic Testing

The increase in genetic knowledge without preventive or therapeutic effects other than for some rare diseases is a problem that has not been adequately discussed. Research into the dispositions for illnesses could even cause more problems, if the increased knowledge of possible future diseases cannot be met with medical therapies. It is conceivable that the health and life insurance industry may become interested in data on the genetic make-up of their clients. Ethically relevant in this case is the balance between the principle of fairness – how much solidarity should a community of insurance holders accept? – and the principle of the individual's right to privacy.

On a more theoretical level, one might ask the question whether the competence to define what counts as disease could have the effect of a possible discrimination. As the complex terms of 'health' and 'disease' cannot be described in objective empirical terms – although these are very important indicators – the hermeneutic background has to be considered in every step that is taken to define a certain genetic anomaly as 'disease'. Otherwise, a questionable reductionist view would be the cause of inadequate conceptions of health.[3] The German Ethical Advisory Group of the Federal Ministry of Health stated clearly: 'Disability is not the same as illness'. Jean Dausset defined 'predictive medicine' as 'the identification of healthy individuals who have a predisposition to develop a given disease' and of 'individuals who have no such predisposition or are protected by special resistance genes'.[4]

The right or the duty to know and the right not to know are relevant even on the level of basic research. The individual right to information or the question whether there could even be a duty to information has to be balanced against the definite right not to know everything about one's own genetic make-up. This individual right must be seen in the context of a socially influenced definition and interpretation of 'health' and 'disease'. The more knowledge of the genetic structure of humans we gain, the more an individual is concerned, as they are confronted with demands to know even in contexts where no direct connection to the individual's health exists. This is the case in possible screenings in the workplace or in screening programmes for all pregnant women in a specific area or of a specific age or in other applications of genetic screening related to specific populations that are now being proposed.

Since the Bioethics Committee of the UNESCO has presented the 'Declaration on Human Rights and the Protection of the Human Genome' (1997, extended to 'Universal Declaration on Bioethics and Human Rights' in 2005), there has been a discussion about to whom the individual genome belongs. Is it a 'common heritage of mankind?' Does it fall under human solidarity in the use of all special information about genetic specialities of populations? Can this information be collected for commercial interests? Population screening is not only a programme of different pharmaceutical companies, but also the approach of a special committee of experts, which until 2004 were responsible for European research. In these committees, the companies were well represented (five members among thirteen; eight were independent ethicists, who were from a more liberal background). The results of this committee's deliberations were published in May 2004 and there are 25 recommendations which in general support the implementation of genetic testing, including population screening under the condition of free and informed consent. The committee took a position against what they called 'genetic exceptionalism', in which human genetic engineering is seen as a set of technical options that is to be monitored with more caution than other medical technologies.

The difference between conventional and genetic diagnostic tests is important for an ethical discussion. One may say that there is only a gradual difference between genetic and so-called conventional testing. A first line of objections to this position is that genetic testing will lead to an acceleration of knowledge for a

---

[3] Cf. E. Beck-Gernsheim "Health and Responsibility – From Social Change to Technological Change and Vice Versa". In: EHGA, 199–216. CF. Also the studies of Dirk Lanzerath (Bonn) and Monika Bobbert (Tübingen), 2001.

[4] LC, 58.

person's private life for which personal responsibility will not accelerate at the same time; it will lead to a variability of diagnosis and choices, to a monoculture of genetic approaches to diseases and to the question how to balance the degree of insecurity with the degree of security regarding its effects in life. It thus seems that we need more time to establish a 'reflective equilibrium' between applications and their integration into counselling and lifestyles as well as into institutions.

The most dramatic difference between conventional and genetic diagnostic tests is the number of persons potentially affected by the result. For if a genetic disease or disorder is diagnosed, other family members or relatives may be affected as well, directly or indirectly – in the present or in the future. Therefore, the nature of decision-making also changes: how can we take the interests of other family members into consideration? How is their right to privacy to be weighed against their possible interest in knowing their genetic status, and especially their possible interest in preventive or prophylactic measures (where are they applicable)? Up to now, ethicists or medical professionals have been quite vague in their formulations:

> *Confidentiality of the results of the test is an ethical imperative. Genetic data should not be released, except with the free and informed consent of the woman or couple. If the genetic data are relevant to the interests of other family members, the woman or couple should be strongly recommended by the genetic counsellor to allow the release of such data to these family's members.*[5]

Genetic testing and 'individualised' medicine is also a theme for ethics. The question of the testing of individuals is used to open the door to more diagnostic and predictive information which can, on the one hand, promote genomic drugs and, on the other hand, influence the lifestyle of the individuals. 'The right not to know' has to be protected against these challenges. This will not be easy if a person's genetic knowledge will influence their family and their family planning. The question of handing on such information to third parties (not only to relatives) such as insurance companies and employers is not only about the pressure they might exert, but also a question for personal decision-making, if, for example, a person wants to negotiate better contracts with these companies based on his/her negative results in genetic testing.

Research for Health Purposes on Supernumerary Embryos

Research on supernumerary embryos is established in several European countries that have unused embryos created in fertility treatments. Not all of these countries have legislation about this practice. But in all countries, even if there is a lack of law and guidelines, there is a restriction corresponding to the Biomedical Convention: it must be research for health purposes. On the other hand, the ethical

---

[5] Quoted from the opinion of the Group of Advisors on the Ethical Implications of Biotechnology to the European Commission (GAEIB) No. 6 on "Ethical Aspects of Prenatal Diagnosis" (Sécrétariat Géneral, Brussels).

problem consists of the fact that all embryonic research destroys the embryo. How is this kind of research being justified?

The definition of health purposes is not so clear. What is clear is the imperative to serve − immediately or in the long run − the health of concerned patients. Research on supernumerary embryos includes research for the improvement of in vitro fertilisation (IVF) of pre-implantation genetic diagnosis (PGD) and for the construction of embryonic stem cells and stem cell lines. The first application is to help IVF treatment. The purpose of this practice can be considered to be an improvement in health, although only if one accepts the World Health Organisation's definition of undesirable infertility, accompanied by the suffering this undoubtedly can bring, as an illness. The second application is to help future parents who are carriers of a genetic disease, with the desire for a healthy child, who suffer from the possible or given experience of a child who has that disease. The recognition of this desire by law and in practice is the background of the promotion of research for improvement of PGD.

In both the cases, a sensibility for the ethical significance of the destruction of the embryo is taken into account by restricting the procedures and the institutions, which are allowed to do this research. The moral status of the early embryo is seen as a status 'between' the understanding of the embryo as a part of 'human life' and as a human person with human rights. The 'between' of this status is the result of an evaluation from two perspectives: the perspective of potentiality, identity and continuity in human development and the perspective of a certain gradualism of this development. Because a decision between these two perspectives is difficult, this ambiguity leads to the principle, 'respect for human life', which is weaker than 'right to life', and stronger than its identification as a part of a human body or as a collection of cells.

This principle allows policy makers to balance the 'respect for life' with the 'good' of health. The fact that this is a balancing of rights reinforced by the fact that supernumerary embryos which are no longer a parental project will have to die. In research, they die, supporting the health objectives which have helped to create them, so that the whole purpose is integrated into a medical service for health (even if the need to die applies to all humans, the decision to use them for research can be seen as an instrumentalisation of the human person).

If this applies to fertility treatment, we can ask, is this also the case in research on supernumerary embryos for embryonic stem cells? The health objective in this case is only an option and not immediately connected with the goals of assisted reproduction. The balancing happens between the 'goods' of a human's life, the 'good' of freedom of research and the 'good' of a perhaps not-yet-existing but imaginable patient. The last good may be seen very differently, even in a scientific discussion without ethical perspectives.

The distinction between 'health purposes' and 'basic research' is not so sharp. 'Research' in a broader sense includes the motifs and the options for improving health but in a strict sense research is distinct from these aspirations, because they are not 'scientific' in themselves. There is an input of hope which transforms the scientific purpose into positively evaluated 'health purposes' which may be unattainable.

Ironically, although the connection between research and biomedical applications is not so intertwined, the destination of the supernumerary embryos — having no alternative than to die — is taken more into account by those who want to promote this kind of research. It is still necessary, however, to evaluate the chances of this kind of research for future health.

A philosophical and legal question is whether safeguards for the embryo can be outweighed by other 'goods' and therefore allow 'embryo-wasting research'? This does not seem to be thinkable if behind the 'good' of the embryo there is a right derived from the dignity of humans as persons. Some lawyers and philosophers who claim the dignity of personhood for the embryo admit that between such dignity and the right derived from it there is a difference: dignity can be maintained even if the right is treated as a 'good' in relation to other 'goods', because dignity has to be seen at a fundamental level which cannot be touched, but rights are always in competition with other rights, goods or values. But in this case, the burden of proof for a 'higher' right in opposition to a 'basic' right like the right to life should be very heavy. It is a discussion that will go on even if legislators must decide.

In contrast to the regulations and the practices in these European countries, the German Embryo Protection Act (1990) states that supernumerary embryos shall not be at the disposition of research. Because there is no provision for embryo freezing but only for pronuclear freezing, few such cases exist. The first reason for this restrictiveness is that when we as humans ourselves use and modify the natural programme of reproduction, we take over a responsibility for reproductive teleology which nature does not have. The second reason is that human dignity cannot be divided between humans, and so it includes also the early embryo as the first appearance of a human. It shows how a tradition of ethical thinking based on human dignity comes to different practical conclusions than one based on empirical criteria for personhood for which the embryo does not qualify.

Good Clinical Practice

I mention in passing the main problem of the directive of good clinical practice which has to be adopted by the 15 of 25 member states and has now been adopted by many countries, including Germany (2005). Up until now, the paradigm that clinical trials had to be exclusively for the benefit of the participants of the trial had been favoured. But now under certain conditions — more or less following the European Convention on Biomedicine — these trials can be performed without direct advantages for the participating persons but only for the group to which they belong, e.g. for children of the same age.

People unable to give consent are affected by these kinds of trials. The justification for clinical trials only by consent or only for the benefit of the participating persons has been widened to the advantage of a group. In the place of individual rights of protection against interventions, the question of an ethical principle such as 'solidarity without consent' is promoted. How can any exception to the central norms of clinical trials be limited so strictly that a change in the ethical paradigm of medicine can be avoided? The problem is that there may be a failure to impose very strict limitations on exceptions, for example, in the case of children, where trials on adults are not sufficient to avoid the dangers of drugs that are not specifically tested by and for children. The problem is that the ethical justification through the advantage for a specific group remains ambiguous.

If the personal benefit for every participant is included, there is no ethical problem; but if only a part, a majority or a minority, of the tested group will have the potential advantage, then the consequence is an instrumentalisation of people unable to give consent in the name of solidarity with others. A crucial question is: does solidarity need free and informed consent? Under what conditions can solidarity without consent be claimed? These questions have not been sufficiently answered by the GCP-Directive of the European Commission nor by its transcription into national laws, e.g. in German law (AMG-Novelle).

In conclusion, a sliding transition from protection based on the principle of non-instrumentalisation to a Utilitarian neglect of basic rights can be observed under the label of 'solidarity'. The weakening of protection for the most vulnerable in society, in international, including European conventions, calls for an awareness among citizens that ethics cannot be left to international biomedical agreements, governments and professional bodies but needs moral reflection and initiative at a more democratic and participative level.

The Demand for Transparency in Research

One way of making the protections for human dignity operational in the processes of research is to elaborate clear guidelines for what transparency in research requires. First, I will begin with some examples of the lack of transparency and I shall close with a list of specific criteria for dealing with the question of transparency.

In gene therapy, there has been great expectation that diseased organs could be cured by genetically modified materials. Less consideration was taken of the opposite assumption that the modifications could alter the course of the disorder or disease in a negative way. Efforts were concentrated on peripheral goals such as monitoring and reducing the aggressivity of viral material of so-called 'gene ferries'.

In some cases, as for example when Ritalin, a psychostimulant, was given to reduce distress in stressful situations (school, exams), the claims for its applicability were widened without any transparent justification. Demand is generated. Subsequent negative individual experiences are diagnosed such that its use becomes reinforced and in fact the medication becomes trendy.

Another example of this is in the undifferentiated widening of the diagnosis of burn-out syndromes. Frequently in the area of sports, the need for quick regeneration after prime performances, as well as a weak diagnosis of a predisposition, was used to justify giving a medication that was normally under suspicion and in any other situation would constitute doping. The justification then consists in an action having two effects, one of which is sought, while the other is based on what is only accepted now as a convention. The question this raises is whether the intention is to give priority first to that which is permitted over that which is prohibited.

A well-known example of intransparency is scientific lobbyism both for public funds and to influence the strategies of their distribution. This happens especially when a new paradigm of research is propagated in public as necessary so that projects under this flag are deemed to be more deserving of funds than others. Here, the argument of competitiveness between countries often plays an important role.

Transparency means more than that, it implies the most extensive and optimal process of information about means, risks, opportunities/chances for success and consequences. This demand arises, for sound scientific reasons, in the sciences themselves. Beyond this, transparency is both a question of societal, political and legal responsibility for the institutional area of science to safeguard its scientific character, and it is a question about how to order our application of science in aiming to solve the problems that pose themselves as old and new challenges to society.

The demand for transparency, which is internal to the objectives of the science itself, is often reiterated in words and documents without its implications being made fully explicit. This acceptance is based first of all on the recognition of the freedom of academic research (exemplary in the German Constitution), on the preference for 'value-free' (Max Weber) science or science that abstains from value judgements. In addition, it is recognised that research networking needs transparency. Such transparency becomes much more open for peer review if there is a requirement to publish research efforts. Wrong behaviour becomes easier to identify. Moreover, the freedom to participate, especially for young scientists, is made possible through transparency. Finally, the power of self-regulation of the scientific community (e.g. through a moratorium) depends on established and functioning transparency.

Transparency is a good that has to be delivered by the sciences. It should be taken over freely and not be forced. But society does not function in this simple manner. That is why there is a need to classify science legally in the name of transparency. Yet, often this external requirement of transparency, in relation to politics, the public and the participation of citizens, is contested. It is contested, for example, in the name of the independence of science from 'incompetent' influences that could be promoted by transparency. This is an argument that tries to set in stone the asymmetry between science and society. Thus, expert groups often try to insulate themselves from what are seen as excessive disclosures: do neurosurgeons, for example, disclose how many failures are the counterpart of their successes? Does IVF supply information about the cases which do not result in the birth of a baby?

On the other hand, there is the need for controversy in the sciences to be made explicit in order to prepare the ground for societal decision-making, for instance about the necessity of embryonic stem cell research. There is, significantly, a serious lack in the area of science journalism, which is essential to democratic debate but does not exist to the extent required. It is often restricted to national high-quality newspapers.

In the name of transparency, biomedicine has to be asked: does scientific progress, for instance in the area of IVF, serve as a substitute for the solution of social issues (infertility through delayed reproduction, education and professional work with children, disability mainstreaming)? The establishment of citizens' fora, which exist to some extent in the United Kingdom also belongs to transparency.

For the media that occupy themselves with science, the demand for transparency should lead to a more critical view of accounts of successful 'solutions' that filter out risks, burdens and failures. They would have to be complemented by accounts of the failures which are often more numerous. This is made more difficult by the fact that people are more prepared to speak in public about successes rather than about failures. Who would want to talk about having been able to have a child in the usual way after unsuccessful IVF fertility treatment? I have heard about such cases privately, but not through the media.

The demand for transparency also puts high demand on the character of the individual. In reference to Kant's distinction between duties of law and duties of virtue, these are duties of virtue. They are socially embedded in the sense that they can flourish much more in a favourable context of respect between humans. In this sense, they are not at all a matter of pure individual choice.

In relation to virtue and character of the researcher, it should be possible to have the courage not to submit to an 'arcane discipline' of secrecy of results imposed by the 'churches of science'. Truth and truthfulness should not have to stop at the door of scientific progress. They are not to be substituted by the language of advertising for projects. Also, scientists need self-control, courage, resistance, when it comes to insinuations, as for example from the delivering and requesting companies with which they may work. This is why the willingness to respect the demand of transparency should become a selection criterion in the appointment of new colleagues to scientific groups.

Beyond the claims addressed to scientists and to the scientific community, the legal framework also needs to be in place such as the obligation to offer a complete description of the projects, their context and their risks when a project is presented at the agencies of distribution. Moreover, there is an obligation to be comprehensible, for each project, appendices are required that make it possible for a wider public to grasp it. There should also be a legal safeguard that nobody should be disadvantaged in their career if she/he refuses to take part in projects that are against her/his conscience. It is also the task of institutions in society to strengthen informal opportunities for deliberation with new institutions for the information/enlightenment of citizens, media initiatives and engagement in civil society.

Finally, I offer a summary of the principles for research ethics that were developed by the Enquête Committee of the German Bundestag as a guide for analysing the implications of any research in the life sciences. These are as follows:

1. Medical research, being research on the human person as distinct from other research, has to satisfy special criteria.
2. Medical research is under the criterion never to violate human dignity. Respect for the rights to life, freedom, bodily and psychological integrity as well as the protection of the

private sphere of the research subject always have to take first place. Special protection is due to vulnerable and dependent people and people unable to consent.

3. The central goal of medical research must be to improve the treatment of sick and disabled people. In the case of conflict, other aims have to take second place. Medical research is required to improve the treatment of illnesses. If human beings are used as research subjects, it has to be justified in that the aim of improving treatments cannot be reached in other ways.

4. Nobody can be forced directly or indirectly to take part in medical research. As a principle medical research is permissible only if research subjects have given their voluntary and informed consent. The research subject has the right to withdraw their consent at any time. If a person is not capable, or only capable in a restricted way, to give their own consent, this consent has to be given by a person authorised to do so. The presumed will of the research person as well as verbal and non-verbal utterances that allows to conclude a refusal to participate have to be taken into account. This means: proxy/vicarious consent has to be bound as far as possible to the presumed agreement and to the expression of the will of the research subject who is unable to consent.

5. Benefit and the potential for damage of medical research have to be in an adequate relationship to each other. A corresponding assessment has to be supplied and based on scientific references.

6. Research for the benefit of self, of a group and of others has to be clearly distinguished. To the benefit of a group is classified as for the benefit of others.

7. Medical research that includes research subjects must satisfy the highest standards of quality. Multiple and parallel research has to be avoided. It has to be safeguarded so that references to potential for damage and burdens are made known.

8. Medical research on and with research persons must be evaluated and monitored by an independent, qualified and legitimated agency (ethics commission).

9. The individual researcher's freedom of research has to be safeguarded against external influence. Freedom does not untie a researcher from responsibility but is a presupposition/condition for taking it over.

10. Responsibility in research has internal and external dimensions. Internal scientific responsibility means that the rules of fairness and of scientific honesty/integrity are kept and are controlled by the scientific community through internal rules, so that the freedom of conscience of the individual researcher is safeguarded. External scientific responsibility means that the means and consequences of research towards all who are directly or indirectly affected can be ethically supported and *are open to being examined by society'*.[6]

Bibliography

Clarke A. *The Genetic Testing of Children*. Washington, DC: Oxford; 1998.

Beyleveld D. "The moral status of the human embryo and fetus". In: Haker H, Beyleveldt D, editors. *The ethics of genetics in human procreation*. Aldershot: Ashgate; 2000. p. 59–100.

Baumgartner C, Mieth D, editors. *Patente am Leben? Ethische, rechtliche und politische Aspekte der Biopatentierung*. Paderborn; 2003.

[6] Working group of the Enquete Commission of the German Parliament 2003–2005, unpublished final report.

Beck M, Mensch-Tier-Wesen. *Zur ethischen Problematik von Hybriden, Chimären, Parthenoten.* Paderborn; 2009.

Bobbert M. "Ethical Questions Concerning Research on Human Embryos, Embryonic Stem Cells and Chimeras". *Biotechnology* 2006;1:1352−69.

Bundestag D, Öffentlichkeitsarbeit R, editors. *Enquete-Kommission Recht und Ethik der modernen Medizin: Stammzellforschung und die Debatte des Deutschen Bundestages zum Import von menschlichen embryonalen Stammzellen* [Zur Sache 1/2002] [Available in German, English and Japanese].

Duewell M, Rehmann-Sutter C, Mieth D, editors. The Contingent Nature of Life. Bioethics and the Limits of Human Existence. Springer; 2008.

Englert Y. Gamete Donation: Current Ethics in the European Union. Oxford; 1998.

Ford NM, Herbert M. *Stem Cells.* Strathfield, NSW; 2003.

Hermeren G. "Patents and Licensing, Ethics, International Controversies". In: Murray TJ, Mehlmann MJ, editors. Encyclopedia of Ethical, Legal and Policy Issues in Biotechnology. Wiley and Sons; 2000.

Hottois G, Missa JN, editors. *Nouvelle Encyclopédie de Bioéthique. Médicine, Environnement, Biotechnologie.* Bruxelles; 2001.

Graumann S. *Die somatische Gentherapie. Entwicklung und Anwendung aus ethischer Sicht* (Ethik in den Wissenschaften Bd. 12) Tübingen; 2000.

Haker H, Beyleveld D. *The Ethics of Genetics in Human Procreation.* Aldershot; 2000.

Haker H, Hearn R, Steigleder K, editors. *Ethics of Humane Genome Analysis.* Tübingen; 1993.

Haker H, Beyleveld D, editors. *The Ethics of Genetics in Human Reproduction.* Aldershot, GB/Burlington, WI: Ashgate; 2000 [The status of the Embryo 59−100, Legal regulations 215−294].

Hildt E, Mieth D, editors. *In vitro Fertilisation in the 1990s. Towards a medical, social and ethical evaluation.* Aldershot, GB/Brookfield, WI; 1998.

Junker-Kenny M, editor. *Designing Life? Genetics, Procreation and Ethics.* Aldershot, GB/Brookfield, WI; 1999.

Hildt E, Mieth D, editors. *In vitro Fertilisation in the 1990s. Part 7: The status of the embryo.* Aldershot, GB/Brookfield, WI/Vermont; 1998. p. 237−78.

Hildt E, Graumann S, editors. *Genetics in Human Reproduction.* Aldershot, GB/Brookfield, WI; 1998. p. 141.

Koertner UH, Kopetzki C. *Stammzellforschung. Ethische und rechtliche Aspekte (Schriftenreihe Ethik und Recht in der Medizin, Band 2.* Springer; 2008.

Hilpert K, Mieth D, editors. *Kriterien biomedizinischer Ethik. Theologische Beiträge zum gesellschaftlichen Diskurs.* Freiburg-Basel-Wien; 2006.

Höffe O, Honnefelder L, Isensee J, Kirchhof P, *Gentechnik und Menschenwürde.* Köln; 2002.

Hoedemaekers RHMV. *Normative Determinants of Genetic Screening and Testing.* Wageningen, the Netherlands; 1998.

Honnefelder L, Streffer C, editors. *Jahrbuch für Wissenschaft und Ethik.* Bd.7, 2. Berlin; 2002.

Mieth D. *Was wollen wir koennen? Ethik im Zeitalter der Biotechnik.* Freiburg-Basel-Wien 2002. Ital.: Che cosa vogliamo potere? Brescia; 2003.

Mieth D. "The Ethical Relevance of 'Justified Interests' as an Hermeneutical Problem in Genome Analysis." In: Haker H, Hearn R, Steigleder K, editors. *Ethics of Human Genome Analysis, European Perspectives.* Tübingen; 1993. p. 272−89.

Mieth D. "Stem Cells: The Ethical Problems of Using Embryos for Research". *J Contemp Health Law Policy* 2006;22:439–47.

Nordgren A, editor. *Gene Therapy and Ethics*. Uppsala; 1999.

Eberhard-Metzger C, Stollorz V, Mieth D. *Gentherapie*. Berlin; 2003.

Rehmann-Sutter C, Duewell M, Mieth D, editors. Bioethics in Cultural Contexts. Reflections on Methods and Finitude. Springer; 2006 [International Library of Ethics, Law, and the New Medicine 28].

Walters L, Palmer JG. *The Ethics of Human Gene Therapy*. New York, NY; 1997.

Walters L. "The Ethics of Human Gene Therapy." In: Beauchamp TL, Walters L, editors. *Contemporary Issues in Bioethics*, 3rd ed. Belmont, CA; 1989. p. 523.

Wimmer R. "Ethics of Research on Human Embryos." In: Hildt E, Graumann S, editors. *Genetics in Human Reproduction*. Aldershot, GB/Brookfield, WI; 1998. p. 141.

5 Ethics as Consensus Management in Expert Cultures — or Through Civic Debate in the Public Sphere?

Dietmar Mieth

Max Weber Center for Advanced Cultural and Social Studies, University of Erfurt, Germany

Abstract

Ethics as practiced in expert committees has an ambiguous status: the appointing institution may expect support and the delivery of a consensus on its existing bioethical options, while ethicists see themselves as giving independent advice that contributes to public deliberation on crucial questions. I begin my reflections with an analysis of dilemmas between science and society: Science in its location between a pure quest for knowledge and being driven by interests, as well as between trust and uncertainty in a media-dominated society; society facing increasing individual options that make solidarity hard to achieve unless faced by major disasters. With a concept of tolerance that often fails to define itself against what is intolerable, the only consensus achievable seems to be one of less restriction. This creates a political dilemma regarding the promotion or restriction of controversial new technologies. On the background of a critical diagnosis of shifts in the semantics of life, I treat the arguments put forward in expert commissions from different viewpoints relating to the European Patenting Directive, and the civil society initiative Greenpeace took against patents using embryonic stem cells that was recently decided by the European Court of Justice. I conclude with the paradox that arises when pluralism and tolerance become the only relevant values which seem to make any further argumentation in ethics unnecessary.

Key Words

Ethics committees, scientific, social and political dilemmas, life, prejudice, embryonic stem cell patenting, European values, repressive tolerance

The alternative indicated in the title between allowing expert cultures to decide on the ethical permissibility of new technologies, and engaging citizens in the public sphere, will be explored in the following four steps. Beginning with a brief

Ethics for Graduate Researchers. DOI: http://dx.doi.org/10.1016/B978-0-12-416049-1.00002-7

description of the expectations with which members of ethics committees are confronted, I will analyse some dilemmas that arise in general between (bio-)science
and society.[1] In the second part, I will discuss how Ivan Illich, guided by a hermeneutics of suspicion, highlights recent shifts in the meaning of 'life'. The
third part treats the issue of patenting and the controversy about patenting
embryonic stem cells in which Greenpeace mounted a protest against the
European Patenting Office, a private enterprise in Munich, as an example of
civic initiative and debate. I will conclude these analyses with an examination
of the European recognition of the 'diversity of views' and of 'mutual respect
as leading values in Europe.

My experience in ethical advisory groups is that those who nominate the
members try on the one hand to combine different interests and representations
of ethically relevant options, and on the other hand to safeguard a certain majority for the support of the biopolitical mainstream. So, these expert committees
can also be seen as a political instrument for the implementation of biopolitical
options. But this aspect, the expectation of consensus management on behalf of
the appointing institution, cannot totally suppress the other aspect: independent
advice for the public and for the public discussion of crucial questions. This is
true at national and European levels. For the task of moving to a European public sphere, it will be necessary for the EU to promote and support a European
press initiative. Up to now, events in Europe have been discussed far more
extensively than the details of European politics. Because bioethics is becoming
more and more an instrument of societal transfer, a European civil society needs
to be built that is able to reflect on this instrument in open public discourse.
This begins with analysing the role given to science and technology in society
under the competitive conditions of a global marketplace, and with the need to
critically   assess   the   element   of   prejudice   in   our   practices   and   self-
understandings.

Dilemmas Between Science and Society

Science as a Quest for Knowledge and as Driven by Interests

On the one hand, science wants to contribute to knowledge as a goal in itself. On
the other hand, science tries to be socially useful and has a covenant with society.
Modern (biological) science intervenes into nature and devises instruments to do
so. The technical preparation and organisation of research is not only a result but
also a presupposition for the practice of modern science. Freedom of knowledge,
the first goal, finds its limits in the social acceptance of these instruments, as well
as in the theoretical aims of knowledge, and of its practical application. The

---

[1] See D. Mieth, "Conflicts between Bioethics and some Aspects of Traditional Ethics and Religion," in
D.J. Roy, B.E. Wynne and R.W. Old (eds.), Bioscience – Society. Report of the Schering Workshop
on Bioscience (Chichester: Wiley, 1990), vol. 2, 293–304.

scientific dilemma between the insistence on freedom of knowledge and the necessity of control by society will be illustrated later on with examples from biomedicine that show how science is never only science in itself. The promotion of science has political implications, moral options and individual as well as social preferences embedded in it. The dilemma is that science is not neutral and not above given interests. But all scientists are seen in the role of experts, even if they are only experts for their own paradigm of research and its application. They are not experts for contexts, assessments, ethics or education. But in contemporary society, which has an irreversible contract with science, technology, economy and their development, the scientific expert is often accepted for all kinds of expertise, and this may be a temptation for scientific lobbies. One can easily imagine that a group of scientists proposes a specific development as beneficial for society, but one cannot imagine, for example, a group of sociologists proposing their findings as a scientific method. Scientists are at the same time members of the scientific community, and, as high-ranking experts, distinguished citizens. Therefore, it is absolutely necessary to bring societal and ethical discourse into the scientific community and not only an alliance of scientific and economic lobbyism into society.

Science Between Trust and Uncertainty in a Media-Dominated Society

Contemporary society has entered into an alliance with science, technology and economic forces for its own progress and well-being. This alliance cannot be disengaged without the damage for all being greater than the benefit. Retrogression is not a responsible option; the only possibilities are the revocation of particular scientific advances which have not promoted well-being, and a conscious choice between various options within scientific progress. To what extent this choice actually exists, in what values and principles it finds its orientation and how it can seek a universal consensus belong to the most pressing questions of the twenty-first century. Progress is desired, but it is also ambivalent. This ambivalence can only be curtailed if life-promoting aspects are distinguished from life-negating ones at the scientific source of progress. It is difficult to make this choice retrospectively, as one can see with the attempted retraction or reversal of environmentally hazardous technologies and economies as well as with the debate on nuclear energy. This is why an early debate is preferable as a preventive measure. Benefits, as the history of progress shows, also create risks and disadvantages. Which of them are acceptable and will be so in the future?

The intense preventive trust of a society that is oriented towards progress is directed towards science, and within scientific progress, particularly towards progress in medicine. Many people think that while health may not be everything, without health everything else is nothing. While this view does not stand up to empirical verification in the lives of disabled, chronically ill and elderly fellow citizens, it does express a current blend of preferences, defensiveness and preventive trust. Contributing to the trust of a knowledge-oriented society is a media-dominated public transfer of information and opinion.[2] However, it is conceivable that today's highly celebrated scientific advance may well be a monster that needs to be combatted tomorrow. The capacity for memory of the various news media is poor, and their interest in the coherence of news is often scarce. The same holds true for their audiences.

Public opinion is often based on ostensibly scientifically based knowledge and achievements in which options are marketed as truths. The underlying question here is to what degree this depends on a media-dominated transfer of scientific knowledge, or to what degree it is inherent in science itself to create such a socially relevant state of expectation. It is not a matter of journalistic prejudices, which undoubtedly abound, but of a prejudice in science itself, which co-determines its activity within the social alliance mentioned earlier. Yet, science – under the banner of enlightened scepticism and critique – purports to do away with prejudices in society. With noticeable regularity, books are published which fight religious, anthropological and moral prejudices in the name of science. Prejudices are combatted in science like excess pounds in a diet. Doping, too, is fought in sports yet appears to be inherently ineradicable. This dramatic comparison may seem disrespectful but, as the corrections and retractions regularly published in serious scientific journals reveal, is not out of place.

We need to consider the usage of the term prejudice in science, its various meanings and nuances, as well as comprehend the social conditions informing prejudice as a specific form of a hermeneutically inevitable prejudgement, which, as we will show, also extends into scientific practice.

Prejudice became a pre-eminent topic of rational science during the Enlightenment.[3] The prevailing opinion was that if the human being were to make use of his or her capacity of reason and were to collect scientific insights with precise and verifiable methods, he or she could dispel traditional prejudices. These were purportedly due to a lack of courage to fully use one's own powers of reason. Above all, religious prejudices were not only the target but also prejudices against human beings. In a second phase, there was a greater development of what the Enlightenment, particularly Immanuel Kant, also envisioned: a critique of reason. It became increasingly evident that in rational discourse, too, prejudices would have to be taken into account. The initial focus was on prejudices as social ills arising in conjunction with religious convictions or social conventions which were to be overcome by the faculty of reason. In a second step, reflection on the conditions of the possibility of knowledge, including the knowledge produced in the sciences, gradually caused a shift in emphasis to the question of whether prejudices might be conceivable within science. A depressing historic example of such

---

[2] See S. Graumann, "Die Rolle der Medien in der Debatte um die Biomedizin," in S. Schicktanz, C. Tannert, P. M. Wiedemann (eds.), Kulturelle Aspekte der Biomedizin: Bioethik, Religion und Alltagsperspektiven (Frankfurt: Campus, 2003), 212–243; as well as S. Graumann, "Die Situation der Medienberichterstattung zu den aktuellen Entwicklungen in der Biomedizin und ihren ethischen Fragen" (Berlin, 2002), a formal opinion commissioned by the Max-Delbrück-Center of Molecular Medicine.

[3] See A. Pelinka, K. Bischof and K. Stögner, Handbook on Prejudice (New York: Cambria Press, 2009).

prejudices are the widespread and far-reaching differentiations between 'desirable' and 'undesirable' genetic constellations in eugenics in the first half of the last century.

Prejudice, in its negative meaning, that is, in its capacity to produce and reproduce polemics and exclusion, is a prereflective state of a preconception towards facts or towards persons that is critically unaware of its prejudice and thus incapable of correction, a state of preconception that continually feels affirmed, even under adverse conditions. We know that we all have prejudices. Dealing with the prejudicial structure of our consciousness is a distinguishing feature of human processes of maturing. Dealing with the prejudicial structure of our consciousness is called self-reflection in philosophy. Self-reflection is the ultimate emancipatory concept dating from the Enlightenment. People who have prejudices in the sense of a pre-reflective pre-conception, prejudices which are no longer examined and thus remain incapable of being corrected, which constantly seem re-affirmed, are human beings who are not capable of attaining self-reflection in its central sense.

One of the most dangerous prejudices is the coupling of one's own prejudice with one's own purported lack of prejudice. The negative figure of the 'authoritarian personality' exemplifies this image. Frequently a danger with scientists, scholars, politicians, teachers, physicians and so forth, it is to be found in those areas in which self-affirmation is a professional imperative. Coming to terms with the tendency for prejudice in the sense of a negative force, specifically, in the sense of an incapacity for correction, entails, first, the acceptance of the inevitable prejudicial structure of one's own consciousness and, secondly, an open process of experience, which continually puts oneself on the line.[4] The right attitude is an attitude critical of prejudice, not an attitude free of prejudice, just as one must cautiously seek the right approach towards violence not in an illusion of non-violence but in support of a minimalization of violence.[5]

How can it be explained that lack of prejudice is often asserted but not practiced in science? One possible explanation lies in the particular capacity of exacting scientific inquiry to extract problems from their contexts and isolate them. This demand for scientific or scholarly 'exactness' is often a problem for reflection in the humanities due to the severe limitations of the 'laboratorial' nature of strategies for insight and the repeated pressure to re-contextualize its 'laboratory findings' in a multi-factorial reality. Paradoxically, empirical methods are non-empirical in that they do not simply record a parameter, an observation, a datum or a physical phenomenon, but first place it in a conceptual framework, where it appears as one part. The temptation is great to take these partial understandings for the whole. One could call this the *pars pro toto* temptation. As long as the scientific discourse

---

[4] For Gadamer, the inevitable confrontation with one's own prejudice (*'Vor-urteil'*) is related to the realisation that our knowledge is finite. We can only try to cope with this condition, not ignore it. If we do ignore it, we arrive at a destructive prejudice.

[5] Jürgen Habermas reproaches Gadamer for precluding prejudice from criticism. However, this criticism should begin with elucidating the individual's prejudgment.

remains within its boundaries and keeps its experimental conditions transparent as limitations for conclusions – and this is a customary practice – this temptation does not arise. If, however, this discourse is embedded in social discourse, then it must take the given structures of prejudice into account or it will lose its precision. Exactness is thus attained through the reduction of the constellations of the problem and through a methodological framework.

Societal Dilemmas: Increasing Individual Options, Pluralism, Tolerance and the Lack of Restrictive Consensus

Modern and even more so, post-modern societies are based on individual rights and on their protection by institutions. The liberal state corresponds to a pluralistic society that includes very different options. Yet, choices that are made are not always authentic ones but can conform to social trends. Conformity to the leading concept of 'authenticity' is one example, namely of the paradox that the more an atomistic concept of individualism is promoted, the more conformity in concepts of individualisation emerges. People want to be authentic and original but they take the same objects (clothes, travels, behaviour) to express this claimed authenticity. Pluralism in society is, and this may be a paradox, its own greatest enemy. The same paradox is true of tolerance: post-modern tolerance even has problems to exclude intolerance from tolerance. Because solidarities are based on a pluralistic foundation, the achievement of societal solidarity which integrates some differences seems to be possible only in times of great counter-experiences and pressure by negative facts (Chernobyl, Fukushima). But in most cases, the distinction between good and evil depends on a person's experiences and on individual or societal options which can be quite different. A solidarity that would be able to connect pluralistic options can only be reached by transparency of interests and argumentation, and by a shared understanding built on narration and memory in which convictions are formed.

The Political Dilemma Between Promotion and Restriction

In the same simplifying manner in which Snow[6] spoke of the two cultures of science and humanities (*Geisteswissenschaften*), one can also speak in a heuristic sense of two mentalities in questions of biomedicine. The biomedical mentality involved in the link between experimentation and clinical application is a mentality of hope of promotion and acceleration. Limits are seen as given by our self-understanding, for example, that it is forbidden to voluntarily create human monsters, or restrictions are seen as limited to the present social context, or as arising from individual specific options, e.g. of religious groups. As experts who feel responsible for the promotion of the interests of health or other great aims of a constantly developing society, members of the culture of science often see in political opposition that promotes restrictive guidelines nothing but a mixture of ignorance, conservatism

[6] C.P. Snow, Science and Government (Harvard: Harvard University Press, 1962).

and fundamentalism. On the opposite side, bioethics undertaken by scientific experts and by their philosophical servants is considered to be a conspiracy against the needs and values of the people.

Shifts in the Concept of Life

Against this polarisation, it is helpful to begin by clarifying basic concepts that have shaped cultural self-understandings, such as the concept of life. The Greek understanding of *zoe* as self-movement found a counterpart in the monotheistic conception of life as a gift, as something relational and bestowed. As an example of a hermeneutics of suspicion that uncovers the recent loss of this history of meaning, I will analyse a lecture given by the cultural critic Ivan Illich to the Lutheran Church in America in Chicago; in 1989 on 'The Institutional Construction of a New Fetish: Human Life.'[7] Ivan Illich started with the following thesis:

> *'Human Life' is a recent social construct, something which we know and take so much for granted that we dare not seriously question it. I propose that the Church exorcise references to the new substantive life from its own discourse.*

For Illich, the new notion of life, which is so essential for modern ecological, medical and ethical discourses, in the Western tradition is 'the result of a perversion of the Christian message'. In this message life (*bios, zoe, vita*) means something moved by an internal teleology of the soul (vegetative, sensitive or intellectual). Under contemporary conditions, the notion of life no longer belongs to the world of such sacred and contemplative feelings. It is a word that belongs to the field of modern management, to the language of planning so-called human resources. Following a Cartesian dualism, life is an objectivisation and a field of experimental intervention and manipulation with the intention of improvement. The context of epistemic presuppositions to be included in a unquestioned mentality of progress makes the idea of a better life into a new fetish. This turn has created a struggle between two contradictory options, between pro-life and pro-choice. Pro-life means *pro vita*, and pro-choice means the best preference in using the biological material for a better quality only of the self-determined life of individuals. The life of individuals means *vita*, but restricted to an anthropocentric view. But this discourse neglects the connotation of non-objectivisation, which was primarily given with the gospel of life. The gospel of life is personal, expressed in the message, 'I am life', from Moses to Jesus. The modern notion is a value, a good, which must be either preserved or destroyed for social options.

Illich offers five observations of the history of life which we should not forget. 'First, life, as a substantive notion, makes its appearance around 1801.' Instead of the religious and philosophical tradition of *psyche, bios* and *zoe*, the term biology

[7] I. Illich, In the Mirror of the Past (New York/London: Marion Boyars, 1992).

means 'a science of life' (Jean-Baptiste Lamarck). Life is from now on a construct of organic phenomena like reproduction, genetic development and so on.

'Second, the loss of contingency, the death of nature and the appearance of life are but distinct aspects of the same consciousness.' The loss of contingency here is the loss of a dependent and actual connection with the breath of creation. A mechanistic model replaces the creative-relational model.

'Third, the ideology of possessive individualism has shaped the way life could be talked about as a property.' It can easily be demonstrated in the discourse on patenting life that life is being discussed in its 'elements' not as a matter of 'discovery' but as a matter of human 'invention' even if it remains identical to its natural state. On the other hand, the instrumentalisation of human life, which can be seen in options of cloning, is clearly a result of this 'possessive individualism'.

'Fourth, the fetitious nature of life appears with special poignancy in ecological discourse.' To think of life as a system of correlations between living forms and their habitat is a reduction of imagination. It delivers life over to all kinds of empirical and also virtual objectivisation.

'Fifth,' the pop-science fetish of life tends to empty the legal notion of a person. 'The distinction between "human life" and "human person" created the notion of a "human non-person," which is not a member of the so-called "moral community". 'The new discipline of bioethics', this is Illich's conclusion, 'mediates between pop-science and law by creating the semblance of a moral discourse that roots personhood in the qualitative evaluation of the fetish, life'.

I refer to these critical observations by Illich as an important perspective of so-called bioethical questions because we are seldom aware that before beginning an ethical discourse, we have to exorcise a language and a language politics which only allows the semblance of an ethical approach. Bioethics is an invention of the scientific language of biology and its derivations. This paradigm dominates ethical, legal and social responsibilities. It is clear that there is also an interdisciplinary approach to ethics and that interdisciplinarity makes sense in the ethics of sciences and new technologies. Nevertheless, the perception is not inadequate that the paradigm of life as a fetish of a scientific paradigm is strongly present in this kind of discourse.

Maybe some of Illich's claims are a caricature of the more pluralistic world of biology and medicine. However, this experimental approach that questions the basis of political power as well as the paradigm of scientific progress may be helpful to reflect on motivations, presuppositions and conventions, and to come up with alternative assessments.

Controversies in Expert Cultures and in Civil Society About Patenting Embryonic Stem Cells

To summarise a longer history, a turning point occurred when patent applications involving living organisms began to be filed on a regular basis. Although there was already a predisposition to regard patenting biological resources as no different from patenting anything else, the decisions of the US Supreme Court in the landmark *Chakrabarty* case established a principle that 'the relevant distinction was not between living and inanimate' things but whether living products could be seen as 'human-made inventions'. This was part of a major but invisible cultural change, expressed by a senior UK patent expert, Crespi:

> *Historically, the patent system came to birth to meet industrial needs. Industry was perceived as activities carried on inside factories... Manufacture was the key word. Agriculture was felt to be outside the realm of patent law. Living things were also assumed to be excluded as being products of nature rather than products of manufacture... This restricted view no longer persists in most industrialised countries. Thus the European Patent Convention of 1973 declares agriculture to be a kind of industry.*[8]

In almost all ethical systems, however, a vital distinction is made between how we treat what is living and what is not. The Directive on Biopatenting of 1998 (EU) gave an example that some biological 'materials' (i.e. the language of the directive) are prohibited to be patented, even if those patents cannot permit any process or use that is against existing laws and regulations. Patents based on embryo research for industrial or commercial purposes are prohibited in the directive. Thus, the European Patent Office (EPA for *Europäisches Patentamt*) in Munich, challenged by Greenpeace and others, withdrew in 2002 a special part of the so-called Edinburgh Patent which included a human embryo cell collection. The EPA repeated this negative decision for other biopatents that included embryo research (one of them from the German researcher Oliver Brüstle in 2006). At the end, the European Court of Justice in Luxembourg decided on 18 October, 2011, that embryonic stem cells and their derivates cannot be patented.

On the other hand, a serious problem of biopatenting remains: the absolute protection of the biological entity itself, not only of the inventive method or process which is needed for its commercial use. There are many objections against such an absolute property right which may create difficulties for academic research, as well as for farmers in the Two-Thirds World. Such materials, e.g. the whole model of a mouse, are not themselves invented.

The EU Biopatenting Directive strongly affirmed the principle of patenting almost anything biological. It merely added a set of exclusion clauses for applications such as human cloning known to be politically sensitive to the European Parliament. It did not respond appropriately to the full range of relevant ethical concerns and made clear that its prime concern was European economic growth and competitiveness. This drive to patent anything biological makes the commercial paradigm into the only relevant imperative.

---

[8] Cf. R.S. Crespi, "Patents in Biotechnology: The legal background," in Proceedings of the International Conference on Patenting Life Forms in Europe (Brussels: unpublished, February 1989), 7–8. Cf. International Cooperation for Development and Solidarity (CIDSE) (ed.), Biopatenting and the Threat of Food Security – A Christian and Development Perspective (Brussels, 1999), 16.

A second distinction concerns what has been invented. Where genetic modifications to an animal or plant are at issue, the addition of two or three genes to an animal with perhaps 100,000 genes does not turn the animal into a human invention. The inventive step is to add the new gene construct to the animal. The novel construct, or the inventive application of a modified animal to a specific purpose, might be awarded with a patent.

The same applies to a gene. It may take great intellectual effort to decipher a gene and identify its function, but the gene is just as much a product of nature as the animal is. Despite the considerable investment involved, the identification of a gene's function does not give an ethical ground for claiming inclusive rights. Even though intellectual effort has been used, it is of the nature of a discovery, not of an invention. However, the EU wanted to find a premise to patent human genes. The Biopatenting Directive states that genes are patentable inventions because they have to be copied, using bacteria or chemicals, to be isolated and identified.

The Church of Scotland put its opposition to patenting living organisms as follows:

> *Living organisms themselves should therefore not be patentable, whether genetically modified or not. It is wrong in principle. An animal, plant or micro-organism owes its creation ultimately to God, not human endeavour. It cannot be interpreted as an invention or a process, in the normal sense of either word. It has a life of its own, which inanimate matter does not. In genetic engineering, moreover, only a tiny fraction of the makeup of the organism can be said to be a product of the scientists. The organism is still essentially a living entity, not an invention.[9]*

I am sure that a scientist in favour of patenting will answer: Is it the inventive step in processing a product which gives the reason for patenting? Genes for example are only 'products by process'. And so they are not considered a creation, they are only included in the term invention.

This may be an example why a top-down argumentation in theological ethics, arguing from God's act of creation, as in the example cited, does not reach the real complexity of the problem. The decisive question is whether patents on the process and patents on living resources can be separated. And they can.

If this is the case, then the living resource in itself gives the reason for financial gain. And this is what meets with ethical objection, taking into account the recognised principle of the non-commercialisation of the human body and its parts. This is an application of the respect for human dignity, the real reason for rejecting biopatents on human genes. This argument is reinforced by a monotheistic belief in creation, but it does not need this belief; the ethical concept of human dignity is sufficient. In continuing research, one has to keep in mind that progress in one dimension does not guarantee progress for the destiny of humanity in general.

In this discussion, the question of how core notions are used depends on one's conception of language: if one has a nominalistic conception of language, all

---

[9] Cf. CIDSE (ed.), Biopatenting, 12.

notions are only conventions between those who use the word. As a consequence, there are no problems with an interpretation of a discovery as an invention, if this makes practical sense. But if one insists on a conception of coherence of signification in a language system or on a correspondence between language and reality, it is not possible to use the word invention for what is a discovery of what already exists.

Conclusion: A Final Remark on Pluralism and Tolerance as Leading Values

In the Opinion of the European Group on Ethics (EGE) 12, on *Ethical Aspects of Embryo Research*, published on 23 November 1998, one can read the following about the diversity of ethical positions:

> *1.23 The diversity of views regarding the question whether or not research on human embryos in vitro is morally acceptable, depends on differences in ethical approaches, theories and traditions, which are deeply rooted in European culture...*
>
> *1.25 The diversity in policies and regulations concerning embryo research in the Member States of the EU reflects fundamentally differing views... and it is difficult to see how, at these extremes (cf. embryo as human life or as a human being), the differences can be reconciled.'*

This kind of introduction of an opinion often leads to the result that a substantial restriction will not be acceptable.

'Mutual respect' is also mentioned in the EGE Opinion (cf. 2.5):

> *1.27 Pluralism may be seen as a characteristic of the European Union, mirroring the richness of its tradition and asking for mutual respect and tolerance.*

In other papers, 'mutual respect' is precisely focused on 'moral choices. Therefore, the more liberal positions always have a political advantage. They cannot be trumped because, if they are, respect for different approaches and moral choices no longer seems to be granted. This is what the critical theorist Herbert Marcuse has called 'repressive tolerance'. One can always suppress substantial restrictions but not a substantial liberalisation.

Ethical discourse on pluralism, tolerance and compromise seems to be quite underdeveloped. Most members of bioethical committees speak of these attitudes but the words remain without clarification. If pluralism is not 'laissez-faire', then what is its meaning? If pluralism is not the same as the lowest restrictive level, then how can it be precisely defined? If pluralism has a tendency to compromise, then what distinction is to be made between a practical compromise and an ethical judgement? I am speaking from a concrete experience, which I have made as a member of a European Project on Pluralism. There is an ethical paradox when one takes pluralism as the *norma normans*; one does not need any ethics at all because all argumentation can be stopped by the norm of pluralism. But if there are no limits for pluralism, then the so-called position (reclaiming pluralism) risks turning into a kind of fundamentalism.

If one tries to initiate a moral discourse with the goal of consensus, one should begin by doubting one's own moral position and reflecting on the conditions necessary to work towards reaching consensus: not to be dominated by a power of definition led by the politics of language or by repressive tolerance. We must also understand that disagreement and conflict in moral arguments does not mean that respect for persons is being violated. If it is true that ethicists have to learn about scientific specialisations and the scientific use of language, the same is necessary for scientists in public debate. In both the cases, there is a danger of too little education of public opinion for the conditions of a moral discourse.

As an ethicist, when dealing with the high hopes and great promises of biomedical advances, I cannot help wondering about a breakthrough mentality that will not take into account essential factors of the human constitution. Humans are prone to error. Often, we attempt to rationalise our motives and ignore the danger of instrumentalising others. Debate in the public realm can draw on traditions of reflection in which human finitude is accepted and shared in solidarity, and fallibility is met with critical alertness.

Bibliography

Beyleveld D. "The Moral Status of the Human Embryo and Fetus". In: Haker H, Beyleveld D, editors. *The Ethics of Genetics in Human Procreation*. Aldershot: Ashgate; 2000. p. 59–100.

Crespi RS, "Patents in Biotechnology: The legal background," in *Proceedings of the International Conference on Patenting Life Forms in Europe* (Brussels: unpublished, February 1989).

Bundestag D, Öffentlichkeitsarbeit R, editors. *Enquete-Kommission Recht und Ethik der modernen Medizin: Stammzellforschung und die Debatte des Deutschen Bundestages zum Import von menschlichen embryonalen Stammzellen*. Zur Sache 1; 2002. This report is also available in English.

European Group on Ethics in Science and New Technologies (EGE), Opinion 12: *Ethical Aspects of Embryo Research*; 1998.

Graumann S. "Die Rolle der Medien in der Debatte um die Biomedizin". In: Silke Schicktanz Christof, Tannert, Wiedemann PM, editors. *Kulturelle Aspekte der Biomedizin: Bioethik, Religion und Alltagsperspektiven*. Frankfurt: Campus; 2003. p. 212–43.

Graumann S, Die Situation der Medienberichterstattung zu den aktuellen Entwicklungen in der Biomedizin und ihren ethischen Fragen. Report Max Delbrück Center of Molecular Medicine. Berlin; 2002.

Hildt E, Graumann S, editors. *Genetics in Human Reproduction*. Aldershot: Ashgate; 2000.

Hildt E, Mieth D, editors. *In Vitro Fertilisation in the 1990s: Towards a Medical, Social and Ethical Evaluation*. Aldershot: Ashgate; 1998.

Honnefelder L, Lanzerath D, editors. *Cloning in Biomedical Research and Reproduction. Scientific Aspects − Ethical. Legal and Social Limits.* Bonn: Bonn University Press; 2003.

Honnefelder L, Streffer C, editors. *Jahrbuch für Wissenschaft und Ethik*, vol. 7. Berlin: De Gruyter; 2002 [With a documentation of international and national regulations and ethical opinions on embryonic stem cell engineering.].

Hottois G, Missa J-N, editors. *Nouvelle Encyclopedie de Bioethique, Medicine, Environnement, Biotechnologie.* Brussels: De Boeck Universiteé; 2001.

Illich I. *In the Mirror of the Past.* New York/London: Marion Boyars; 1992.

International Cooperation for Development and Solidarity. CIDSE, editor. *Biopatenting and the Threat of Food Security − A Christian and Development Perspective.* Brussels; 1999. p. 16.

Mieth D. "Conflicts between Bioethics and some Aspects of Traditional Ethics and Religion". In: Roy DJ, Wynne BE, Old RW, editors. *Bioscience − Society. Report of the Schering Workshop on Bioscience*, vol. 2. Chichester: Wiley; 1990. p. 293−304.

McLaren A. *Ethical Eye: Cloning.* Strasbourg: Council of Europe Publishing; 2002 (Coordinator).

Mieth D. "Science under the Spell of Prejudice: The Example of Biosciences". In: Pelinka A, Bischof K, Stoegner K, editors. *Handbook on Prejudice.* New York, NY: Cambria Press; 2009. p. 345−74.

Pfleiderer G, Brahier G, Lindpaintner K, editors. *GenEthics and Religion.* Basel: Karger; 2010.

The President's Council of Bioethics. *Human Cloning and Human Dignity. An Ethical Inquiry.* Washington, DC; 2002.

Snow CP. *Science and Government.* Harvard: Harvard University Press; 1962.

Voeneky S, Wolfrum R, editors. *Human Dignity and Human Cloning.* Leiden/Boston, MA: Martinus Nijhoff Publishers; 2004.

6 Nanomedicine and European Ethics — Part One

Hille Haker

Theology Department, Loyola University Chicago, Chicago, IL, USA

Abstract

In this chapter, I ask what the role of ethics is or could be with respect to science and the new technologies, turning particularly to nanomedicine. I argue that while the current so-called ethical, legal, social aspect methodology offers important insights, it needs to be complemented by a distinct social–ethical methodology that enables ethics to address new technologies as social practices whose categories, goals and means are open to philosophical and societal deliberations. This chapter addresses ethical questions concerning the diagnostic and therapeutic prospects of nanomedicine and presents the recommendations of the European Group on Ethics in Science and New Technologies.

Key Words

Ethics, bioethics, nanomedicine, European Group on Ethics

One of the striking characteristics of new technologies is their ability to be 'applied' in rather diverse contexts, which in nanotechnologies — the technology I will address here — includes health-related applications in diagnostics, the development of new pharmaceuticals and drugs, therapies and medical devices, cosmetics, energy and/or environmental-related organisms and tools, military devices, food ingredients or household products. Nanotechnology can be applied in almost infinite ways, using different existing technologies and scientific sub-areas (hence, e.g. the label of converging technologies). While each of these applications needs thorough examination, in this chapter I will focus on the methodological deliberations with which any ethical analysis of new technologies is confronted. Prior to this, I will look briefly at the historical developments that have led to the demand for a new approach in the 'ethics of new technologies' is briefly described.[1]

---

[1] Parts of this article contain a revised version of another article: "Ethical Reflections on Nanomedicine," in Johann S. Ach, Beate Lüttenberg (eds.) *Nanobiotechnology, Nanomedicine and Human Enhancement*, Berlin Lit Verlag, 2008, 53–75.

Ethics for Graduate Researchers. DOI: http://dx.doi.org/10.1016/B978-0-12-416049-1.00006-4

Since the 1970s, offices or institutes of technology assessment were assigned in several countries with the task to assess the future impact, including the costs and benefits, harms and risks of emerging technologies.[2] The reports issued by these institutes were an important tool in the overall evaluation of new technologies, but they were certainly not designed to offer a more 'comprehensive' social or ethical evaluation. With the rise of bioethics as an academic discipline in the 1980s − an approach that in the beginning included animal ethics as well as environmental ethics but was quickly equated with biomedical ethics − seemed better equipped to bridge the gap between technology assessment and ethics. Bioethicists not only succeeded in establishing clinical ethics committees, they also re-worked the guidelines of research ethics, they continue to contribute to the drafting of ever-new guidelines in medical fields and have established medical ethics courses as part of the medical curricula. In addition to these tasks, bioethicists also co-authored reports in national commissions about new technologies, particularly the so-called life sciences, mainly in areas related to health care or medicine, increasingly addressing new technologies that go beyond the medical application. Up to the present, medical ethics boards or national ethics committees have been established in most of the countries, designed to assess the impact, risks or social and ethical concerns of new technologies. They are not only meant to assist political bodies in their governance and legal regulations, but also meant to communicate between the sciences and the society.[3] So far, however, no 'common' methodology has evolved that these committees could apply; rather, it seems that some committees more often apply the technology assessment methodology that offers mostly risk assessment, while others apply the bioethical methodology that was developed in view of ethical decision-making in clinical contexts.

Can we really turn to the bioethical methodology that evolved in the biotechnological and biomedical field, and implement and/or adjust it to the new technologies − in this case to nanomedicine? More precisely, should we assess the visions and potential risks and hazards of new technologies, for example, in light of the principles Beauchamp and Childress? They have introduced, albeit with much criticism, the main principles associated with bioethics (autonomy, non-maleficence, beneficence, justice). Or should we interpret the prospects of new technologies in light of the one and overarching principle, human dignity, spelled out as respect for human rights, as it is this that is the cornerstone of European and United Nations policy papers addressing biomedical concerns the so-called Oviedo Convention and the so-called UNESCO Bioethics Convention?[4] What methods do we have to reasonably speak about hierarchies and the balancing of moral rights and values, e.g. the values of freedom of research, technological innovation and economic competition, over

---

[2] One significant institute is the US Office of Technology Assessment that was established in 1972 but subsequently closed in 1995.

[3] Cf. for further information the International Bioethics Meeting organised by the EU Commission; and the EGE that has convened three times since 2009: http://ec.europa.eu/bepa/european-group-ethics/bepa-ethics/ec-international-dialogue-bioethics/index_en.htm.

[4] Council of Europe *Convention for the Protection of Human Rights and Dignity of the Human Being with regard to the Application of Biology and Medicine: Convention on Human Rights and Biomedicine* (1997) and UNESCO Universal Declaration of Bioethics and Human Rights (2005).

and against the human rights to health care, to privacy or the protection against environmental or medical hazards? Should we follow a Kantian or a Utilitarian approach in our ethical evaluation, or should we rather work on a case-by-case basis and apply a framework of medical–ethical decision-making that is context sensitive and does not carry with it too much baggage from foundational ethical reasoning? Or should we follow system theory, as Khushf argues, with respect to nanoethics,[5] or proceed self-reflectively and analyse the power enacted through the very definition of what counts as 'ethical issue'?[6] Should we, in the assessment of nanomedicine, too, distinguish between the internal and the external ethical issues to distinguish between different levels of accountability: 'internal' issues include the ontological status of nanoparticles or nanostructures and 'external' issues, such questions as a social apocalyptic view of complete loss of privacy or control over one's private life or the totalizing control of nature by the success of instrumental reason?[7] None of these questions are new within bioethical reflection and academic discussions, but they need to be addressed newly in view of current developments: in view of the possibility that nanotechnology will change not only our health care system or the ways we produce and use energy and any products of our daily lives, but also our self-understanding, the way we interact with 'machines', and, last but not least, the way we interact with others, including the environment and nature as such. Finally, new technologies cannot but be seen in light of the social and political problems we face today: when we take global poverty into account and take seriously that over a billion people lack a minimal standard of living, and when we consider the energy crisis, climate change and the deficits in global health.

Ethics – which is the reflection on actions and practices, on agency and the necessary dispositions to moral agency, and the reflection on the normative orders accompanying social, political and legal institutions – is necessarily reflective. It does not set up values, principles or norms but rather 'extracts' them from specific actions, social practices or institutions who have established more or less abstract systems of values and norms. Ethics is a set of theories which analyse the different moral dimensions of a question or action to articulate them or, depending on its own frameworks of reasoning, to criticise or strengthen them. Reflecting on ethical methods is part of a meta-ethical enterprise that is yet further detached from practice but is necessary as the current system is no longer regarded as sufficient. From this perspective, we need to acknowledge that no ethical theory aiming at the assessment of new technologies starts from the scratch; rather, it needs to reflect upon the following:

> the normative framework (principles or guiding values) that informs the analysis of the practices under scrutiny;

---

[5] Khushf, G. "Systems theory and the ethics of human enhancement: a framework for NBIC convergence" *Annals of the New York Academy of Sciences* (2004), 1013124–49.
[6] Lewenstein, B. V "What counts as a 'social and ethical issue' in nanotechnology?" *Hyle* 11 (2005), 5–18.
[7] Gordijn, B. "Nanoethics: from utopian dreams and apocalyptic nightmares towards a more balanced view" *Science and Engineering Ethics* 11 (2005), 521–533. and Robinson, W. "Nano-Ethics," in *Discovering the Nanoscale* Baird, D., Nordmann, A., (eds.), (Amsterdam: IOS, 2004) pp. 285–300.

the constitutive categories of the practices which are analysed, namely their epistemological concepts, goals and methods of new technologies;
the cultural and social origins and the contexts of these constitutive categories, particularly of the goals and their underlying values, and the priorities they express; and
the moral agents/institutions that take up (or must take up) the responsibility for the actions and practices that are envisioned.

In the Section 'Ethics in Nanosciences: The ELSA Approach', I will take up the current ELSA approach and demonstrate it with respect to nanomedicine as an example of a new technology that has been examined by the European Group on Ethics in Science and New Technology. In the Section 'Ethics, Policy and Society: The Role of the EGE', I will summarise the role of the EGE and quote the recommendations it presented to the European Commission, ending with a short overview of how the European Union responded to the challenges of nanotechnology.

Ethics in Nanosciences: The ELSA Approach

The common methodical approach in ethical analysis regarding new technologies stems from the time of the Human Genome Project. The US and European public funding in the 1990s was given on the condition that research gave consideration and time to what were labelled the 'ethical, legal and social implications' (later this was exchanged with the term 'aspects') of the Human Genome Project. Since then, ELSA has become the default method and is considered sufficiently comprehensive to embrace research and development of new technologies. It implies that these three areas can adequately re-situate the goals, means and implications of new technologies. The ELSA approach, however, may be called a technology-oriented ethical analysis (i.e. the first strategy in an ethical analysis of new technologies), because it is the technologies that shape the analysis with their epistemological frameworks. The technologies emerge and are then complemented with the assessment of their legal, social or ethical implications as external factors. In contrast to this methodology, I will later argue that a different approach is necessary, because otherwise ethics is simply imitating or even repeating what technology assessment can do better than ethical analysis. I therefore argue (as the second strategy of an ethical analysis of new technologies) that ethics should also challenge underlying assumptions alongside the technology assessment and partial strategy of the so-called ELSA approach. In this part, however, I will take the nanosciences as an example of a new technology that is analysed currently mainly following the ELSA approach.

Nanomedicine is health-related nanotechnology, making use of the size, structure and properties of the material it applies to the different fields of intervention: the development of new diagnostic systems, such as chips, arrays and imaging techniques; biomaterials and synthetic material, such as synthetic drugs containing nanoparticles or nanostructures, or drug delivery systems based on synthetic molecules, 'biosynthetic' tissue or nanobased implants; therapeutic systems, such as targeted drug delivery systems making use of the surface, property, sensitivity and size of nanostructures, implants and cell regeneration systems, or material used in surgery. Taking the clinical–medical categories, nanomedicine is expected to have a major impact in four relevant fields: prevention, diagnosis, therapy and post-therapeutic monitoring.[8] By way of example, I will take a short look at these fields and comment on them in a preliminary, technology-oriented ethical interpretation, subsuming diagnosis, prevention and monitoring under one heading, and therapy under the other.

Prevention via Pre-Symptomatic Testing, Diagnosis and Monitoring

In the twentieth century, diagnosis of physical health became more and more dependent on 'technology' in contrast to the practitioner's perception and doctor–patient communication. Since the 1970s, the focus shifted to laboratory analysis and diagnosis of biochemical processes and, with the development of imaging techniques, to a highly sophisticated imaging technology. Two different forms of diagnosis must be distinguished in the nanomedical field: *in vitro* diagnosis improving, for example, DNA analysis and the development of chips or sensors used outside the human body and *in vivo* diagnosis using nanoparticles and/or sensors and targeted devices to diagnose which part of an organ, tissue or other parts of the body is affected.

Diagnosis may become the most interesting field for nanomedical research in the next years: the development of better imaging techniques, bio-nanosensors and targeted devices will certainly enable more precise and better targeted diagnosis. Using the structure of DNA, the so-called lab-on-the-chip technology is no longer science fiction but rather a vision scientists aim to put into reality. Obviously, the distinction between pre-symptomatic and diagnostic tests may be almost irrelevant for this application, as both types of *in vitro* tests depend on the same technique.

Modern medicine aims not only at the diagnosis, but more and more at the prevention of diseases, e.g. using pre-symptomatic tests and health-related lifestyle measures. Many of these, like cancer screening, are well established and do not raise profound ethical questions; although, on the level of individual ethics, issues with compliance and the motivation of specific population groups to make use of these preventive (as diagnostic) screenings, are issues not yet solved satisfactorily.

For the last decades, however, one type of screening has indeed been debated in the ethical community, namely pre-symptomatic genetic tests and screening for conditions where no therapy can be offered. If nanomedicine, as is predicted, improves *in vitro* pre-symptomatic test methods, it may provide a time-saving and location-independent service to those who choose to be tested, and become a major step forward to a personalised medicine. As discussed earlier, all preventive measures in medicine are dependent on the compliance of (or welcoming by) individuals who are not (or not yet) patients but who should consider certain activities or a certain lifestyle as unfavourable for their health condition. Nanomedicine itself does not solve the problem of interpretation, compliance and motivation.

---

[8] European Technology Platform. *Strategic Research Agenda* (2006).

Nevertheless, it is hoped that better, easier and finally also cheaper tests might have an impact on the individuals' attitude towards their future health. Whether this holds true will not depend on the technology itself, but rather on a social atmosphere of trust. This can only be built up if scientists are able to make their argument that the tests indeed serve the interests of individuals, that they will improve their health condition, and that society is well advised to cover these tests by health insurance. Trust certainly has become a major issue in modern medicine, as Onora O'Neill rightly states, but especially with regard to bio/nanotechnology, it is not always clear whether economic interests correspond with health-related interests of individuals.[9] This is the argument scientists have to make, without concealing their genuine interests to gain patents, or to maintain or become competitors in the global market.

Second, the categorical ethical concerns about predictive and diagnostic tests do not change with the advent of nanotechnology, but with the almost all-embracing, fast and cheap tests available, the social and ethical problems (who will get which information for what reason with what effect) will certainly intensify and increase for the persons concerned. Personalised preventive medicine may evolve as the driver of a major shift in medicine as such – most significantly shifting responsibility to the individuals who must decide what they want to know and how to interpret the medical data they gain. Medical professionals may more and more serve as translators of medical information – in contrast to their current authority and competence which is to not only to translate but also to interpret the data in light of the patient's health status. This more important step may be left to the patients or clients themselves.

At first sight, this might be a desirable shift from paternalism to individual autonomy and responsibility; a shift that in fact has taken place already over the last few decades.[10] However, if there is almost 'complete' information, much more selection between irrelevant and relevant information is needed. The inherent value of necessary selective interpretation of medical data does not exclusively depend on medical expertise, rather it is mediated by social norms and values; self-reflective reasoning within medicine is needed to secure patients' autonomy. Again, extension, acceleration, cost-effectiveness and independence of a medical setting may merely intensify a tendency we experience already in genetic testing and diagnosis. What can be learned from the past, however, is that the moral standards for responsible genetic testing were not thoroughly debated and reflected upon before the tests were established. Take, for example, pre-natal predictive genetic testing: Why should the genetic condition of a late-onset disease like Chorea Huntington count as a moral reason to terminate a pregnancy, if this condition does not affect the prospective parents in their responsibility to care for their

---

[9] O'Neill, O. *Autonomy and Trust in Bioethics*. Gifford lectures 2001, (Cambridge: University Press, 2002).

[10] Autonomy is not only a principle that needs to be respected; it is also an ideal based upon the value of sovereignty and 'control over one's life' that is characteristic in Western approaches to self-fulfilment cf. O'Neill, *Autonomy and Trust in Bioethics* and Faden, R. R. and Beauchamp, T. *A History and Theory of Informed Consent*, (New York; Oxford University Press, 1986).

child? Ethicists have argued that we can assume the future child's interest not to live with this condition − but in this case, as in other late-onset diseases, this decision could be left to the future person itself.[11] In line with this example, if all known genetic conditions come with a risk to develop into a disease and can be tested, who assists the members of society to make 'responsible choices'? It becomes clear that to offer more information in a quicker and cheaper way does not solve the problems of ethical decision-making. Certainly, this problem does serve as an overall argument against the introduction of predictive tests based on nanomedical tools, but the analysis directs us to the social and ethical dimensions of the decision to develop and introduce them.

In addition to these *in vitro* applications, *in vivo* diagnosis raises questions that go far beyond traditional biomedical ethics. Whereas it can be assumed that it is desirable to get a diagnosis as quickly and precisely as possible, not much is known about the behaviour of nanoparticles *in vivo* and, perhaps even more important, about their possible substantial changes in property over a period of time. Insofar as nanobased devices will be applied to improve imaging techniques, e.g. in screening for cancer or neurodegenerative diseases, ethical analysis is dependent on risk assessment and on prognostic scenarios to exclude currently unknown harms.

Monitoring after positive predictive testing may become much easier with nanomedical technologies. Especially, when imaging techniques are further developed, it will be easier, quicker, more extensive, hopefully cost-saving and personalized.[12] As is well known from the field of DNA testing, it is hard to confine information technology to the medical field. Hence, monitoring may easily turn into health-related surveillance if it is made easy to transgress the narrow context of medical research and clinical application. For the ethical analysis, this easy and possible transgression is relevant exactly because the information may be desired by insurance companies or other agencies. In keeping with the distinction already made between the internal and the external effects of nanomedicine, the impact on health insurance might well qualify as a borderline case. Even though scientists cannot be held accountable for the external effects, they need to reflect upon (or make clear) how they expect to keep the information in control.

The gap between diagnosis and possible therapeutic action is an issue well known from the field of biomedicine. How exactly it can be bridged, cannot be answered by bio- or nanomedicine alone. However, and significantly, handling of the gap requires psychosocial assistance to develop coping strategies, and ethical frameworks to preclude discrimination and stigmatisation. This medical and social competence is not automatically in place and needs to be acquired and engendered

[11] For a broader discussion on reproductive decision-making cf. Haker, H. *Ethik der genetischen Frühdiagnostik. Sozialethische Reflexionen zur Verantwortung am menschlichen Lebensbeginn* (Paderborn; Mentis, 2002) and Haker, H. "Selection through prenatal diagnosis and preimplantation diagnosis," in *Genetics in Human Reproduction* Hildt, E. and Graumann, S. (eds.) (Aldershot: Ashgate, 1999) pp. 157−168.

[12] Leary, S.P., Liu, Charles Y., Yu, Cheng, Appuzo, Michael L.J. "Toward the emergence of nanoneurosurgery: Part II − Nanomedicine: Diagnostics and Imagining at the nanoscale level" *Neurosurgery* 58 (2006), 805−822.

with an infrastructure that does not fall into the medical realm but rather into the realm of public health education. And all this needs to happen before major changes in the diagnostic field should take place. The implementation of diagnoses for which therapies are not available might not be accepted, may even be resisted, by individuals, and, ethically more importantly, patients may not be in themselves socially responsible unless information, education and counselling centres are established where professionals address the personal issues in this new 'era' of personalised medicine.

Therapy

While predictive testing and diagnosis may be applied in different areas in a short time, therapy is much more difficult, although the first therapeutic implementations have already begun, as in cancer therapy.[13] The aim is to design targeted drugs, targeted delivery agents and implants that maximise control and minimise the intervention both locally and temporally. Surgery could make use of imaging techniques, and adult stem cells in connection with implants could cause cells and tissue to regenerate. Using the characteristics of nanoparticles to cross the blood—brain barrier may have an impact on the treatment of neurodegenerative diseases, and nanosensors may be able to control psychiatric conditions. Post-therapeutic monitoring is envisioned to become more effective and more sensitive.

Although therapies are the natural aim of new medical research, not every therapy is as 'good' as another. Normally, alternative ways are assessed, and the one that causes the least harm as a side effect for the patient is chosen. With nanomedicine, however, therapeutic interventions must be evaluated in face of the lack of knowledge, and in face of unknown risks of nano-sized particles and their effect within an organism. Decisions must be made on the basis of medical—ethical guidelines and legislation to protect the individual from harm. However, to set up these guidelines is a difficult task for the scientific community because we are not only dealing with an emerging technology but also with a complex system of risks and safety concerns for which a framework does not yet exist. In addition, the legal challenge − to set up and modify the existing rules − so that it can cope with the implications of new technology, is only slowly being recognised.

Safety in Nanotechnology and Nanomedicine

Safety and risk-related implications analysed by technology assessment need to be integrated in ELSA studies. As stated in the introduction, technology and risk assessment do not belong to ethical analysis as such, but rather need to be integrated.

---

[13] Cf. Arayne MS, S. N. "Review: nanoparticles in drug delivery for the treatment of cancer" *Pakistan Journal of Pharmaceutical Science* 19 (2006) 258−268. And Leary, S. P., Liu, Charles Y., Yu, Cheng, Appuzo, Michael L.J. "Toward the emergence of nanoneurosurgery: Part III − Nanomedicine: Targeted nanotherapy, nanosurgery, and progress toward the realization of nanoneurosurgery" *Neurosurgery* 58 (2006), 1009−1026.

The International Risk Governance Council (IRGC) published its second White Paper in June 2006.[14] In this paper, a framework for risk and technology assessment is set up that could pave the way to an international endeavour to address the health-related risks accompanying nanotechnology and nanomedicine.[15] In the authors' view, governance should include not only the assessment but also the management and communication of risks; they urge that networking (instead of 'top-down' models of technology assessment) and international collaboration needs to be intensified.[16] They argue for an approach that is 'adaptive and corrective', and therefore flexible with respect to the knowledge gaps of current research on nanotechnology, instead of the cause-and-effect approach that has been widely applied in 'traditional' risk assessment. Furthermore, they propose to include what they call 'contingency plans' that leave room to adapt the risk assessment to different economic or political situations. In their temporal framework, the authors distinguish between the development of passive nanostructures (which has been the case from c. 2000); active nanostructures (from c. 2005); complex nanosystems (from c. 2010) and molecular nanosystems (from c. 2015). For each of these phases, they recommend different strategies of social, legal and ethical analysis, and different forms of public participation. Whereas in the first phase self-regulation was dominant, this should be transformed in the next three phases into formal regulation and public participation in decision-making by using known and developing new forms of public discourse. Of particular concern is the attention the report pays to the 'active' structures of nanomaterial, namely its potential to change its properties under different conditions, which is probably dependent also on their life cycle. Nanoparticles cross the blood—brain barrier. This characteristic is applied for the developments in diagnosis as well as in therapies. From the perspective of risk assessment, however, this raises some major concern, namely in the case that nanoparticles affect the nervous system in uncontrollable and unpredictable ways. Prospective and proactive risk assessment is certainly needed and to be funded.

The IRGC emphasises another point that is of special importance for ethical analysis: It claims that the interface of science and policies is so underdeveloped

---

[14] International Risk Governance Council. *White Paper: Nanotechnology Risk Governance.* Renn, O., Rocco, M., Litten, E. 2 June 2006.

[15] These are the main risks the report identifies concerning health on the level of organs: toxic response due to high reactivity, penetration of nerve axons, increased level of toxicity, unknown characteristics whose behaviour cannot be predicted, with similar characteristics to known high risk materials at the microscale. For all these risks, precautionary measures must be taken and finally legally be regulated. In 2007, the same group published the conclusion of the report addressing specific policy recommendations, cf. http://www.irgc.org/IMG/pdf/PB_nanoFINAL2_2_.pdf.

[16] 'The current regulatory measures generally deal with a single event and its cause-and-effect, and do not consider the life cycles of products, secondary effects of interactions with other events. Regulatory organisations and measures are fragmented by the area of jurisdiction, type of regulation (product, process, etc.) intervention levels and national and international harmonisation of assessment and management procedures (or the lack thereof). An integrated governance approach for anticipatory and corrective measures is necessary for an emerging technology that will have trans-boundary and global implications.' This paragraph is followed by a list of 'specific societal infrastructure deficits.' Ibid.

that serious proactive technology assessment seems to be almost impossible. Technology assessment must be a companion to responsible research and ideally synchronized with the development and establishment of a new technology. Done well, it will not only result in structures that enable information, education and communication among the different actors and institutions but, moreover, it will be a part of governance that scientists – as moral agents – should consider not as constraints but rather as a safety net against irresponsible research. This seems to be crucial especially because the development of 'science and technology' consists of multiple agents, research groups from all over the world, different disciplines and different institutions. They all share a responsibility that is difficult to account for by the individual agent. If societies, however, are to promote the concept of responsibility, accountability and liability,[17] we have no alternative to scrutinised ethical analysis. Hence, together with a prospective technology assessment, ethical analysis serves to enable scientists to act responsibly or at least share the load of responsibilities, and to assure the members of societies that relatively autonomous-working sectors such as science and technology have been thoroughly evaluated, to protect or promote their rights.

Ethics, Policy and Society: The Role of the EGE

As mentioned earlier, most countries have established ethics committees that compile reports aimed at bridging the gap between science and society, and also providing political bodies with recommendations of how to embrace the new technologies. The dynamic can be explained as a circle (Figure 6.1).

The European Group on Ethics in Science and New Technologies, which is the ethics committee of the European Commission concerning new technologies, has exactly this role: to bridge the gap between science and society in issuing reports that explain new developments for the general public and in addition to that it recommends specific policies for the European Commission. The EGE is an inter-disciplinary body, consisting of scientists, lawyers and ethicists from the discipline of both philosophy and theology.[18] With respect to nanomedicine, the EGE issued an 'Opinion' in 2007, with the following recommendations:

> The EGE confirms that European Policies must be based upon the respect for dignity, human rights and recognition of European values, in accordance with Millennium Development Goals.

---

[17] Responsibility can be considered as a required attitude of an agent whose actions may have considerable effects on others. Accountability is the way this responsibility is considered (and morally judged) within a given social context. To be held 'accountable' means that *others* can address the obligations an agent has with respect to the effects of his/her actions on others. Liability is a legal term that translates responsibility and accountability into legal sanctions in the case of violation of rules.

[18] All opinions of the EGE can be found at http://ec.europa.eu/bepa/european-group-ethics/publications/opinions/index_en.htm.

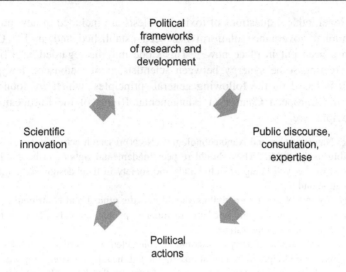

Figure 6.1 The science and society interaction.

With respect to safety, research on new models of risk assessment is needed, most urgently toxicity tests.

Risk assessment needs to be further emphasised and implemented at national and EU level, fostering cooperation between the different institutions, the EGE promotes prospective technology assessment that integrates societal developments.

As regards legal instrument no specific new regulations are called for, rather, the implementation needs to be enforced and overlaps be studied, patient consumer rights must be given highest priority.

Re-assessment of intellectual property rights and the international patent system is called for, the EGE recommends reform that re-establishes a proper integration between intellectual property rights and patients' right to access to health-related products or devices.

The EGE calls for the implementation of all medical–ethical principles in research on nanomedicine.

The EGE calls for European funding not only in accordance with the Framework Programme but also in accordance with Millennium Development Goals.

The EGE recommends that public participation and science and society dialogue be intensified, for example, as academic and public debates on problems and potential benefits of present and near-future nanomedicine. These debates should be designed as two-way communication, not just information for the public.

The EGE proposes interdisciplinary research on the ethical, legal, and social implications of nanomedicine.

The EGE proposes the establishment of a European Network on Nanotechnology Ethics. This should be aiming at the coordination and information exchange.

The EGE recommends research into the blurring and overlap of medical and non-medical use of nanotechnology, e.g. cosmetics and enhancement technologies.

In the case of nanomedicine, responses and follow-ups to the EGE Opinion are already in evidence. Here are a few examples of what has been achieved on the

European level: ethical questions of toxicology tests are included in new proposals; an international governance platform has been established and an EC Code of Conduct has been put in place now.[19] This Code may be regarded as a first step aimed at creating some synergy between scientists, policy advisers, lawyers and ethicists. It is based on the following general 'principles' which are founded and related to the European Charter of Fundamental Rights of the European Union. These principles are:

Meaning: Nanosciences and Nanotechnologies (N&N) research activities should be comprehensible to the public. They should respect fundamental rights and be conducted in the interest of the well-being of individuals and society in their design, implementation, dissemination and use.

Sustainability: N&N research activities should be safe, ethical and contribute to sustainable development. They should not harm or threaten people, animals, plants or the environment, at present or in the future.

Precaution: N&N research activities should be conducted in accordance with the precautionary principle, anticipating potential environmental, health and safety impacts of N&N outcomes and taking due precautions, proportional to the level of protection, while encouraging progress for the benefit of society and the environment.

Inclusiveness: Governance of N&N research activities should be guided by the principles of openness to all stakeholders, transparency and respect for the legitimate right of access to information. It should allow participation in the decision-making processes of all stakeholders involved in or concerned by N&N research activities.

Excellence: N&N research activities should meet the best scientific standards, including integrity of research and good laboratory practices.

Innovation: Governance of N&N research activities should encourage maximum creativity, flexibility and planning ability for innovation and growth.

Accountability: Researchers and research organisations should remain accountable for the social, environmental and human health impacts of their work.

While the example of nanoethics shows that ethics clearly plays an important role in the social and political debate, I will argue in the complementary chapter that a social–ethical methodology is needed to embrace the broader questions that the new technologies raise for and in societies.

Bibliography

Arayne MS, Sultana N. "Review: nanoparticles in drug delivery for the treatment of cancer". *Pak J Pharm Sci* 2006;19:258–68.

Council of Europe Convention for the Protection of Human Rights and Dignity of the Human Being with regard to the Application of Biology and Medicine; 1997.

European Commission. Recommendation of 07/02/2008 on a code of conduct for responsible nanosciences and nanotechnologies research; 2008.

---

[19] European Commission. Recommendation of 07/02/2008 on a code of conduct for responsible nanosciences and nanotechnologies research (2008) The complete text can be found at http://ec.europa.eu/nanotechnology/pdf/nanocode-rec_pe0894c_en.pdf.

European Group on Ethics in Science and New Technologies. *Opinion 21: Ethical Aspects of Nanomedicine*; 2007.

European Technology Platform. *Strategic Research Agenda*; 2006.

Faden RR, Beauchamp T. *A History and Theory of Informed Consent*. New York, NY: Oxford University Press; 1986.

Gordijn B. "Nanoethics: from Utopian dreams and apocalyptic nightmares towards a more balanced view". *Sci Eng Ethics* 2005;11:521–33.

Haker H. *Ethik der genetischen Frühdiagnostik. Sozialethische Reflexionen zur Verantwortung am menschlichen Lebensbeginn*. Paderborn: Mentis; 2002.

Haker H. "Selection through prenatal diagnosis and preimplantation diagnosis". In: Hildt E, Graumann S, editors. *Genetics in Human Reproduction*. Aldershot: Ashgate; 1999. p. 157–68.

International Risk Governance Council. *White Paper: Nanotechnology Risk Governance*; Renn O, Rocco M, Litten E. 2 June 2006.

Khushf G. "Systems theory and the ethics of human enhancement: a framework for NBIC convergence". *Ann N Y Acad Sci* 2004;1013:124–49.

Leary SP, Liu CY, Yu C, Appuzo MLJ. "Toward the emergence of nanoneurosurgery: Part II — Nanomedicine: Diagnostics and Imagining at the nanoscale level". *Neurosurgery* 2006;58:805–22.

Leary SP, Liu CY, Yu C, Appuzo MLJ. "Toward the emergence of nanoneurosurgery: Part III — Nanomedicine: Targeted nanotherapy, nanosurgery, and progress toward the realization of nanoneurosurgery". *Neurosurgery* 2006;58:1009–26.

Lewenstein BV. "What counts as a 'social and ethical issue' in nanotechnology?" *Hyle* 2005;11:5–18.

Maehle AH, Geyer-Kordesch. J. *Historical and Philosophical Perspectives on Biomedical Ethics: from Paternalism to Autonomy?* Ashgate: Aldershot; 2002.

O'Neill O. *Autonomy and Trust in Bioethics*. Cambridge: Cambridge University Press; 2002 [Gifford lectures 2001].

Robinson W. "Nano-Ethics". In: Baird D, Nordmann A, editors. *Discovering the Nanoscale*. Amsterdam: IOS Press; 2004. p. 285–300.

UNESCO. Universal Declaration on Bioethics and Human Rights; 2005.

7 International Agreements on the Prohibition of Human Cloning as a Test Case for Limits in Research

Sigrid Graumann

University of Applied Sciences, Bochum, Germany

Abstract

Research has become more and more internationalised, and the regulation of research has to do justice to this fact. This is one reason why there is an international discussion concerning biomedical research on the issue of cloning. This debate, however, has not resulted in producing binding international regulations, due to disagreement on the distinction between cloning for reproductive purposes and cloning for research purposes. At a European level, in theory, there is already a ban on cloning in the *Charter of Fundamental Rights* which prohibits cloning for reproduction purposes. It does not, however, prohibit cloning for research purposes. As a result, there are several European countries, such as the United Kingdom, where cloning for research purposes takes place. This recognition that cloning has two objectives, but is a single technology, also dominated the United Nations discussions whose goal was to develop a convention on cloning some years ago. These talks resulted only in a declaration but not in an internationally binding convention. The negotiations revealed one central problem: many delegations were focused more strongly on their national discussions and interests than on the need for international regulations.

The public debates concerning cloning are less polarised than one would assume. The main ethical arguments against embryonic stem cell and cloning research relate on the one hand to the protection of human embryos and to the protection of women's rights on the other. Women are in danger of being exploited in their capacity for reproduction because of the numbers of egg cells needed for cloning with the 'Dolly' method, particularly because these eggs can only be procured in a risky procedure. The objection to using human embryos for research shows the deep-reaching socio-cultural significance of protection for the vulnerable. It is shared by a variety of groups in society, by people with a religious world view and by explicit non-believers, by disability activists and by feminists critical of the commercialisation of human life. New possibilities for consensus could emerge if

Ethics for Graduate Researchers. DOI: http://dx.doi.org/10.1016/B978-0-12-416049-1.00007-6

the socio-cultural resonances underlying and joining both aspects – protection of embryos and of women – were to be explored.

Key Words

Reproductive cloning, research cloning, international regulation, UN declaration, egg cells, moral status of the embryo, risk to women's reproductive capacity, Korean stem cell lines

The Birth of Dolly and the Cloning Debate

Since the birth of Dolly, the cloned sheep, in 1996, it has become clear that it is also possible to clone human beings. Ever since the debate surrounding 'baby cloning', this question continues to rage and resurges each time a new attempt to clone is announced. Italian gynaecologist Severino Antinori, his US colleague Panayiotis Zavos and members of the Raël sect, through their company Clonaid, have succeeded in grabbing the headlines by announcing their intention to clone babies or even by announcing that they have already managed to do so. Reputable scientists such as Wilmut, the 'creator' of Dolly, have frequently condemned these endeavours as being 'inhumane' and 'criminal'. By contrast, many of the more reputable scientists are in favour of allowing cloned embryos to be used to produce embryonic stem cell lines to develop cell replacement therapies.[1]

This distinction between cloning for reproductive purposes and cloning for research purposes[2] has been influential in political and public debates. Normally, an embryo is created when an egg cell and a sperm cell fuse. In the case of cloning, the nucleus is removed from a somatic cell and transplanted into an egg cell from which the genetic material has previously been removed. The cell now containing the new diploid genetic material is capable of splitting in the laboratory. Once the cloned embryo is transferred to the uterus of a woman, it can develop into a child. This would be a very rare event. This child would then be the genetic twin of the human being from whom the nucleus of the cloned egg cell originated.

For the purpose of developing therapies, however, the cloned embryos are used to produce embryonic stem cell lines. The cloned embryos are left to develop for a few days in the laboratory until the time when the actual embryonic state forms inside a hollow ball of cells (blastocysts). These embryonic stem cells are then removed and cultured separately. Under the appropriate culturing conditions, it is theoretically possible to grow a variety of tissue such as muscle and nerve tissues from the cloned embryonic stem cells in the same way this is achieved using

---

[1] Wilmut, Ian, *After Dolly: The Uses and Misuses of Human Cloning* (New York: W.W. Norton, 2006)

[2] I have opted to use the terms 'cloning for research purposes' and 'cloning for reproduction purposes' instead of the established terms 'therapeutic cloning' and 'reproductive cloning' so as not to create the impression that the debate today is already focusing on developed therapeutic options. Cf. Mieth, Dietmar, *Die Diktatur der Gene. Biotechnik zwischen Machbarkeit und Menschenwürde* (Freiburg i. Br.: Herder, 2001)

'normal' embryonic stem cells. This is the research objective; however, it is not yet possible in practice. The estimated advantage compared with ordinary embryonic stem cells would be that the cloned embryonic cells would be genetically compatible with the patient's immune system. This is exactly the advantage of adult stem cells for which successful treatments have been generated for some time.[3]

However, the semantic distinction between two types of cloning, one for research, the other for reproduction, has obviously borne fruit. The first country to permit cloning for research purposes was the United Kingdom, and this practice has continued to prevail since August 2004. Other states have followed this example. Furthermore, this distinction also proved to have great impact on the political efforts for an international ban on cloning.

Efforts for an International Ban on Cloning

At a European level, the Charter of Fundamental Rights (European Parliament, Council and Commission of Europe 2000) in theory already contains a ban on cloning. The wording of the document was agreed by the European Parliament, the Council of Ministers and the European Commission. However, as the Charter had been incorporated into the draft Constitution for Europe, it did not have legal force until the ratification of the Treaty of Lisbon on 1 December 2009. The Charter prohibits cloning for reproduction purposes but does not prohibit cloning for research purposes. However, an additional protocol to the *Convention for the Protection of Human Rights and Dignity of the Human Being with regard to the Application of Biology and Medicine*, which the Council of Europe passed in 1998, states: 'Any intervention seeking to create a human being genetically identical to another human being, whether living or dead, is prohibited' (Council of Europe 1998, Section 1). Notwithstanding the prohibition however there are different interpretation in different member states about the point from which life needs to be protected – and thus the decision on the admissibility of cloning for research purposes – has been transferred to the responsibility of national legislation. This shows that the matter is rather complicated.

The fact that cloning has two objectives, but is one technology, has also dominated the UN talks on a cloning convention. In 2003, the German and French governments had elaborated a joint strategy paper. Based on the assumption that it would be almost impossible to convince all countries to implement a 'total ban' on cloning, a compromise strategy was developed. This strategy was to implement a ban on cloning for reproductive purposes and to oblige the signatory states to pass national regulations on cloning for research purposes. The Franco-German partners hoped to reach a consensus as a result. It was expected that states which had yet to pass any regulations would implement comprehensive bans due to the ensuing

---

[3] Adult stem cells are undifferentiated cells that reproduce daily to provide certain specialised cells in the body. Since they can be harvested from the patient, immunogenic rejections are averted. But this is not the only advantage of adult stem cells in my view. Most importantly, it does not raise the ethical problems that are connected with embryonic stem cell research and cloning.

debate in their own countries. Among other things, this strategy focused on those states that, whilst advocating a total ban at the United Nations, did not yet have any national regulations in place. This also includes the United States, which, under President George Bush, officially supported a total ban on the one hand, but on the other, tolerated extremely unregulated domestic research practices at the same time. Both from within and from without, the United States had been accused of pursuing a dual strategy in certain instances: that of resolutely calling for a total ban as a response to the demands made by influential Christian-conservative circles on the one hand, while, at the same time, catering for their equally influential corporate free-market friends by blocking an agreement based on consensus and thus avoiding pressure to have to pass national regulations. The example of the strategy taken by the US government also illustrates just how misleading the impression given by nationally uniform positions can be. Consequently, it can be presumed that in the majority of countries – at least in those states where an open discourse on cloning is taking place – this is a heated debate.

During the talks on the UN Cloning Convention, two 'blocs' formed, one led by Costa Rica and the other by Belgium. Costa Rica called for a ban both on cloning for research purposes and on cloning for reproduction purposes. Ultimately, this motion would have been backed by no less than 56 states, among them Spain, Italy and the United States. The German Foreign Office opted not to join this bloc, but stuck to the consensus strategy agreed with France.

To everyone's surprise, Belgium adopted the contents of the Franco-German paper in its formulation of a counter-motion. This motion sought to ban cloning for reproductive purposes but to allow cloning for research purposes to be decided by national regulations. This motion was to have been backed by Great Britain, China and 30 other states. In the end, however, the call for a vote was vetoed by Germany. The talks in the General Assembly were initially suspended for a period of 2 years in keeping with the proposal of a group of Islamic countries led by Iran, and the task of drafting a convention was transferred to a working group.

In November 2004, the UN negotiations aiming at an internationally binding convention against human cloning failed. Neither the supporters of a comprehensive ban, nor those in favour of a ban on reproductive cloning only, had been able to achieve the critical majority in the General Assembly of the United Nations. But what looked like the end of a convention against human cloning has not been the end of UN negotiations on that issue. The idea emerged to reach at least a UN declaration against human cloning. Italy, supporting a comprehensive ban on human cloning, took the lead and submitted the draft of a declaration the wording of which was 'pro-life' and divisive. In February 2005, the UN Legal Committee adopted by majority decision a declaration entitled 'United Nations Declaration on Human Cloning'. By this declaration, the United Nation calls on member states to adopt urgent legislation outlawing all cloning practices 'as they are incompatible with human dignity and the protection of human life'. The declaration seemed to mark the end of 3 years of a UN deadlock over human cloning. But this impression might turn out to be an illusion.

Countries were divided mainly over the question of whether to protect 'human life' or the 'human being'. Costa Rica, Uganda, the United States, Italy and others who sought to ban all forms of human cloning supported the term 'human life'. Countries including Belgium, Singapore and the United Kingdom, that wanted to only ban the type of cloning that would result in the birth of human beings, insisted on protecting the 'human being', which according to some international legal documents would protect only those already born.

The declaration also calls on countries to 'prevent the exploitation of women'. Cloning requires the harvesting of eggs from women, and delegates from developing countries feared the women of their countries might be regarded as inexpensive 'egg farms'. The declaration calls on wealthier nations to direct attention and funding to pressing medical issues such as HIV/AIDS, tuberculosis and malaria rather than being focused on the promotion of such technologies. It also condemns all applications of any genetic engineering techniques that threaten human dignity.

Though the resolution aimed at being inclusive, its 'pro-life' wording proved to be less than helpful. There are more countries that abstained from the resolution or rejected it than countries that voted in favour of it (71 in favour, 35 against, 43 abstentions). Thus, the resolution left the international community split and incapable of joint action. Remarkably, even countries with a relatively strict and comprehensive regulation of human cloning such as Canada voted against the submitted resolution because they simply did not want to join the 'pro-life' camp.

The negotiations of an international convention on cloning have highlighted a central problem, many delegations obviously focused more strongly on their national discussions and interests than on the need for international regulations. The political process, however, has not been terminated forever. We may soon be confronted with a new effort for a legally binding regulation. Therefore, it would be important to pay greater attention to the debates led within civil society and to assess the arguments made by the research side more critically.

Understanding the Arguments Made in Public Debate

The main ethical arguments against embryonic stem cell and cloning research in political and public debates refer to the protection of human embryos on the one hand and the protection of women's rights on the other. I shall first investigate the pro-life arguments and then the feminist arguments – defending both of them on the basis of their socio-cultural significance – in search of the possibility to prevent polarisation.

Violation of Human Dignity

At least in many countries with a Christian cultural background – but increasingly also in countries with an Islamic background – the question of whether human dignity and the rights derived from it should be applied to human life from conception onward is one of the crucial questions in the public debate on cloning research. However, it is remarkable that pro-life positions are not restricted to people who come from a religious world view. This is particularly true in the German debate. There are also many others, including explicit non-believers, disability activists and feminists who defend pro-life positions. The reason for this – as I interpret it – is that the question of the moral status of the human embryo has a deep-reaching socio-cultural significance. This specific sensitivity has been explicitly stated in the debate.

The question discussed in German public debate was not only whether human embryos have a right to live, but also whether the concept of human dignity should be applied to all human beings. Consequently, the major controversial issues are the general implications of the different ethical conceptions in that debate. Those who argue in favour of cloning for research express doubts that human dignity should or can be applied to early human embryos. In some ethical conceptions, the possession of interests is crucial for the attribution of human dignity and rights.[4] However, if the interest in living is tied to self-awareness, then on this basis embryos do not qualify for such rights. The crucial point here, however, is that following this reasoning, newborn babies or people with severe mental disabilities would also have to be denied human dignity and rights.[5] Consequently, the argument against this conceptualisation is that it would mean that no one could rely on their rights being respected because they could simply lose the capacities on which human dignity and human rights are based at any time.

Those who argue against cloning research usually refer to the Kantian concept of human dignity. The Kantian notion of human dignity, however, is also tied to certain criteria, namely to autonomy and thus moral capacity. But the crucial point here is that the characteristics that make up the moral capacity of the human being are inherent in human nature. They need not always be realised at all times in a person's life. Human development is characterised by identity and continuity from conception to death. Consequently, the embryo is not a different person from the individual who is subsequently born. Because of the potentiality of being a moral subject, human dignity is what characterises human beings as human beings. Human dignity is therefore not seen as something that can be acquired with time or lost again; it can neither be divided nor does it have different gradations.[6]

It is easy to see why this concept of human dignity is more attractive to many people, particularly to people with disabilities and their advocates.[7] With the tendency to relativise the protection of human dignity and human rights at the beginning and at the end of life and the increasing pressure of costs on the social and health care systems, adequate protection of human rights, particularly of the weaker and more vulnerable members of society, could become doubtful.[8] Further,

---

[4] Harris, John, *The Value of Life. An Introduction to Medical Ethics* (Routledge: London/New York, 1985) and Griffin, James, *On Human Rights* (Oxford: Oxford University Press, 2008).

[5] Cf. Kittay, Eva Feder, "At the Margins of Moral Personhood" *Ethics* 116 (2005) 100–131.

[6] Reiter, Johannes, "Die Probe aufs Humanum – Über die Ethik der Menschenwürde," in Graumann, Sigrid (ed.), *Die Gen-Kontroverse. Grundpositionen* (Freiburg i.Br.: Herder, 2001).

[7] Cf. Hubbard, Ruth, "Abortion and Disability," in Davis, Lennard J. (ed.), *The Disability Studies Reader* (New York: Routledge, 1997), 187–202.

[8] Cf. Schneider, Ingrid, "Embryonale Stammzellforschung – eine ethische und gesellschaftspolitische Kritik," in Graumann, Sigrid (ed.), *Die Gen-Kontroverse. Grundpositionen* (Freiburg i. Br.: Herder, 2001) 128–147.

recognition by society of the rights derived from human dignity requires social conditions in which the protection of these rights is institutionally anchored. It also requires a social climate which promotes moral attitudes of recognition of fundamental rights — including of those people not able to defend their own. If all this is true and if the ethical justification for cloning research implies the need to give up the inclusive Kantian concept of human dignity, it is not acceptable from a socio-cultural point of view.

In the ethical debate about cloning in particular, the main contentious issue is the question of whether the cloning of embryos violates human dignity as well. As the Dolly experiment has made apparent, cloned embryos have the potential, under the right conditions — i.e. in a woman's uterus — to develop into a child. From an ethical point of view, they would consequently have to be treated in the same way as 'normal' embryos.

At a conference on cloning organised by the former German Federal Minister for Research, Edelgard Bulman, in Berlin in May 2003, biologist Rudolf Jaenisch presented the view that cloned embryos should not be afforded the right to live because the majority of them were damaged and could not develop into 'normal' human beings anyway.[9] The answer to Jaenisch from a person in the audience who was quite indignant, was that, whilst it is true that cloning for reproduction purposes should be rejected on the grounds of the principle of non-impairment, it is not tenable to deny damaged embryos the right to live when it is granted to undamaged embryos. If we do so, we could also come to the point where we draw the same distinction between born human beings with or without impairment.[10]

In conclusion, I consider the arguments for defending the Kantian encompassing and non-exclusive concept of human dignity to be more convincing than the empirical understanding espoused, e.g. by John Harris, also in consideration of the socio-cultural implications of other positions for persons who do not fulfil the requirement for showing consciousness, agency or interests. This Kantian argumentation gives a moral status to the human embryo by virtue of his or her human origin with its inherent capability for morality.

Violation of the Rights of Women

A separate ethical argument is the concern for women's rights. Therapeutic cloning would demand a significant number of egg cells, which women would have to 'donate'.[11] We know that donated egg cells are already in short supply for other infertile women — in countries which do allow egg cell donation for IVF.

---

[9] Jaenisch, Rudolf, "Die Biologie des Kerntransfers und das Potential geklonter embryonaler Stammzellen: Implikationen für die Transplantationstherapie," in Honnefelder, Ludger and Lanzerath, Dirk (eds.), *Klonen in biomedizinischer Forschung und Reproduktion. Wissenschaftliche Aspekte — Ethische, rechtliche und gesellschaftliche Grenzen* (Bonn: Bonn University Press, 2003), 221–249.

[10] Cf. Hubbard, *Abortion and Disability*, 1997.

[11] Schneider, Ingrid, "Embryonale Stammzellforschung."

This means that incentive systems will have to be created to gain enough egg cells as 'raw material' for therapeutic cloning.[12]

We could observe such developments in the United Kingdom as well as in South Korea. In both the countries, it was very difficult from the beginning to acquire enough egg cells for research. This was due primarily to the British regulation that egg cell donation was not to be paid for. This was to prevent women from risking their health for reasons of money. Without payment, however, there are very few women willing to donate their egg cells. At first, the main possibility for the British researchers to receive fresh egg cells was to ask women undergoing IVF treatment to donate egg cells which were not used for their own treatment. This is the reason why, for example, in Newcastle, the cloning research group is working under the same roof with an IVF treatment unit. All IVF patients in Newcastle are regularly asked to donate their supernumerary egg cells for research. Nevertheless, British researchers still complain that they do not have access to enough 'high-quality' egg cells and so in the meantime, they have also now been allowed to use egg cells donated by women who went through the egg cell attainment procedure only for research.

It is evident that the South Korean cloning researcher Hwang Woo-Suk also had problems with the shortage of egg cells. In a 2004 *Science* paper, Hwang claimed to have created the first-ever cloned embryonic stem cell line, as well as to have grown 11 patient-specific stem cell lines. This was documented in a follow-up 2005 *Science* article. However, it later emerged that all the data had been faked (*Korea Times*, 4 January 2006). However Hwang's reputation was first tarnished by ethical allegations about the procurement of egg cells, both because of payments made for the donations – a practice not barred by Korean law at that time – and because it came to light that donations were also made by women on his research staff. Seventy-five women had been paid 1.5 million dollars. This amounts to 1500 dollars each for egg donation between 2002 and 2005. Altogether about 1600 eggs provided by 86 women had been used in his studies over 2 years (*JongAng Daily National* 4 January 2006). Hwang is also accused of having coerced a junior researcher of his to contribute eggs by using authorship as an incentive. The young researcher changed her mind at the last minute, but she found she could not break her promise due to the pressure from Hwang, something she later reported to the media (*Korea Times* 4 January 2006). In the media, the South Korean case is dealt with primarily in terms of 'a bad boy' issue. However, in my view, this is not sufficient. What Hwang has engaged in represents more than merely the failure of one irresponsible researcher. It points instead to a general problem of pressure to engage in innovative research under the conditions of increasing academic and economic

---

[12] Berg, Giselind, "Die Eizellspende – eine Chance für wen?," in Bockenheimer-Lucius, Gisela, Thorn, Petra and Wendehorst, Christine (eds.), *Umwege zum eigenen Kind. Ethische und rechtliche Herausforderungen an die Reproduktionsmedizin 30 Jahre nach Louise Brown* (Göttingen: Universitätsverlag Göttingen, 2008), 239–253.

competition. This is of course generally problematic, but in the particular case of cloning research it resulted in a violation of women's rights.

Unlike sperm donation, which harbours no risks whatsoever for the donor, harvesting egg cells is a complex and very invasive and risky procedure.[13] One 'concomitant symptom' of hormone therapy is hyperstimulation syndrome. It can cause accumulation of fluid in the abdomen or the formation of cysts on the ovaries. In its most severe form, hyperstimulation syndrome can have life-threatening effects. These adverse effects, from less to more severe, occur in 0.3−0.6% of women whose ovaries are being stimulated. If one assumes that 10 cycles of superovulation make it possible to gain 10 egg cells each and that those 100 egg cells would be sufficient to create 1 stem cell line, this would mean that to produce 100 stem cell lines, 3−6 women would suffer life-threatening complications. Under such conditions, I think, a potential therapeutic use of cloning would be irresponsible in general. Those who argue in favour of cloning research say that taking into account such risks is ethically justified once a woman has given her free and informed consent. It is doubtful, however, that women are willing to endanger their health voluntarily if they have been well informed and if they are free from social or economic pressure.

Some of those who argue in favour of cloning do not ignore this problem. They agree that to expose women to the risks of egg cells production and retrieval only for research purposes cannot be justified. They want to rule out egg cell trading as well as all forms of social and economic incentives for donation. But they would still argue that it would be ethically justified to use supernumerary egg cells from women who are undergoing IVF because of unwanted childlessness.

Apart from the fact that it is unlikely that it would be possible to gain enough egg cells for cloning research by using supernumerary eggs, I do not share the position that this would be morally unproblematic. In principle, as soon as third-party interests enter IVF practice, it is no longer guaranteed that the well-being of the woman will be the most important norm. Speaking more generally, due to the scarcity of available egg cells for research, the possibility cannot be ruled out that women will be forced by social pressure or financial incentives to provide 'surplus' egg cells or to donate egg cells for research purposes. The demand for egg cell donation may expand IVF in a way that interferes deeply with socio-cultural values and locks women into the role of reproductive suppliers. The use of third-party egg cells propagates the idea that claims can be made on someone else's body parts to treat health problems. This could intensify the ethically based pressure on women, in particular, to fulfil the desires of others.[14] I consider it to be extremely problematic to take advantage of the physical services of another person to fulfil third-party interests. The donor is exposed to a high medical risk for this purpose. Furthermore, the interests of third parties in reproductive medicine will result in increased disrespect for women's dignity and rights. To say it in the words used by persons from African and other developing countries during the negotiation process

---

[13] Berg, *Die Eizellspende.*
[14] Cf. Schneider, *Embryonale Stammzellforschung.*

of the UN convention, cloning research degrades women to the role of 'producers of raw material' for third parties.

Conclusions

Considering the above problems, which are — in my view — unavoidably linked to cloning, research with human clones is not ethically acceptable. As adult stem cell research seems to be an adequate alternative to develop new therapies, and has a track record of success, there is also an alternative way for research. Regarding the arguments used in the public debate treated earlier, I am convinced that it would be possible in principle to reach an ethical consensus — on the basis of human rights — on an international ban on cloning for any purpose. The precondition for this is, however, that a polarisation between pro-life and pro-choice positions is circumvented. In my view, the only reason why it has not been possible until now to adopt a legally binding international ban on all forms of cloning is that there are strong research interests which have considerable influence in national politics and these drive the competition between states to provide the presumed optimum conditions for their researchers.

Bibliography

Berg G. "Die Eizellspende — eine Chance für wen?" In: Bockenheimer-Lucius G, Thorn P, Wendehorst C, editors. *Umwege zum eigenen Kind. Ethische und rechtliche Herausforderungen an die Reproduktionsmedizin 30 Jahre nach Louise Brown.* Göttingen: Universitätsverlag Göttingen; 2008. p. 239–53.

Council of Europe. *Convention for the Protection of Human Rights and Dignity of the Human Being with regard to the Application of Biology and Medicine,* <http://conventions.coe.int/Treaty/en/Treaties/html/164.htm/>; 1997 [accessed 17.06.12].

Council of Europe. *Additional Protocol to the Convention for the Protection of Human Rights and Dignity of the Human Being with regard to the Application of Biology and Medicine, on the Prohibition of Cloning Human Beings,* <http://conventions.coe.int/Treaty/en/Treaties/html/168.htm/>; 1998 [accessed 17.06.12].

European Parliament, Council and Commission of Europe, *Charter of the Fundamental Rights of the European Union,* <http://www.europarl.europa.eu/charter/pdf/text_en.pdf/>; 2000 [accessed 17.06.12].

Griffin J. *On Human Rights.* Oxford: Oxford University Press; 2008.

Harris J. *The Value of Life. An Introduction to Medical Ethics.* London/New York, NY: Routledge; 1985.

Hubbard R. "Abortion and Disability". In: Davis LJ, editor. *The Disability Studies Reader.* New York, NY: Routledge; 1997. p. 187–202.

Jaenisch R. "Die Biologie des Kerntransfers und das Potential geklonter embryonaler Stammzellen: Implikationen für die Transplantationstherapie". In: Honnefelder L, Lanzerath D, editors. *Klonen in biomedizinischer Forschung und Reproduktion.*

Wissenschaftliche Aspekte − Ethische, rechtliche und gesellschaftliche Grenzen. Bonn: Bonn University Press; 2003. p. 221−49.

Kittay EF. "At the Margins of Moral Personhood". *Ethics* 2005;116:100−31.

Mieth D. *Die Diktatur der Gene. Biotechnik zwischen Machbarkeit und Menschenwürde.* Freiburg im Breisgau: Herder; 2001.

Reiter J. "Die Probe aufs Humanum − Über die Ethik der Menschenwürde". In: Graumann S, editor. *Die Gen-Kontroverse. Grundpositionen.* Freiburg im Breisgau: Herder; 2001.

Schneider I. "Embryonale Stammzellforschung − eine ethische und gesellschaftspolitische Kritik". In: Graumann S, editor. *Die Gen-Kontroverse. Grundpositionen.* Freiburg im Breisgau: Herder; 2001. p. 128−47.

Schneider I. "Gesellschaftliche Umgangsweisen mit Keimzellen: Regulation zwischen Gabe, Verkauf und Unveräußerlichkeit". In: Graumann S, Schneider I, editors. *Verkörperte Technik − entkörperte Frau. Biopolitik und Geschlecht.* Frankfurt am Main: Campus; 2003. p. 66−80.

United Nations General Assembly. *United Nations Declaration on Human Cloning,* <http://www.nrlc.org/UN/UN-GADeclarationHumanCloning.pdf/>; 2005 [accessed 17.06.12].

Wilmut I. *After Dolly: The Uses and Misuses of Human Cloning.* New York, NY: W.W. Norton; 2006.

Section 3

Contextualising Ethical Principles in Research Practice in Different Disciplines

Cathriona Russell

Department of Religions & Theology, University of Dublin, Trinity College, Dublin, Ireland

Abstract

Section 3 demonstrates the integrity and creativity with which experienced researchers embed ethical argumentation in their specific disciplines. It recommends a willingness to argue issues, an openness to critique and revision, and the competent and honest documentation of how ethics has been specified in practice.

Key Words

Childhood, dementia care, consent, assent, dissent, narrative ethics, medical humanities, disability, vulnerability, social inclusion and exclusion, personal safety, action research

Two significant and inter-related trends can be traced in the recent history of research ethics: first, a move away from a theory-driven approach in ethics to an emphasis on applied ethics and the contextualisation of principles in practice; and second, a shift in the conceptualisation of the research participant from passive recipient of a researcher's paternalistic objectives, to active agent and collaborator. These both reflect and institutionalise shifts in values towards a respect for the dignity and integrity of the human person not in the abstract but in their concrete lived experience. Ethics is not first and foremost prescriptive but better characterised as integrative, inter-disciplinary and interpretive. The chapters in this section show the integrity and creativity with which experienced researchers articulate and contextualise ethical argumentation in practice in their respective domains, in medicine, in archaeology and the social sciences and humanities.

Ethics for Graduate Researchers. DOI: http://dx.doi.org/10.1016/B978-0-12-416049-1.00032-5

The understanding of appropriate ethical protections for participants of biomedical research has not been static, it has evolved over time, and the evolution of research mirrors as well as institutionalises changes in social values and mandates.[1] Ezekiel Emanuel and Christine Grady outline the significant shifts in paradigms of research and research oversight in the history of research ethics since World War II. They trace the steady drift away from 'researcher paternalism' – where the research subject is understood as a passive participant in research which is directed at the general good and carried out by, it is assumed, a benevolent researcher – to a model in which the subject is an active participant in the enterprise, with some expectation that the process will benefit them or perhaps that cohort of the population to which they belong.[2]

Elizabeth Nixon, in her chapter 'Ethics of Oral Interviews with Children', reminds us of the changing conceptions of children and childhood in anthropology and in the social sciences and how these have influenced the way in which children are understood to be potentially active participants in research but also always require protection. Childhood has been reinterpreted as less an isolatable universal stage in life and more and more as the context of children's lives, a reality which children themselves construct. This understanding of children as agents in that reconstruction and in the determination of their own lives has been embraced by various academic disciplines concerned with understanding the lives and development of children. Children are seen as worthy of study in their own right as children and in relation to matters affecting their everyday lives and indeed can be positioned as 'experts in their own right' and not just in respect of what they will become as adults. Nixon navigates the difficulties of acknowledging that children have the capacity to understand some but not all of the issues required for consent – and so are capable of assent – but at the same time researchers have to integrate the child's right to protection from exploitation with the right to participation and to freedom of expression. As Sigrid Graumann points out in her chapter in the context of seeking the 'co-consent' of persons with intellectual disabilities later in this section, this recognition of the integrity and freedom to assent or dissent should not imply less protection for research subjects but rather a greater scope for their own, albeit assisted, decision-making.

The integration of ethical frameworks and the empirical approaches of the individual sciences, however, are not straightforward. For many researchers, becoming competent in ethical analysis already seems like a specialisation they cannot afford to indulge in as they find their feet in their primary chosen discipline. Ethics seems to require skills in philosophical, historical and sociological analyses that can seem peripheral to the task at hand and especially unrelated to research questions, for example, in the biophysical sciences, in theoretical physics or indeed the life cycle of the European eel. However, as Desmond O'Neill points out, there is a body of

---

[1] These developments have been accompanied by the growth and validation of qualitative research methods, particularly in the social sciences, emerging from under the shade of the dominant quantitative biomedical model – the randomised controlled trial.

[2] Emanuel, E. and Grady, C. "Four Paradigms of Clinical Research and Research Oversight," in *Cambridge Quarterly of Healthcare Ethics* 16 (2006) 82–96, 82.

literature in ethics from which to draw on in every profession, as well as evidence of best practice and failed initiatives from which we can learn. Ethical analysis can help researchers to make explicit the value judgements that they unconsciously accept or critique; and in that way they develop analytical skills that contribute to not just the critique of explicitly ethical questions but also the underlying philosophies at work in their own professional contexts.

O'Neill, in his chapter 'Consent, Assent and Dissent in Dementia Care and Research', frames his approach to ethics in terms of supporting informed decision-making for clinical care and research and proposes to integrate narrative approaches and the relatively new area of the medical humanities into his research and practice. Ironically, in speaking of narrative and the medical humanities, we too often seem to be getting away from the need 'to stick close to people's actual lives'.[3] However, in also considering fictions researchers are presented with 'puzzling cases', as Paul Ricoeur suggests, and with imagination, which is both 'structuring and destructuring'. Literature is enlightening because it is filled with 'slippery disappearing identities' and even with 'a long critique of the search for guarantees'.[4] In the narrative of the wounded Russian soldier, O'Neill observes that literature helps to articulate the experience of illness and incapacity and can in turn assist carers to recognise alternative routes to communication, for example, non-verbal expressions of consent or assent to treatment or research in dementia.

O'Neill also makes the crucial observation that is frequently overlooked, that competence in one's own professional discipline is itself an ethical issue. Here, competence refers to both technical abilities but also competence in articulation and communication as a key ethical requirement for professionalism in practice. This demands that those involved in clinical practice and research should engage in ongoing academic and professional development not only in ethics, but also in new developments in care, including collaborative systematic checks.[5] This combination of knowledge, skills and attitude is necessary, according to O'Neill, to provide the 'equipoise' to ensure that those with impaired capacity, in dementia care, for example, are not prevented from benefitting from the possible advances in the neurosciences but are at the same time protected from exposure to undue hazard.

Ethics is an interpretive process and researchers need to be able to recognise and evaluate different versions of key concepts invoked in biomedical ethics, in the humanities and the social sciences. This includes not only concepts such as dignity and vulnerability, autonomy and trust, but also identity and narrative in their orientation towards cultural and social belonging. For example, vulnerability can be an imposed category that individuals and groups may well resist.[6] In bringing the insights of hermeneutics to bear on bioethical questions, the objective is not to turn

---

[3] Ricoeur, P. "Pastoral Praxeology, Hermeneutics, and Identity," in *Figuring the Sacred* (Minneapolis, Fortress, 1995), 303–314, 311.

[4] Ricoeur, *Pastoral Praxeology*, 313.

[5] Cf. Gawande, A., "How do we heal Medicine?" on *Technology, Entertainment, Design Talks*. http://www.ted.com/talks/atul_gawande_how_do_we_heal_medicine.html.

[6] Graumann, S., "Disability and Moral Philosophy: Difference Should Count" in M. Düwell, C. Rehmann-Sutter and D. Mieth (eds.), *The Contingent Nature of Life* (Springer, 2010), 247–258.

interpretation into 'some sort of alternative to objective science', as Ricoeur warns.[7] Hermeneutics helps us to both recognise conflicting interpretations and to move beyond direct opposition to their underlying premises. The integration of the normative and the empirical is an ongoing task. We cannot simply offer 'stipulative definitions', but also need context-setting narrative to frame subsequent discussions.[8] New technologies have trajectories, pasts and futures. In the philosophy of technology, the concept of trajectory captures the way 'that important philosophical questions about technology cannot be framed when one is too narrowly focused on a specific set of tools and techniques'.[9] Indeed it is

> *only when one has grasped both the way in which a technology does indeed commit humanity to a given future, and also the way in which that future is open to a limited number of possible manifestations that one can truly grapple with technologically significant decisions in a democratic manner.*[10]

In her chapter, 'Research Without One's Own Consent', Sigrid Graumann uses a hermeneutics of comparison examining the 2006 *UN Convention on the Rights of Persons with Disabilities* in relation to previous documents. She reprises the history of development in international conventions beginning with the Nuremburg Code of 1946–1947, showing how the requirement for voluntary and informed consent, as the necessary condition for the permissibility of medical research, made research without consent an abuse of human rights. This was adopted subsequently, in 1964, at Helsinki by the World Medical Association.

Graumann detects a weakening of the explicit protection against the instrumentalisation of persons, in the interests of third parties, in the recent Council of Europe's document (1997) and the Seoul revision of the original WMA code (2008). These guidelines no longer tie the permissibility of research to the benefit of the individual research subject but extend it to a group, for example, of the same age, the same illness or condition to which these individuals belong. This move is not supported by the UN Convention which restates instead the protection given by the UN International Covenant on Civil and Political Rights in 1966. She asks, however, whether the UN Convention's move from designating persons with intellectual disabilities as being 'unable to consent' to enshrining their 'legal capability' and equal rights impacts negatively on their protection against being used in research that does not benefit them as individuals. It is a positive step to set out to grant greater scope for involvement in decision-making, albeit assisted. The Convention insists that this needs to be accompanied by the establishment of binding standards for what constitutes consent, rather than pressure, to come to this agreement with others. The practical outcome of this shift to the recognition of the capacities of those with cognitive disabilities as well as of their right to assistance will have to be seen.

[7] Ricoeur, *Figuring the Sacred*, 304.
[8] Thompson, P., "The Agricultural Ethics of Biofuels," in *Journal of Agricultural and Environmental Ethics* 21 (2008) 183–198, 185.
[9] Thompson, *The Agricultural Ethics*, 186.
[10] Thompson, *The Agricultural Ethics*, 188.

Sensitivities to the asymmetry in relationships of power and political framing of research results are not only crucial in the biosciences but also in the humanities. Deirdre Stritch in her chapter 'Contested Archaeologies: Archaeology in Politics and Identity Formation' shows how modern personal or social identities are affected by the way in which we look at, and interpret, the past, and can be either confirmed or denied by how that past is presented and understood. She illustrates how prevailing political and social norms can be implicit in the interpretation of knowledge in any and all disciplines which lay claim to a degree of objectivity and critical thinking. Stritch looked specifically at the historical background to heritage management and analyses the way in which broad ideological and economic agendas, as mechanisms of social inclusion or exclusion, have impacted on archaeological site conservation and site presentation in Israel and Cyprus. Stritch highlights the need to make epistemological and political prejudices explicit in research to safeguard objectivity and to recognise the value of social inclusion in the presentation and interpretation of archaeological remains.

In a different context, Gladys Ganiel in her chapter, 'Research Ethics in Divided and Violent Societies', develops her concept of 'ethical opportunity' as a guide to safeguarding those would-be researchers who are committed to 'making a difference' to peace and reconciliation after conflict. Ganiel introduces us to 'action' research – which owes a debt to feminist approaches – and which is assessed on its 'transformational validity', locating its worth in its ability to raise consciousness and provoke action to remedy the problems of oppressed peoples. She contrasts action research with the 'notionally value-free' tradition of 'positivist' research' in which the researcher stays out of the research, so as not to contaminate it. Action researchers are therefore not external but fully embedded in the worlds they are researching. Given that this is the case, Ganiel offers invaluable and innovative insights, from her own experience, not only for the management of expectations for a positive outcome to the research but also, crucially, for the safety of everyone involved. In pursuing their goals, Ganiel argues that action researchers need to plan for their own personal safety, plan for participants' personal safety, and plan how they will communicate and disseminate their results negotiating a complex of sensitivities after conflict. She also unapologetically provides a clear lesson for and critique of the formal requirement for signed consent forms. In the interests of safeguarding research participants in conflicted societies, she keeps no written record of participant consent and manages research results with similar objectives.

Charles Bosk has also highlighted the problem of uncritically transferring the need for consent forms in medical settings to other contexts. He points to the dilemma facing researchers in the social sciences whose qualitative research depends on a process of establishing a relationship with participants. They can feel hampered by the formal requirement for a signed consent form for observational research with formal interviews.[11] Ethics committees, Bosk notes, and even publishers, it has been suggested are, in contrast, bothered by their absence. It is true that the consent form provides an auditable trail that helps protect the human

---

[11] Bosk, C., "Bioethics, Raw and Cooked: Extraordinary Conflict and Everyday Practice," in *Journal of Health and Social Behavior* 51 (2010) 133–146, 141.

subject from harm, and insulates the institutions that support and oversee this research from future liability.[12] However, as Ganiel illustrates in her work, protecting vulnerable subjects overrides concerns for ethics governance where it is counterproductive and in danger of creating new vulnerabilities. Ironically, there are situations where the only guarantee of anonymity and confidentiality is in the absence of a signed consent form.[13] Rather than understanding research ethics as compliance with rules, including those taken over from another context, in domain-specific contextualisation researchers should thematise the concerns and argue for a context-adequate procedure. This should be clearly and honestly documented and researchers prepared to argue for their approach, be open to critique and revision and show how ethics have been specified in practice.

Bibliography

Bosk C. "Bioethics, Raw and Cooked: Extraordinary Conflict and Everyday Practice". *J Health Soc Behav* 2010;51:133–46.

Emanuel E, Grady C. "Four Paradigms of Clinical Research and Research Oversight". *Camb Q Healthc Ethics* 2006;16:82–96.

Gawande A. How do we heal Medicine? TED.com Talks. <http://www.ted.com/talks/atul_-gawande_how_do_we_heal_medicine.html/>.

Graumann S. "Disability and Moral Philosophy: Difference should count". In: Düwell M, Rehmann-Sutter C, Mieth D, editors. *The Contingent Nature of Life.* Springer; 2010. p. 247–58.

Ricoeur P. *"Pastoral Praxeology, Hermeneutics, and Identity". Figuring the Sacred.* Minneapolis: Fortress; 1995. p. 303–314.

Thompson P. "The Agricultural Ethics of Biofuels". *J Agric Environ Ethics* 2008;21:183–98.

Captions and links for PODCAST files for this section.

Deirdre Stritch

1. Beginning a PhD in archaeology: broad conceptual underpinnings.
2. Rationale for the choice of case studies.
3a. The 'archaeological' tour and modern cultural identity.
3b. Archaeology and tourism at Caesarea.
4. Ethics in the long-term management of archaeological remains.
5. Interpreting remains along nationalist lines.
6. Dealing with critiques.

Des O'Neill

1. Ethics and ageism in medicine.

---

[12] Bosk, *Bioethics*, 141.
[13] Ibid.

2. Competence as an ethical issue in dementia care.
3. An ethics of care, competence and communication.
4. Research with people with impaired capacity.
5. Assessing capacity: consent, proxy decision-making and assent.

Gladys Ganiel

1. Theoretical framework for social research ethics.

These can be found at http://booksite.elsevier.com/9780124160491

8 Consent, Assent and Dissent in Dementia Care and Research

Desmond O'Neill

Centre for Ageing, Neuroscience and the Humanities, Trinity College, Dublin, Ireland

Abstract

Supporting informed decision-making for clinical care and research for those with dementia and their families represents a subtle and rapidly changing topic of professional and academic debate. In particular, it demands that those engaged in such care and research, including those in the life sciences and advising research ethics committees, should engage in ongoing academic and professional development in not only ethics, but also in new developments in dementia care. These skills are critical to understand the various ways by which those with even quite severe dementia may express their wishes; the possibilities for enhancing participation through an ethics of care, communication and competence; and the nuances of co-decision-making with third parties. This combination of knowledge, skills and attitude is necessary to provide the necessary equipoise to ensure that those with dementia are not prevented from benefitting from the possible advances in the neurosciences, while at the same time protecting them from exposure to undue hazard.

Key Words

Ethics, consent, assent, decision-making, dementia, research, personhood

To be good is noble — to teach others to be good is nobler, and less trouble
Mark Twain

A summer blockbuster film may seem an unusual starting point for a discussion on the ethics of research with surrogates, but complex ideas are often best illustrated by metaphor, and artists often provide us with the most apt and relevant metaphors. In the 2011 film, *Rise of the Planet of the Apes*, we meet a biologist who breaks a range of ethical rules to provide his father with an experimental treatment for Alzheimer disease [1]. So many principles of ethical probity are broken (it is hard to know where to start — theft of the medication, using it on his father without

Ethics for Graduate Researchers. DOI: http://dx.doi.org/10.1016/B978-0-12-416049-1.00008-8

consent or appropriate testing, sequestering a laboratory animal due for destruction) that it might be possible to miss three wider and deeper messages.

The first is the ethical duplicity and corner-cutting by the bio-engineering firm, a concern consistent with increasing concerns about the might of the medical—industrial complex, akin to the concerns that Dwight Eisenhower raised about the undue influence of the military—industrial complex on US society. The second is the enormous potential for damage that the new sciences can wreak and the corresponding need for heightened ethical vigilance. Finally, the protagonist's lack of insight into his ethical illiteracy and naïveté is a reminder of how few scientists receive education in ethics as a core element of their basic or post-graduate education. Although some efforts have been made to remedy this in the United Kingdom [2], in many countries, including Ireland, this remains the exception rather than the rule: and I was struck by the absence of life scientists at the post-graduate module in ethics that I delivered for a national ethics programme for doctoral students. Those attending came from the social sciences and the humanities, and I had the strong sense that they already had a significant awareness of the ethical implications of their research and practice.

If You Design for the Old...

Although the issue of surrogate decision-/co-decision-making can arrive at any stage of life, it is most likely to happen in later life, given the increasing prevalence of illnesses that cause dementia (such as Alzheimer disease, vascular dementia or fronto-temporal dementia), and it is not surprising that the ethics of decision-making for those with impaired capacity is at the heart of the practice, research and education of geriatricians. This competence is a useful basis for developing perspectives relevant to all ages, as older people with cognitive impairment are more likely to suffer from multi-morbidity, sensory impairments (such as impaired vision and hearing) and harmful prejudices (such as ageism) which can impact on their participation in decision-making than are younger people. In addition, in terms of vulnerability, older people are also an important practical and theoretical field of experience. As the eminent geriatrician Bernard Isaacs wrote: if you design for the young, you exclude the old, but if you design for the old, you include the young.

Why Do We Need Ethics?

The lack of engagement by the life sciences with ethics in under- and post-graduate education points to the key challenge that while science students understand clearly that their knowledge of science is sufficiently under-informed to require serious education and study, they feel that they are already ethically formed and do not require significant development in this area. As aptly phrased by Rhodes [3], the first hurdle for professional schools' ethics education therefore is the establishment of its importance and its relevance. An aid to this is an embedding of ethics pro-grammes in the different subject matters of the course at strategic and relevant points so as to engage the students and alert them to the relevance and utility of ethics [4], and in addition, a policy of pairing ethicists and practitioners is likely to pay dividends [5].

The development of appropriate professional ethical standards and practice is a part of the societal contract between society and professional groups such as scien-tists and clinicians. In return for considerable discretion in scope and style of prac-tice in matters that potentially have a huge impact on the well-being of humans, the professions are expected to outline the standards by which its practitioners – geneticists, physicians, physicists or nanotechnologists – exercise that freedom in a responsible way so as to maintain the trust of society and its members. When lapses occur, the invariable societal response is to circumscribe the professional scope of practice by way of regulation, but regulation on its own is insufficient to maintain high standards of practice.

Indeed, one of the earliest commentators on the ethics of clinical research wrote – after outlining 22 instances of unethical experiments involving humans including infants and the mentally impaired – that regulation on its own was insuf-ficient to protect participants in clinical trials and that the presence of an intelli-gent, informed, conscientious, compassionate and responsible investigator offered the best protection for human research subjects [6]. Notwithstanding the develop-ment since then of increasingly widely accepted standards for Research Ethics Committees, the need for ethically sensitised and ethically competent clinicians and researchers remains as important as ever.

This is a challenge already in health sciences: health care ethics, although widely regarded as a pillar of professionalism, is often ill-served by the implemen-tation of adequate academic structures to support it: e.g. in a 2004 survey in the United States and Canada, one-fifth of schools provided no funding for ethics teaching and 52% did not fund curricular development in ethics [7]. In the United Kingdom, a similar survey showed an urgent need for full-time teachers (as most ethics teaching was still by part-time and voluntary staff); funding for books and journals, and additional teaching materials (including further case vignettes, hand-outs and sample exam questions) [8]. Worldwide this situation is paralleled, e.g. in France [9] and Sweden [10]. The situation for those involved in non-clinical life sciences research is almost certainly even more under-developed, and this volume of papers will hopefully act as a catalyst for debate on further development of ethics teaching in the life sciences.

Ethics and Law

One of the first starting points in approaching any issue in clinical and research ethics is to differentiate clearly between law and ethics. While a knowledge of the law is important, the law is anethical – e.g. it is not illegal for a psychiatrist to sleep with a patient, but it is considered to be highly unethical – and in certain jurisdictions, the law may routinely place practitioners in situations that test their professional ethics. Examples include mandatory reporting for driving for many illnesses in all Canadian provinces which raises significant ethical concerns [11] and similar concerns that mandatory reporting of elder abuse in all 50 US states is a counter-productive measure for some.

There are clearly important links between health law and ethics [12], and undergraduate and graduate education needs to be informed by medical jurisprudence, and medical jurisprudence courses have developed in advance of bioethics courses in many universities. Many societal debates on ethical issues are aired and decisions achieved through law, albeit in a setting in which discourse is constrained by legal protocols, and where often decisions may be antagonistic to professional and deeper ethical principles. However, law is a separate discipline, and special skills are needed to clarify the interface between the law, ethics and professional practice [13]. A final concern is the avoidance of 'legalism', whereby practitioners place an undue emphasis on the law [14].

So, a due balance between ethics and medical jurisprudence is needed, which will recognise not only the needs of students and practitioners to acquire and continually develop competence in each of these areas, but also equally important that each discipline has an academic presence of sufficient size for the maintenance of academic credibility, standing and focus of the discipline: 'orphan' middle-level academics embedded in other departments will not facilitate an optimal development of bioethics.

Virtuous Clinician/Researcher or Toolkit for Ethical Analysis?

The aim of teaching health care or life science ethics evokes two major points of view as identified in a major review of clinical ethics teaching – as to whether it is a means of creating virtuous physicians or of providing physicians with a skill set for analysing and resolving ethical dilemmas [15]. The pragmatic answer is that both aspects should be addressed [16]. A key to ensuring that ethical reasoning is incorporated into personal practice is to ensure that the curriculum is relevant to the present and future experience of the students (ideally by ensuring co-working between ethicists and attuned clinicians/scientists [5], and relating the teaching to issues that students encounter [17]) and that imbue a sense of moral agency at even the earliest stages of their career, as evidenced by an interesting paper on the imperative for physicians to speak out if they encounter unethical practice – the challenge of adding *primum non tacere* (first do not be silent) to the venerable Hippocratic principle of *primum non nocere* (first do no harm) [18].

Our own articulation of clinical ethics as encompassing the three aspects of care, communication and competence (both technical and ethical) [19] is an expression of how ethical practice is not just an exercise in moral reasoning but is deeply embedded in professionalism, care and reflective practice. Allying teaching methods to the techniques of narrative medicine can be of assistance. Charon's [20] model of the multiple narratives inherent in the physician–patient interaction is a helpful framework for personalising and reflecting on ethics and our role as clinicians and that the discourse between the patient and the doctor requires empathic engagement is obvious. Less apparent is that needed between the doctor and his/her peers; standards, audit, conscious and unconscious rationing requiring the development of due professionalism. The third discourse is that which the doctor has with him/herself beliefs, fears, prejudices, uncertainties and past experiences mandating reflective practice. Finally, there is the dialogue with society – stigma, rationing, ethics, support/lack of support – an awareness of which is critical to the development of trust. A superb example of combining the narrative approach and the imperative for incorporating ethics into personal practice is Gawande's *Complications* [21], the single 'must-read' text on our ethics module.

Capacity for Research

The developing interest in assessing capacity for decision-making in research among people who may be compromised due to vulnerability draws on an increasingly rich research literature. In part, this development relates to a maturing in our understanding of capacity and consent for medical procedures, and in part to a better understanding of the fact that much of the compromise in capacity may arise from a failure of health and social care professionals to adapt their practices to those who suffer from such compromise.

In addition to intellectual disability, there are many acquired diseases which cause impaired capacity, such as head injury, schizophrenia and stroke. Alzheimer disease and related diseases however are a useful trope for exploring the issues of research with those with impaired capacity. The illness is common, likely to affect about 1 in 10 of us between the age of 65 and the end of our life. Although many of those affected suffer from a mild form of the illness, in its middle and later stages it can cause significant distress to patients, and to an even greater extent to families, as well as an enormous cost to society. It is also an illness where there has been a considerable development in medical ethics [22], with an emphasis on preserved abilities and the challenge to clinicians of recognising and nurturing personhood in dementia [23].

One of the key challenges of the ethics of consent and participation in clinical research with those affected by congenital or acquired conditions that affect their intellectual abilities or alter their consciousness is to provide a due degree of protection of their human rights while not depriving them, and their very many fellow sufferers of illness, of the benefits of advances in medical and biological sciences. And advances there have been, including the development of the first generations of medications with (albeit modest) efficacy in Alzheimer disease, and a range of other therapies and diagnostic tests in the pipeline. In the train of these advances, there have also been some significant negative side effects in some research studies, particularly that of a serious brain condition, encephalitis, with the vaccine against the amyloid protein in Alzheimer disease [24].

A literal reading of the Nuremberg code of 1947, formulated following the excesses of wartime experimentation in Germany and Japan, would exclude the participation of all those with impaired capacity from these advances. In general, there has been a steady evolution in the thinking and practice of how to carry out clinical trials with those with impaired capacity. Indeed, one commentator has posited that it is not morally acceptable to prevent research with vulnerable participants, as these populations could become even more vulnerable and find themselves as 'therapeutic orphans'[25].

This inherent tension has developed further following the very major initiatives arising from systemic malpractice investigated by the Belmont report [26]. This report was prompted by the egregious cases of abuse such as those reported by Beecher in 1966, and in particular by the study allowing African Americans in Tuskegee to go untreated so as to study the course of syphilis infection, and the use of intellectually disabled children at Willowbrook in a similar manner to study the course of hepatitis.

Informed Consent in Research and Practice: A Subtle Concept

The Belmont report was in many ways a milestone in updating the application to research of the famous ruling in 1914 by Benjamin Cardozo in New York. This ruling is widely considered to have established the concept of informed consent. While simple in theory, the reality has always been somewhat more challenging, particularly in terms of the degree and extent to which patients could be, or wish to be informed, about the procedure that they were to undergo. In addition, it is clear that consent is a central part of the doctor−patient relationship, but in many cases it is implied rather than explicit. In general, the key factor deciding whether consent is explicit relates to the potential risk from the intervention [27]. Therefore, for a patient to take an aspirin is a relatively low-risk intervention, and explicit informed consent is usually not invoked. On the other hand, the amputation of the leg or removal of a kidney both have potentially significant side effects and also the likelihood of pain and suffering. It is clear that in terms of the social contract that the patient and doctor should have a discussion about risks and benefits for any procedure with appreciable risk, and this is a difficult area of practice to standardise as patients' perceptions and wishes in this can differ significantly [27].

Patients and their families require support and guidance in clinical medicine to arrive at a decision, and often at a moment where they face significant psychological challenges. The degree to which a patient wishes to acquaint him/herself with the full spectrum of risk arising from any intervention is hugely variable, and this is in evidence in the literature which suggests that it is exceptionally hard to obtain true informed consent in the purest sense of the word [28]. To a certain extent, consent is a negotiated concept, relying on the development of a relationship between the clinician and the patient, and to an understanding as to the degree of information and detail a patient wishes to know. In this, we are assisted by Pellegrino's [29] concept of the clinician assuming the role of a moderate autonomist and of a moderate welfarist. It is not simply a case of laying out facts, and of the patient making a rational choice: even in developments in the science of marketing we understand that such decisions are rarely made on a rational basis in the world of commerce, as evidenced by the Nobel Prize-winning research by the economist Kahneman [30].

The need for supported decision-making was beautifully outlined by the celebrated surgeon Ingelfinger [31] when speaking of his own major illness. One of the world's most distinguished oesophageal surgeons, in a twist of irony he developed cancer of the oesophagus and was alarmed by the extent to which those doctors to which he went laid out the facts in the manner of an intellectual debate, rather than in terms of his needs as a patient. 'I do not want to be in the position of a shopper at the Casbah... A physician who merely spreads an array of vendibles in front of his patient and then says "Go ahead, choose, it's your life" is guilty of shirking his duty...'

Vulnerability: From the General to the Particular

We can identify the concept of a 'universality of vulnerability', and that to a certain extent, vulnerability informs to a greater or lesser degree all discussions on consent. One of the major challenges for the clinician is to detect those who have a predictably increased degree of vulnerability that further challenges their ability to be a partner in this process of negotiation of consent. This is a difficult area of debate in the ethics literature, and in the research arena, it is compounded by a second form of generic vulnerability whereby not only is there potentially an increased risk, but in general with the adoption of placebo-controlled trials as the norm, a participant in a study may not have access to a therapy which proves to be effective and in doing so may be exposed to risk.

In addition, given that much of the research occurs at the cutting edge of therapeutic development, there is a strong likelihood that participants and their families will be less conversant with the medical and technological background of the proposed intervention than with the more standard therapies and interventions.

There is an interesting literature on vulnerability: some commentators deplore an over-generalised use of the term which could dilute its applicability, and useful contributions have been made in this regard in a paper by Silvers [32] contrasting personal vulnerability arising from conditions such as dementia, psychiatric illness or head injury against those forms of vulnerability which are due to political, social or economic circumstances that can make people also vulnerable to caution or deceit; she labels this a contingent vulnerability to exploitation.

Silvers introduces the useful concept of a historical criterion for this contingent vulnerability due to political, social or economic circumstances. By this, she introduces the notion that this vulnerability is historicized and relates to evidence of a past (and possibly ongoing) disregard for the well-being of the populations to which a patient might belong. In the context of a rapidly changing world, this vulnerability can also shift quickly; and it would then be unhelpful to limit access for these populations to the potential benefits of medical research. Nevertheless, the historical criterion imposes an extra obligation on researchers and ethics research committees to be sensitive to such contingent vulnerabilities in targeted populations. This, for example, would apply to populations who are sufficiently socioeconomic disadvantaged as to have low literacy skills, and where consent needs to be tailored accordingly. Kottow [33] refers to such vulnerabilities as susceptibility. A further helpful insight on the danger of a mis-emphasis on vulnerability is granted by Levine's [34] paper whereby negative outcomes for research subjects are shown to have arisen from flaws in study design or oversight although they had initially been misattributed to a 'vulnerability' of the patient group.

There has been wide-ranging debate on this form of contingent vulnerability in terms of research carried out in low- and middle-income countries and this is an area of ongoing concern in terms of globalisation, cost-saving and multi-centre trials. These concerns relate not only to the political, social and economic vulnerability of trial participants, but also to the universality and rigour of ethics research committees and their function in low- and middle-income countries [35].

The Ongoing Evolution of the Research Ethics Committee

In this respect, it is a sobering thought that research ethics committees, now generally an accepted part of the academic and research practice in the developed world, are a relatively new phenomenon, and one that is in continual evolution. In 1968, the World Health Organisation (WHO) convened a scientific group to develop principles for clinical evaluation of drugs. This laid the ground for a further working group in 1975, and the WHO's guidelines for Good Clinical Practice (GCP) [36] for trials on pharmaceutical products was produced in 1995. This process is an international ethical and scientific quality standard for designing, conducting, recording and reporting trials involving the participation of human beings. The GCP provides a range of benefits, including public assurance that the rights, safety and well-being of trial subjects are protected; consistency with the Declaration of Helsinki; and the production of credible data. However, it is noticeable that the body charged with ongoing development of GCP, the International Conference on Harmonisation of Technical Requirements for Registration of Pharmaceuticals for Human Use (http://www.ich.org) covers Europe, Japan and the United States only.

This historical perspective is important in terms of researchers understanding that the nature of research ethics committees is not fixed. There has been massive development in the process and discourse of research ethics committees over the last few decades. A signal change there has been the very clear shift from the use of the term 'subject' to 'participant' in general aiming to signify a partnership rather than a paternalistic relationship. In addition, the development of the principles of GCP have added significantly more rigour to the process of research ethics committee review.

Supporting Decision-Making Capacity

The development of more sophisticated thinking on the protection of vulnerable subjects coincides with an increased interest in how to maximise capacity in those with impaired capacity, facilitate expression of their personhood and support them in decision-making rather than make decisions for them.

The assessment of capacity for any significant therapeutic procedure or research should be expert, appropriately supported in terms of interdisciplinary support such as speech and language therapy and psychology, and facilitated in terms of promoting opportunities for enhancing capacity, e.g. by treating a previously undiagnosed depression, detected thorough preliminary assessment. The 'counsel of perfection' for research studies would be an independent capacity assessment, although this would be challenging in practice. Although some instruments have been proposed as supporting capacity assessments, none as yet has sufficient validity or reliability to take the place of an expert assessment.

Towards a Better Understanding of Life with Dementia

The development of the social model for disability in the 1960s was a potent factor for empowering those with intellectual disability by removing them from institutional care and allowing them to live in the community with support. This in turn has led to models of co-decision-making, most prominently in jurisdictions such as British Columbia and Saskatchewan [37]. Although these have not been as helpful as might have been expected with guardians who are not family members, the concept probably provides a good insight into the extent to which patients consult with family for co-decision-making in practice [38].

A possible difference between those with intellectual disability and those with progress of illnesses such as dementia is that the literature suggests that the capacity to increase understanding remains possible with intellectual disability, given the right environment and stimuli. This has been heretofore assumed not to be the case with dementia. However, the science and practice of dementia care changed radically arising from pioneering thinkers such as the late Kitwood. In his groundbreaking *Dementia Reconsidered*, Kitwood [39] presents a radical vision of ongoing personhood and vitality in those with dementia. He argues that the constraints of memory and language are exacerbated to a significant degree by the failure of those without dementia to adapt the ways of communication to those with dementia. This is a key issue in terms of both clinical care and research for people with dementia, as there is no doubt that adequate dementia-care training can imbue a sensitivity to the wishes and aspirations of those suffering from Alzheimer disease and related disorders.

Such dementia-care training can be augmented through the use of the medical humanities approach using film literature and music to give a vivid picture of the internal life of those affected by dementing illnesses. For example, Maurice Ravel composed both piano concertos and his 'Boléro' while suffering from fronto-temporal dementia [40], Terry Pratchett continues to write into the second decade of the twenty-first century while affected by a form of Alzheimer disease, and the great Dutch American abstract Expressionist Willem de Kooning painted great pictures while suffering from Alzheimer disease [41].

In addition, writers such as Mordechai Richler in his magisterial *Barney's Version* gives his deep insights into what it must be like to be suffering from Alzheimer disease in its early and middle stages [42], and Barbara Kingsolver in *Animal Dreams* portrays a family doctor with Alzheimer disease who continues to work. In cinematic terms, the movie portraying the Alzheimer disease of Margaret Thatcher, *The Iron Lady*, gives a sympathetic and always interesting portrait of the connections that motivates and drive the behaviour of those affected by this illness [43].

And even more vivid insight into what life must be like with dementia is provided by Luria's extraordinary *The Man with a Shattered World* [44]. In this true narrative of caring for a Russian soldier with a serious head wound that affected both his memory and language, we encounter a proxy for similar deficits in dementia and stroke [45]. In terms of insights relevant to capacity and research, there are two important aspects: the first is that Zasetsky, the Russian soldier, could not express himself in the 'standard' manner proposed by the doctors, learning to write by learning the letters one by one. Instead, it was only when left to his own devices in a facilitated way that he began to write, a prime example of the necessity of facilitating communication with those with impaired cognitive function. The second insight is of his vivid understanding of what is going on around him, which is in contrast with his relative inability to express emotions or thoughts in easy manner.

Similar insights come to us from the significant disability of stroke in Jean-Dominique Bauby's [46] *The Diving Bell and the Butterfly*, whereby a young man with locked-in syndrome from a stroke is only able to communicate by moving his eyelids. In many settings, one must worry that neither the skills, perception nor support of an appropriately trained speech and language therapist would be available to someone in his condition, and the richness of their interior lives would not be equally apparent.

From Literature to Real Life

In the clinical-care setting, this awareness of how the modes of communication for those with dementia is significantly altered is of increasing importance. For example, a person with late-stage dementia may no longer tolerate the mild discomfort of a nasogastric tube that most of us would accept in a state of better cognition as a minor evil to be tolerated in the context of a therapeutic good. To a properly trained clinical team, such an action would be appropriately interpreted as a gesture of not consenting from the point of view of the patient in his/her current state. This insight will prevent us from trying to restrain the patient or more securely fix a tube, and instead work on what options remain without further use of a nasogastric tube.

Equally, while many patients with advanced dementia or cerebrovascular disease have a disorder of their swallowing whereby fluid and food will go directly into their lungs (aspiration), they may no longer at this stage understand or be in agreement with strictures either not to drink or to drink thickened fluids or eat a modified diet. In the past, if such patients tried to drink from their neighbour patient's water jug or bottle of carbonated drink, staff may have made efforts to stop them. Hopefully, in an appropriately dementia-attuned setting, the staff will review this desire to drink while the patient is not aware of potential risk of aspiration as a patient choice for which the therapeutic response is to adapt as well as possible with the consequence of aspiration for the patient, family and staff in a palliative manner.

This form of enhanced understanding of non-verbal expressions of assent or dissent must continue to inform clinical and research activity with those with impaired capacity. A number of researchers have proposed that signs of distress or dissent should be monitored throughout any trial with those affected by dementia and that data collection and interventions should cease at this point [47].

However, in a condition where behavioural and psychological symptoms occur commonly, it can be difficult to be sure as to whether it truly is dissent, without an expert review. Ethicists such as Post [48] have argued that, in the context of exceptional circumstance where there is a very high potential benefit-to-risk ratio available only through the research study, it can be correct to proceed without the assent of the person with dementia.

This evolving discourse forms a valuable context for the deliberations of family or next of kin. In the clinical setting, if we reach a point at which we determine that the patient no longer has capacity, in the absence of a formal health care proxy, decisions are usually taken in consultation with family, next of kin or friends. In effect, what is being sought is usually a combination of a values history for the patient [49]; a review of whether the patient had spoken of their wishes should this particular combination of clinical circumstances arise; whether they had made either an advanced care plan or an advance directive; and a sense of the dynamics of co-decision-making between family members. This has been described as a relationship-based approach that integrates principles of personal equality, social justice and an ethic of caring [50].

In general, these factors are used to support a decision based on substituted judgement (an estimate of what is considered the patient would have wished in the circumstances) and best interests (what is considered in the clinician's opinion after consultation to be the standard medical practice in such cases, a mixture of beneficence and Utilitarianism in most instances). The Irish legal precedent has been helpful in this regard in establishing that the doctor should make a decision in consultation with the family and that should this prove not to be consensual, that a second opinion should be offered [22].

Third Party 'Consent' or 'Assent'?

For procedures and treatments that usually require written consent, the practice occurs in many countries whereby 'consent' is sought from next of kin or chief co-decision-maker in the absence of a legally defined health care proxy. In reality, this would be better described as 'assent' and represents recognition of the need for formal consultation with the patient's key co-decision-maker(s) and is generally a protection for the patient with impaired capacity and the clinician alike.

This principle of third party 'consent' or 'assent' is widely prevalent in recommendations for research with participants who do not have capacity for informed consent on their own. There is quite considerable variability in how this is exercised in the United States, with an endorsement by US federal regulations of informed consent by a legally authorised representative. However, many states do not provide clear policy guidance on this: There is considerable heterogeneity and little, if any, of the state law appears to directly address the issue. The law should trail ethical practice is not hugely surprising, but a failure to have adequate congruence can mean that research may be unduly restricted for important uncontroversial research, as outlined by Kim et al. [51].

Among the factors that are important, in terms of the protection required for the patient are the degree of intervention and risk, the likelihood of an invasive procedure such as a lumbar puncture, and the structure of the study in terms of monitoring risk. Federal regulations in the United States for children spell out risk in terms of four levels that give an indication of the sort of risk that might be considered by researchers and research ethics committees: (i) research that does not involve greater than minimal risk; (ii) research that involves greater than minimal risk but presents the prospect of direct benefit for the individual subjects; (iii) research that involves greater than minimal risk and no prospect of direct benefit to individual subjects but that is likely to yield generalisable knowledge about the subject disorder condition; and (iv) research otherwise not approvable (Code of Federal Regulations, Title 45, Section 46, Subpart D), with increasingly stringent risk—benefit analysis at each stage.

The discussion in relation to consent should take place with both participant with impaired capacity and the next of kin and it should be made clear to both of the role of the other. The congruence between patient's preferences and the surrogates may not be strong; however, in a major survey of 246 first-degree relatives of Alzheimer disease patients, the majority (almost 90%) stated that they would be happy for family members to consent for them if no advance directive existed. In addition, four-fifths would endorse a family member over-riding an advance directive if they considered the research to be potentially of benefit for themselves, should they develop a dementia [52].

A further protection for those with impaired capacity should be heightened vigilance by research ethics committees in ensuring that research involving human subjects, and particularly those with impaired capacity for consent, has been designed with the primary goal of social value. The research ethics committee should ensure independent review of protocols by an expert in the area if the committee does not already have such expertise among its membership. Randomised controlled trials should be included in the CONSORT database to facilitate scrutiny of results should the trial be unsuccessful, and the research ethics committee should have a low threshold for preventing studies that unnecessarily replicate previous studies, or are tailored to meeting regulatory approval without adding to informing clinical practice. Research ethics committees should also ensure that assessment and recruitment of subjects with impaired capacity is only undertaken in settings where there is sufficient expertise to provide an appropriate level of assessment, facilitation and support, as well as the ability to monitor continuing consent in the research study [53].

Summary

The undertaking of research with participants who have impaired capacity is a sophisticated and increasingly important area of activity for clinicians, basic researchers and research ethics committees. Each of these groupings needs to ensure that they keep abreast of the advances in the ethics literature that appropriate under- and post-graduate ethics training is a core part of the curricula of their profession, with due regard to the issues of care and research for those with dementia and other conditions that predispose to impaired capacity to consent for treatment and research. In this task, they will be aided by advances in the understanding of the personal experience of dementia and person-centred care in dementia, an emphasis on maximising residual capacity and an emphasis on care, communication and competence that will support the inclusion of those with impaired capacity in research studies that afford them due protection.

References

[1] O'Neill D. "Primates at the Pictures". *BMJ* 2011;343:d5486.
[2] Downie R, Clarkeburn H. "Approaches to the Teaching of Bioethics and Professional Ethics in Undergraduate Courses". *Biosci Educ E-Journal* 2005;5:c1.
[3] Rhodes R. "Two concepts of medical ethics and their implications for medical ethics education". *J Med Philos* 2002;27(4):493–508.
[4] Rhodes R, Cohen DS. "Understanding, being, and doing: medical ethics in medical education". *Camb Q Healthc Ethics* 2003;12(1):39–53.

[5] Russell C, O'Neill D. "Ethicists and clinicans: the case for collaboration in the teach-
     ing of medical ethics". *Ir Med J* 2006;99(1):25—7.
[6] Beecher HK. "Ethics and clinical research". *N Engl J Med* 1966;274(24):1354—60.
[7] Lehmann LS, Kasoff WS, Koch P, Federman DD. "A survey of medical ethics educa-
     tion at U.S. and Canadian medical schools". *Acad Med* 2004;79(7):682—9.
[8] Fulford KW, Yates A, Hope T. "Ethics and the GMC core curriculum: a survey of
     resources in UK medical schools". *J Med Ethics* 1997;23(2):82—7.
[9] De Saint Martin L, Tanguy-Latouche B, Pasquier E, Henry A, Baccino E. "[Teaching
     ethics in French medical schools: evolution or revolution?]". *Presse Med* 1998;27
     (20):968—70.
[10] Jacobsson L. "[The faculties should have units of medical ethics]". *Lakartidningen*
     1998;95(25):2964—6.
[11] McLachlan RS, Starreveld E, Lee MA. "Impact of mandatory physician reporting on
     accident risk in epilepsy". *Epilepsia* 2007;48(8):1500—5.
[12] Dickenson DL, Parker MJ. "The European Biomedical Ethics Practitioner Education
     Project: an experiential approach to philosophy and ethics in health care education".
     Med Health Care Philos 1999;2(3):231—7.
[13] Madden D. *Medicine, ethics and the law.* Dublin: Butterworths; 2002.
[14] Appelbaum PS. "Legalism, postmodernism, and the vicissitudes of teaching ethics".
     Acad Psychiatry 2004;28(3):164—7.
[15] Eckles RE, Meslin EM, Gaffney M, Helft PR. "Medical ethics education: where are
     we? Where should we be going? A review". *Acad Med* 2005;80(12):1143—52.
[16] Pellegrino ED, Thomasma DC. *The virtues in medical practice.* New York, NY:
     Oxford University Press; 1993.
[17] Kushner TK, Thomasma DC. *Ward ethics: dilemmas for medical students and doctors
     in training.* Cambridge: Cambridge University Press; 2001.
[18] Dwyer J. "Primum non tacere. An ethics of speaking up". *Hastings Cent Rep* 1994;24
     (1):13—8.
[19] Russell C, O'Neill D. "Developing an ethics of competence, care, and communica-
     tion". *Ir Med J* 2009;102(3):69—70.
[20] Charon R. "The patient—physician relationship. Narrative medicine: a model for empa-
     thy, reflection, profession, and trust". *JAMA* 2001;286(15):1897—902.
[21] Gawande A. *Complications: a surgeon's notes on an imperfect science.* London:
     Profile; 2003.
[22] O'Neill D. "Cogito ergo sum? — refocusing dementia ethics in a hypercognitive soci-
     ety". *Ir J Psychol Med* 1997;14(4):121—3.
[23] Post SG. *"The moral challenge of Alzheimer disease".* Baltimore, MD. Johns Hopkins
     University Press; 1995.
[24] Orgogozo JM, Gilman S, Dartigues JF, Laurent B, Puel M, Kirby LC, et al. "Subacute
     meningoencephalitis in a subset of patients with AD after Abeta42 immunization".
     Neurology 2003;61(1):46—54.
[25] Slaughter S, Cole D, Jennings E, Reimer MA. "Consent and assent to participate in
     research from people with dementia". *Nurs Ethics* 2007;14(1):27—40.
[26] National Commission for the Protection of Human Subjects of Biomedical and
     Behavioural Research. *The Belmont Report: Ethical Principles and Guidelines for the
     Protection of Human Subjects of Research.* Washington, DC: National Commission for
     the Protection of Human Subjects of Biomedical and Behavioural Research; 1978
     [Report No.: DHEW Publication No. (OS) 78-0012].

[27] Easton RB, Graber MA, Monnahan J, Hughes J. "Defining the scope of implied consent in the emergency department". *Am J Bioeth* 2007;7(12):35−8.

[28] Breitsameter C. "Medical decision-making and communication of risks: an ethical perspective". *J Med Ethics* 2010;36(6):349−52.

[29] Pellegrino ED, Thomasma DC. "The conflict between autonomy and beneficence in medical ethics: proposal for a resolution". *J Contemp Health Law Policy* 1987;3:23−46.

[30] Kahneman D. *Thinking, fast and slow.* 1st ed. New York, NY: Farrar, Straus and Giroux; 2011.

[31] Ingelfinger FJ. "Arrogance". *N Engl J Med* 1980;303(26):1507−11.

[32] Silvers A. "Historical vulnerability and special scrutiny: precautions against discrimination in medical research". *Am J Bioeth* 2004;4(3):56−7 [discussion W32].

[33] Kottow MH. "The vulnerable and the susceptible". *Bioethics* 2003;17(5-6):460−71.

[34] Levine C, Faden R, Grady C, Hammerschmidt D, Eckenwiler L, Sugarman J. "The limitations of 'vulnerability' as a protection for human research participants". *Am J Bioeth* 2004;4(3):44−9.

[35] Klitzman RL, Kleinert K, Rifai-Bashjawish H, Leu CS. "The reporting of IRB review in journal articles presenting HIV research conducted in the developing world". *Dev World Bioeth* 2011;11(3):161−9.

[36] World Health Organization. *Guidelines for good clinical practice (GCP) for trials on pharmaceutical products.* Geneva: World Health Organization; 1995 [Report No.: No. 850, 1995, Annex 3].

[37] Gordon RM. "The emergence of assisted (supported) decision-making in the Canadian law of adult guardianship and substitute decision-making". *Int J Law Psychiatry* 2000;23(1):61−77.

[38] Ho A. "Relational autonomy or undue pressure? Family's role in medical decision-making". *Scand J Caring Sci* 2008;22(1):128−35.

[39] Kitwood TM. *Dementia reconsidered: the person comes first.* Buckingham: Open University Press; 1997.

[40] Alonso RJ, Pascuzzi RM. "Ravel's neurological illness". *Semin Neurol* 1999;19(Suppl. 1):53−7.

[41] Espinel CH. "Memory and the creation of art: the syndrome, as in de Kooning, of 'creating in the midst of dementia'". *Front Neurol Neurosci* 2007;22:150−68.

[42] Canavan M, O'Neill D. "Barney's Version". *BMJ* 2010;341:c4561.

[43] O'Neill D. "How dementia tests Thatcher's mettle". *BMJ* 2012;344:e378.

[44] Luria AR. *The man with a shattered world; the history of a brain wound.* New York, NY: Basic Books; 1972.

[45] O'Neill D. "The man with a shattered world". *BMJ* 2010;340:c1315.

[46] Bauby J-D. *The diving bell and the butterfly.* 1st U.S. ed. New York, NY: A.A. Knopf: Distributed by Random House; 1997.

[47] Berghmans RL, ter Meulen RH. "Ethical issues in research with dementia patients". *Int J Geriatr Psychiatry* 1995;10(8):647−51.

[48] Post SG. "Full-spectrum proxy consent for research participation when persons with Alzheimer disease lose decisional capacities: research ethics and the common good". *Alzheimer Dis Assoc Disord* 2003;17(Suppl. 1):S3−11.

[49] Rich BA. "The values history: restoring narrative identity to long-term care". *J Ethics Law Aging* 1996;2(2):75−84.

[50] Dewing J. "From ritual to relationship: a person-centred approach to consent in qualitative research with older people who have dementia". *Dementia* 2002;1:157−71.

[51] Kim SY, Appelbaum PS, Jeste DV, Olin JT. "Proxy and surrogate consent in geriatric neuropsychiatric research: update and recommendations". *Am J Psychiatry* 2004;161 (5):797–806.

[52] Wendler D, Martinez RA, Fairclough D, Sunderland T, Emanuel E. "Views of potential subjects toward proposed regulations for clinical research with adults unable to consent". *Am J Psychiatry* 2002;159(4):585–91.

[53] Mueller MR, Instone S. "Beyond the informed consent procedure: continuing consent in human research". *Cien Saude Colet* 2008;13(2):381–9.

9 Research Without One's Own Consent? Consequences of the New United Nations Disability Rights Convention for Research

Sigrid Graumann

University of Applied Sciences, Bochum, Germany

Abstract

The new United Nations (UN) Convention on the Rights of Persons with Disabilities traces changes in international conventions that have become corner-stone documents in the protection of individuals from being used in research. Since the Nuremburg Code of 1946/47 and confirmed by the UN Covenant on Civil and Political Rights in 1966, research without consent had been judged internationally as an abuse of human rights. However, more recent documents such as the EU Convention on Human Rights and Biomedicine (1997) and the recent revision of the Declaration of Helsinki (2008) show considerable deregulation: according to these documents research is no longer restricted to the benefit of the individual but expanded to a group, for example, of the same age, the same illness or condition to which the individual belongs. Against these developments, the 2006 UN Convention restates the binding limit set by the UN Covenant on Civil and Political Rights. However, the point of normative reference has been changed. The 2006 UN Declaration has moved away from the concept of 'unable to consent' and states a right to the acknowledgement of 'legal capability' for all persons with disabilities. As a consequence, the way to protect persons from research in the interest of third parties should no longer consist in attesting to their inability to consent, but in establishing binding standards for how effective consent to an agreement with others may and may not be reached.

Key Words

UN Convention, disability, research without consent, legal capacity, Declaration of Helsinki, Nuremberg Code

Ethics for Graduate Researchers. DOI: http://dx.doi.org/10.1016/B978-0-12-416049-1.00009-X

In research, there is always the danger that persons with and on whom research is carried out will be harmed. This is especially problematic when research is not in the research persons' own interests, and when they belong to vulnerable groups such as prisoners, seriously ill patients, children or persons with disabilities. From an ethical and legal perspective, research with and on persons is only permissible when the free and informed consent has been given by the research subject. In the first international regulations of research, the conclusion was drawn that the inclusion of persons who had been testified as being 'unable to consent', such as children or persons with cognitive disabilities, had to be prohibited as a matter of principle. Yet, this prohibition has been increasingly softened as it constitutes a considerable obstacle to medical research.

The new United Nations (UN) Convention on the Rights of Persons with Disabilities (UN-RPD, the Convention) has created a new situation. To classify a person as 'unable to consent' means denying his/her legal capability for action. Yet, this contradicts Article 12 of the Convention, which states that 'persons with disabilities enjoy legal capacity on an equal basis with others in all aspects of life'. This is why the question arises as to whether the special regulations of protection for persons with cognitive disabilities have to be given up? In my view, this is not the case; on the contrary, the UN Convention protects members of vulnerable groups in an encompassing and effective way from being instrumentalised through research. The key for this interpretation is that Article 15 UN-RPD consciously takes over the exact wording from Article 7 of the International Covenant on Civil and Political Rights (1966) (Civil Covenant); according to it, scientific or medical experimentation on a person is permissible only under the condition that he/she has given his/her informed and voluntary consent to it.

The Controversial Prohibition of Research in the Interest of Third Parties with Persons 'Unable to Consent'

The existing ethical and legally codified norms for protecting the rights of patients and of research subjects originated on the historical backdrop of human rights violations in medical research that cost many of those affected their health and their lives. This historical experience — in particular the cruel human experimentation that was carried out in German concentration camps — has profoundly shaken the trust in the moral integrity of physicians and researchers.[1] Universally valid ethical and legally codified norms that would protect research subjects from instrumentalisation and abuse have turned out to be indispensable. Since the Nuremburg trials against physicians, the protection of research subjects in scientific experimentation has been based primarily on the concept of voluntary and informed consent.

[1] Katz, Jay: "Menschenopfer und Menschenversuche. Nachdenken in Nürnberg." In: *Medizin und Gewissen. 50 Jahre nach dem Nürnberger Ärzteprozeß — Kongressdokumentation.* Frankfurt am Main: Mabuse-Verlag 1998, 233.

The Nuremburg Code, as is well known, was written by the American Military Tribunals that conducted the Nuremberg trials against physicians in 1946–1947.[2] With it, the action of doctors was measured by internationally recognised standards of human rights. For the first time and in the most prominent place, i.e. as the first point of the Code, the voluntary and informed consent of the experimental subject was established as a necessary condition for the permissibility of medical trials. Since then, research on and with human beings that was conducted without voluntary and informed consent has been considered internationally to be an abuse of human rights.

The concept of voluntary and informed consent acquires a double function in the regulation of research with and on human subjects: it consists, on the one hand, in the protection of the experimental person's right to self-determination as such, and on the other, in putting him/her into a position of him/herself being able to claim and realise respect for his/her rights. Thus, voluntary and informed consent constitutes the linchpin in the protection against potential instrumentalisation in the interest of third parties.

It took 17 years after the Nuremburg doctors' trials for the World Medical Association to bring itself to follow suit by establishing comparable standards for the protection of vulnerable groups in research in the Declaration of Helsinki. At the eighteenth meeting of the World Medical Association that took place in 1964 in Helsinki, ethical guidelines for medical research on humans were finally adopted. In it, the concept of voluntary and informed consent acquires a central role among the 'Basic Principles' of the Helsinki Declaration. It states:

In any research on human beings, each potential subject must be adequately informed of the aims, methods, anticipated benefits and potential hazards of the study and the discomfort it may entail. He or she should be informed that he or she is at liberty to abstain from participation at any time. The physician should then obtain the subject's freely given informed consent, preferably in writing.

The Helsinki Declaration is certainly the document most cited in ethical discussions about research on and with human beings. As to the question how legally binding it is, however, the corresponding regulation in the Civil Covenant is more significant because it is binding in international law. The Universal Declaration of Human Rights (1948) does not yet contain any specific regulation for the protection of experimental subjects in research. Article 5 only states: 'No one shall be subjected to torture or to cruel, inhuman or degrading treatment or punishment'. In the Civil Covenant, this sentence is supplemented with the following addition in Article 7: 'In particular, no one shall be subjected without his free consent to medical or scientific experimentation'. This means that – corresponding to the Nuremberg Code – with only one sentence any research with and on human beings without their voluntary consent has been prohibited as a matter of principle.

---

[2] Mitscherlich, Alexander/Mielke, Fred (2001): *Medizin ohne Menschlichkeit. Dokumente des Nürnberger Ärzteprozesses.* Stuttgart: Fischer-Verlag (15th ed.).

When considering the protection of members of vulnerable groups, it is important to note that the voluntary nature of consent can be questionable for two different reasons: due to the capabilities for self-determination of the person him/herself
who is to be included into a research project (1), or due to his/her living situation
which can reduce his/her possibility for self-determination (2).

1. Reduced Capacity for Self-Determination: Not all people are in the position to estimate
adequately the consequences of participation in research for their physical and psychological integrity (at least not on their own). Children and adolescents can only do so in the
course of their development, many seriously ill people have lost the capability for it tem-
porarily and some people with cognitive impairment are not able to do so on a permanent
basis. To safeguard the protection of their rights in research, it was considered sufficient
up until recently to take recourse to the concept of 'proxy consent'. In it, the authorisation
of a proxy to consent to a research project is closely tied to the welfare of the experimental person. Proxy consent, however, can constitute an open door for possibly relinquishing
the rights of those affected. In giving proxy consent, one is obliged to decide on the basis
of the presumed consent of the person who has been testified to be 'unable to consent'.
The measure for this that has gained international recognition is that proxy consent has to
be directed towards the best interests of the person represented.[3] In this context, the distinction between research in one's own interest and in the interest of third parties is essential. In relation to participating in a research project, it can only be presumed that only
his/her own physical welfare is in the best interest of the person represented, not, however, a contribution to scientific progress. Proxy consent can thus only be given to
research which are to the own benefit from the perspective of the person represented. In a
more extensive view, clinical research is 'also to one's own benefit', when diagnostic,
preventive and therapeutic measures in the framework of scientific studies serve the treatment of the patient.[4] Research is considered to be 'purely to the benefit of third parties'
when it pursues exclusively scientific questions from which the individual experimental
person derives no benefit.[5] Research that is purely to the benefit of third parties carried
out on persons whose 'inability to consent' has been attested therefore is impermissible in
the view of all three of the named documents: the Nuremberg Code, the Helsinki
Declaration and the Civil Covenant.

2. Reduced Capability for Self-Determination: When persons live in situations in which
their freedom is severely restricted and in which they are exposed to particular conditions
of dependency, they are especially in danger of being instrumentalised in research.
Inmates of prisons belong to these groups, as do persons who live in institutions or
homes. In the discussion leading up to the adoption of the Helsinki Declaration, the question was asked whether truly voluntary consent for participating in a research project
could be expected from persons who live under such conditions. It was pointed out that
the consent of persons in particular situations of dependency could be easily manipulated;
they could be hoping for better treatment or fearing disadvantages or even sanctions if

---

[3] Kopelman, Loretta (1997): "The Best-Interests Standard as Threshold, Ideal, and Standard of
Reasonableness," in *The Journal of Medicine and Philosophy* 22, 271–289.
[4] Hirsch, G. (1995), "Heilversuch und medizinisches Experiment: Begriffe, medizinische und rechtliche
Grundsatzfragen." In: Kleinsorge, H./Hirsch, G./Weissauer, W. (Hg.), *Forschung am Menschen*,
Springer, Berlin, Heidelberg 1995, S. 13–17.
[5] Eser, Albin/von Lutterotti, Markus/Sporken, Paul (1989), *Lexikon Medizin, Ethik, Recht*. Herder,
Freiburg 1989, 170 ff. and 487 ff.

they refused to consent. This is why the permissibility of research in the interest of third parties under such conditions was fundamentally put into question.[6] A general prohibition, however, of research in the interest of third parties with 'dependent persons', comparable to the international regulation of such research with persons 'unable to consent' could not gain acceptance. Yet, the aspect of manipulation or influence on decision by dependencies is always virulent in medical research. I will return to this at the end of this chapter.

Trends Towards Liberalisation and the Invention of 'Benefit to a Group'

The formulation of requirements for the permissibility of medical research on and with persons has always been controversial when they collide with research interests. This can be shown with great evidence in the ongoing development of the Helsinki Declaration. Originally in 1964, it said: 'The subject of clinical research should be in such a mental, physical, and legal state as to be able to exercise fully his power of choice'. In relation to persons unable to consent, the most recent revised version adopted in 2008 in Seoul contains a new regulation: 'These individuals must not be included in a research study that has no likelihood of benefit for them unless it is intended to promote the health of the population represented by the potential subject, the research cannot instead be performed with competent persons, and the research entails only minimal risk and minimal burden'. Thus, the controversial concept of 'benefit to a group', which since the adoption of the European Convention on Human Rights and Biomedicine, has been taken over into more and more national and international documents has also entered the Helsinki Declaration.[7]

In the Convention of the Council of Europe of 1997, Article 17 regulates the 'protection of persons not able to consent to research'. Their participation in research projects is deemed permissible when a benefit is expected for 'the person concerned or to other persons in the same age category or afflicted with the same disease or disorder or having the same condition' and when 'the research entails only minimal risk and minimal burden for the individual concerned'. Especially in Germany, this regulation was taken as a relativisation of the protection of persons unable to consent in medical research and led to hefty political debates. Disability organisations and the churches have spoken vehemently against softening up the prohibition against research with persons labelled 'unable to consent'.[8]

---

[6] Graebsch, Christine: "Medizinische Versuche mit Gefangenen und anderen Unfreiwilligen."

[7] Eser, Albin (1999): *Biomedizin und Menschenrechte. Die Menschenrechtskonvention des Europarates zur Biomedizin – Dokumentation und Kommentar*, Verlag Josef Knecht Frankfurt a. M. 1999.

[8] Klinnert, Lars (2009): *Der Streit um die europäische Bioethik-Konvention. Zur kirchlichen und gesellschaftlichen Auseinandersetzung um eine menschenwürdige Biomedizin.* Edition Ruprecht Göttingen.

A Change of Presuppositions Through the UN Convention on Persons with Disabilities

As mentioned at the beginning of this chapter, the UN Convention chose in Article 15 the identical formulation of Article 7 of the Civil Covenant for the regulation of research. According to it, the permissibility of scientific and medical experiments on humans is, as a matter of principle, tied to their voluntary consent. This may be considered to be surprising. It will hardly have escaped the attention of the negotiating parties that the concept of 'benefit to the group' has increasingly become accepted in international and national regulations for research. It thus has to be assumed that the negotiators have consciously opted for a return to the original position in international law and thus for confirming the prohibition of proxy consent to research projects that are purely for the benefit of third parties or of groups.

In addition, as distinct from the Council of Europe's Convention on Biomedicine and from the Bioethics Declaration of the UNESCO, the UN Convention abstains from using the term 'unable to consent'. According to Article 12 of the Convention, it would be problematic in terms of human rights to attest to a person or to a group of persons their 'inability to consent'. It presupposes instead their 'legal capacity' independently of the type or degree of their disability. Moreover, it is important to note that the binding character of the UN Convention as an international treaty is higher than that of other agreements, such as those of the Council of Europe including all the European and national regulations that build on it, or indeed of the revised Helsinki Declaration of the World Medical Association.

Article 12 of the Convention, 'equal recognition before the law' belongs to those regulations that were discussed at length and controversially in the Ad hoc Committee in which the text of the treaty was worked out. A consensus was reached that all persons with disabilities have to be recognised as bearers of equal rights and that equal access to support has to be safeguarded for people with disabilities. This constitutes a turn away from the principle of proxy consent towards a paradigm of assisted decision-making.

Article 12 acquires a key role for those who represent the concerns of people with cognitive or psycho-social impairments. It is true that worldwide still 'many people with disabilities are being restricted in the exercise of their rights by being made a ward of court being put under legal guardianship or tutelage, by restrictions for consent and by using legal categories such as "contractual incapacity" or "restricted contractual capacity."'[9] The negotiators shared the will to end such conditions and to realise 'equality before the law' without exception for all people with disabilities throughout the world. This intention is reflected in Article 12, paragraph 1 which states: 'States Parties reaffirm that persons with disabilities have the right to recognition everywhere as persons before the law'. With Article 12,

---

[9] Lachwitz, Klaus (2008): "Übereinkommen der Vereinigten Nationen über die Rechte von Menschen mit Behinderung," 145.

paragraph 2, the positive definition is added that they have full *legal capacity* to be exercised on the same basis with others: 'persons with disabilities enjoy legal capacity on an equal basis with others in all aspects of life'. What this does not imply, however, is that people with cognitive or psycho-social impairments can do without assistance in the exercise of their rights. However, the concrete implementation of this claim was not uncontroversial in the Ad hoc Committee that drafted the text of the Convention. Some members rejected the provision of legal representation fundamentally as amounting to disenfranchisement and as tutelage, whereas others wanted to ensure through appropriate regulations that representatives could not abuse their power. The rejection of the model of legal representation finally prevailed in the negotiations. The originally intended term, 'personal representative' no longer appears in the final version of the Convention. Article 12, paragraph 3 states instead: 'States Parties shall take appropriate measures to provide access by persons with disabilities to the support they may require in exercising their legal capacity'.

The question this raises is how a person who is allegedly unable to consent can reach the ability to consent through support. It follows from the cited regulation that, in the future, care and guardianship regulations have to be replaced by regulations oriented towards the concept of legal assistance and keep the full legal capacity of persons with disabilities untouched. Concretely, the regulations adopted make provision that measures of such legal assistance have to respect the will and the preferences of the person affected, have to be free of conflicts of interest and tailored to the concrete conditions, be used for the shortest time possible and be strictly monitored.

Also under debate is whether regulations that restrict consent in national legislation are compatible with Article 2, paragraph 2 of the Convention.[10] This could ultimately mean that persons with cognitive impairment cannot be generally assumed not to be able to consent to participating in research projects. Proxy decisions foreseen by international documents to regulate research with and on children and on persons and with persons with cognitive impairment thus would have to be critically examined and may have to be replaced by 'co-consent' regulations.

Assistance Instead of Representation

If the same rights are to be guaranteed to all people with disabilities, as the UN Convention demands, it follows that no one can be denied legal capacity in principle. The crucial question then is whether it is necessary to also give up specific regulations of protection against instrumentalisation, as for example in the context of research.

The insight that a separate UN Convention is needed for persons with disability arises from the experience that respect for formally equal rights is not sufficient for

---

[10] Lachwitz, Klaus (2008), "Übereinkommen der Vereinigten Nationen über die Rechte von Menschen mit Behinderung," 147, refers to the German Code of Civil Law, § 1903 Bundesgesetzbuch (BGB).

them to be able to use these rights equally. Despite this the Convention consistently supports an orientation of human rights towards freedom and develops them in a new perspective of the ethics of human rights that I would designate as 'assisted freedom'. This means that no new human rights are created for people with disabilities but that the universal human rights are concretised and specified in view of the particular dangers to which they are exposed. The Convention achieves this on the one hand by strengthening human rights – civic and political as well as the economic, social and cultural rights – as freedom rights; on the other, it formulates human rights not primarily and exclusively as negative rights of protection, but connects them with the duties of the state to offer support of social services and benefits. The concept of 'assisted freedom' that is new in the complexity in which the UN Convention develops can be justified in the perspective of a human rights ethics.[11]

If we want to maintain freedom and equality as universal norms, we also have to safeguard that they are valid for all human beings with and without disabilities. From here, a binding claim to assistance in relation to individual needs and life situations can be justified. Representation by proxy is to be replaced by assistance. These roles differ in that the assistant does not decide *for* the person, keeping him/her in tutelage, but grants the assistance he/she needs to decide responsibly him/herself, confirming this by giving 'co-consent' as an assistant. For consenting to participating in a research project this means that it is not decided by the proxy, but by the person him/herself in his/her own personal capacity, which may happen with the support and confirmation of the assistant. It follows that ultimately such research cannot take place if the affected person's own consent cannot be obtained, even with assistance.

Yet, a normative re-orientation of this kind may lead not only to restrictions for research but also to dangers for the persons who can consent aided by assistance. It might be the case that they could be persuaded, pressurised or forced to consent although they cannot estimate the consequences of their participation due to internal or external conditions, or due to personal dependencies and fears of rejection if they refuse.

Effective consent, however, is based on the general condition that the consenting person can judge the essence, significance and extent of his/her decision and can make it free of pressure and coercion.

This is exactly what the new concept of protection of members of vulnerable groups from instrumentalisation through research is based on. The starting point is to renounce attesting an 'inability to consent' to particular persons, to protect them from research for the benefit of third parties and to establish standards for effective consent instead. Because the point of reference is not a judgement on the capabilities of the person in question but a judgement on the quality of the agreement he/she makes with others, discrimination can be excluded. What is decisive is that binding standards for effective consent to the participation in a research project are

---

[11] Cf. S. Graumann, *Assistierte Freiheit. Von einer Behindertenpolitik der Wohltätigkeit zu einer Politik der Menschenrechte* (Frankfurt a.M.: Campus, 2011).

formulated. These specify in particular, on the basis of evidence and confirmed by 'co-consent,' first, that consent was given by the person him/herself; second, that she understood the essence, significance and extent of his/her decision; and third, consent was given free of pressure and coercion. Assistance can serve to help the person to give effective consent according to these criteria. Only if these conditions are met, can consent be legally valid. This regulation also would have the advantage that by attesting an 'inability to consent' no blank cheque for proxy decisions against the will of the person is given. The responsibility for having received effective consent remains on the side of the researchers as well as the risk that subsequently may not be able to prove in a way that is generally convincing.

But what does this mean in practical terms? Regarding research for the benefit of third parties and for the recent new category, the benefit of so-called groups, this regulation effectively seems to establish the highest possible measure of protection of experimental subjects, albeit at the price of restricting research. For persons with strong cognitive impairment, this largely corresponds to the original prohibition of research for the benefit of third parties with persons 'unable to consent'. Some persons, however, with less pronounced cognitive impairment who up to now counted as 'unable to consent' might be able to be included in research if on the basis of good assistance the demanding conditions for effective consent can be fulfilled. A 'small window' that was closed in previous UN documents might here be opened for research. In addition, experimental subjects who are restricted in their possibility of self-determination due to dependencies are to be much better protected against instrumentalisation through research. Only if it can be guaranteed that their consent is really free of any direct or indirect constraint, can they be included in research.

Bibliography

Eser A, von Lutterotti M, Sporken P. *Lexikon Medizin, Ethik, Recht*. Freiburg: Herder; 1989, 170 ff and 487 ff.

Eser A. *Biomedizin und Menschenrechte. Die Menschenrechtskonvention des Europarates zur Biomedizin — Dokumentation und Kommentare*. Frankfurt am Main: Verlag Josef Knecht; 1999.

Council Europe. "Covenant on Human Rights and Biomedicine." In: Honnefelder L, Streffer C, editors. *Jahrbuch für Wissenschaft und Ethik*, Bd. 2, Berlin; 1997. p. 285–303.

Graebsch C. "Medizinische Versuche mit Gefangenen und anderen Unfreiwilligen. Anmerkungen für eine kontextorientierte Ethikdebatte und einige Fragen aus kriminologischer Sicht". In: Joerden JC, Neumann JN, editors. *Medizinethik 3 Ethics and Scientific Theory of Medicine*. Peter Lang; 2002. p. 153–200.

Hirsch G. "Heilversuch und medizinisches Experiment: Begriffe, medizinische und rechtliche Grundsatzfragen". In: Kleinsorge H, Hirsch G, Weissauer W, editors. *Forschung am Menschen*, 1995. Berlin, Heidelberg: Springer; 1995. p. 13–7.

Katz J. *"Menschenopfer und Menschenversuche. Nachdenken in Nürnberg"*. Medizin und Gewissen. *50 Jahre nach dem Nürnberger Ärzteprozeß — Kongressdokumentation*. Frankfurt am Main: Mabuse-Verlag; 1998, 233.

Klinnert L. *Der Streit um die europäische Bioethik-Konvention. Zur kirchlichen und gesellschaftlichen Auseinandersetzung um eine menschenwürdige Biomedizin.* Edition Ruprecht Göttingen; 2009.

Kopelman L. "The Best-Interests Standard as Threshold, Ideal, and Standard of Reasonableness". *J Med Philos* 1997;22:271–89.

Lachwitz K. "Übereinkommen der Vereinigten Nationen über die Rechte von Menschen mit Behinderung. Auswirkungen auf die Rechte von Menschen mit geistiger Behinderung und/oder psychosozialen Problemen". *BtPrax* 2008;4:143–8.

Lederer SE. "Research without borders: The origins of the Declaration of Helsinki". In: Roelke V, Maio G, editors. *Twentieth Century Ethics of Human Subjects Research. Historical Perspectives on Values, Practices, and Regulations.* Wiesbaden: Franz Steiner Verlag; 2004. p. 199–217.

Mitscherlich A, Mielke F. *"Medizin ohne Menschlichkeit". Dokumente des Nürnberger Ärzteprozesses.* 15th ed. Stuttgart: Fischer-Verlag; 2001.

UNESCO. Universal Declaration on Bioethics and Human Rights; 2005.

United Nations. Universal Declaration of Human Rights; 1948.

United Nations. International Covenant on Civil and Political Rights; 1966.

United Nations. Convention on the Rights of Persons with Disabilities; 2006.

World Medical Association. Declaration of Helsinki. Ethical Principles for Medical Research Involving Human Subjects. Revised Versions of 1964; 1996; 2002; 2008.

10 Contested Archaeologies: Archaeology in Politics and Identity Formation

Deirdre Stritch

National Qualifications Authority of Ireland

Abstract

The subject of ethics and the role of the archaeologist have attracted increasing amounts of attention in recent years not least in relation to nationalism and its impact on archaeological practice and interpretation. It is now widely accepted that modern personal or social identities are affected by the way in which we look at, and interpret, the past, and can be either confirmed or denied by how that past is presented and understood. Those who control and represent the past are in a powerful political and social position. Thus archaeologists, as professionals, must not separate knowledge from the context in which it is produced; archaeological narratives are not immune to contemporary political and economic idioms.

Key Words

Archaeology, politics, identity formation, ethics

The subject of ethics and the role of the archaeologist have attracted increasing amounts of attention in recent years, not least in relation to nationalism and its impact on archaeological practice and interpretation. It is now widely accepted that modern personal or social identities are affected by the way in which we look at, and interpret, the past, and can be either confirmed or denied by how that past is presented and understood. Those who control and represent the past are in a powerful political and social position.[1] Thus archaeologists, as professionals, must not separate knowledge from the context in which it is produced; archaeological narratives are not immune to contemporary political and economic idioms.[2]

---

[1] Bond, G.C. and Gilliam, A. eds. *Social Construction of the Past: Representation as Power* (London; Routledge, 1994), 1.

[2] Whitelam, K. *The Invention of Ancient Israel: the Silencing of Palestinian History* (London; Routledge, 1996), 26.

Ethics for Graduate Researchers. DOI: http://dx.doi.org/10.1016/B978-0-12-416049-1.00010-6

The broader research underpinning this chapter[3] examined the factors determining archaeological practice and archaeological heritage management in the Republic of Cdyprus and in Israel. It looked specifically at the historical background to heritage management and at the relevant infrastructural and policy environment in each country. While policy and practice in this area are constantly evolving, the broad ideological and economic agendas driving and constraining policy were analysed and evaluated in terms of their impact on archaeological site conservation, site presentation and with regard to their role as a mechanism of social inclusion or exclusion.

My research placed the development of the discipline of archaeology in Israel and Cyprus in historical, cultural and intellectual contexts. Nationalism and archaeology made a simultaneous appearance in the Eastern Mediterranean at the end of the nineteenth and beginning of the twentieth centuries.[4] Archaeology had entered this arena as a tool, first of colonialist and later of nationalist policy. Archaeology, through its concern with time, culture and identity has proved invaluable in a region thought to host the roots of Western civilisation and religion. Later in the new states of Israel and the Republic of Cyprus, the birth pangs of nationalism necessitated the presentation (both internally and externally) of a historic, homogenous identity rooted in the land. Through time, this nationalist agenda has been enlarged to incorporate economic concerns related to the development of cultural heritage tourism.

Archaeology (and images derived from it) therefore not only informs us about the rise of Western civilisation, but those same images are the symbols of modern nations and peoples. In economic terms, these symbols are valuable commodities in an international tourism market. My research studied the impact of these factors on the practice and interpretation of archaeology in Israel and the Republic of Cyprus today, and the consequences for minority cultures not represented by nationalistically inspired, archaeologically derived symbols. In this chapter, I will present my research first by outlining my rationale in selecting Israel and the Republic of Cyprus as case studies and my analysis of the relationship between archaeology, ethnic identity and nationalism. Second, I will focus on two sites in particular in Israel, describing my fieldwork and methodology. The two archaeological sites, Jerusalem Archaeological Park and Caesarea, are representative of the way in which ideological and economic agendas drive and constrain heritage management practice, and their public presentation is analysed and evaluated in terms of its impact on archaeological site conservation and with regard to its role as a mechanism of social inclusion or exclusion. Finally, the ethics of practice in relation to such contested archaeologies is explored.

---

[3] This research is based on my PhD thesis entitled *Archaeology and the State: An Examination of Archaeological Practice and Official Interpretation of Archaeological Remains in Israel and the Republic of Cyprus* (2007). The fieldwork which informed this research was conducted in 2005. Alterations to the archaeological sites referenced in this article may have taken place since that time.
[4] Mouliou, M. "Ancient Greece, its Classical Heritage and the Modern Greeks, Aspects of Nationalism in Museum Exhibitions." in: Atkinson, J. Banks, I. and J. O'Sullivan, eds. *Nationalism and Archaeology/Scottish Archaeological Forum* (Glasgow; Cruithne Press, 1996) 174–175.

Israel and the Republic of Cyprus as Case Studies

Israel and the Republic of Cyprus were chosen for this study on the basis of their close geographic proximity and because they share a number of common elements in their respective pasts and present. The archaeological heritage of each place testifies to the numerous invasions and conquests endured by both. In the modern period, power was transferred from first Ottoman to British to finally Israeli and Cypriot self-rule. The archaeological infrastructure of both countries is indebted to this Ottoman and particularly British colonial past; the result being highly centralised heritage management systems centred on government antiquities departments or authorities. Since independence, the archaeological profession and academia in these two countries have been both driven and constrained by similar factors, ranging from questions of ethnogenesis to the problems caused by rapid development and urbanisation. Both countries faced enormous external and internal pressure on their territorial and ethnic integrity from the time of their formation. This resulted in an intense need or desire to confirm the Jewish or Greek character of each and professional archaeologists played a significant role, either consciously or unconsciously, in this quest. Furthermore, in both countries, tourism forms a crucial element of the local economy and the archaeological heritage of each country has been commandeered as an essential component in this industry.[5]

This close relationship between archaeology and the state has a number of consequences; archaeology has contributed to national identity and, conversely, selectivity in the practice of archaeology and heritage management has contributed to social exclusion. For example, as will be demonstrated in the studies later in this chapter, in the case of Israel, the presentation of many archaeological sites encompasses multiple topographies of memory and identity, from the shaping and articulating of official Israeli identity, to the confirmation of the visitors' Jewish or Christian identity. By contrast, the Arab and/or Islamic past and present of the country is, at best, downplayed and at worst, silenced or demonised. Israel's archaeological heritage, as presented to the public, therefore functions as a mechanism of social and historical exclusion; for the way in which a heritage item, site or place is managed, interpreted and understood has a direct impact on how those people associated with that heritage are themselves understood and perceived. The particular form in which nationalism was manifested in the countries in question was largely determined by the specific colonial environment already in place. It was also at this time that Westerners, with varying concerns and interests, brought the emergent discipline of archaeology to bear on the remains of Cyprus and Palestine. The flourishing of foreign travel in the Renaissance period profoundly affected the development of archaeological research. Scholars were exposed to the remains of

---

[5] Stritch, Deirdre, *Archaeology and the State: An Examination of Archaeological Practice and Official Interpretation of Archaeological Remains in Israel and the Republic of Cyprus.* Unpublished PhD thesis, Trinity College Dublin (2007).

classical antiquity, thus broadening the parameters of classical study to include art and architecture.[6] In the same vein, increased travel on the part of Westerners to Cyprus and Palestine from the late eighteenth century onwards contributed significantly to the development of the discipline of archaeology in those countries. Travellers brought words and artefacts home that inspired explorers, antiquarians and treasure hunters to seek out the physical remains of the past. As the fully fledged discipline of archaeology emerged news of exciting discoveries in their turn increased travel to the countries in question. The accounts left by early travel writers are significant for the insight they provide into the intellectual and cultural milieu in which early archaeological activity took place. Attitudes to native Cypriots and Palestinians and the perceived inferior nature of the modern culture to antique culture, as detailed in these accounts, are reflected in archaeological interpretation, and set the agenda for future national interpretative trends.[7] These trends, in turn, either confirmed or attempted to refute the original colonial narratives. The parameters thus set ensured that breaking the interpretational mould would prove difficult.

Nationalism and Archaeology

The modern nation-state, since the nineteenth century, has sought to bind groups of people together in a geographically and culturally defined political unit in which ethnic identity is synonymous with national identity.[8] To nurture a sense of unity within, and loyalty to, the state, the notion of the cultural distinctiveness and homogeneity of the group is fostered.[9] Frequently, this cultural particularity is linked to, or indeed presented as the direct result of, the relationship between a people and their physical environment. In this way, the land, the people and the nation-state are tied firmly together in an organic entity born of 'nature' and as such above and beyond question or reproach. The fact that nationalism in its ideological development equated modern state political legitimacy with group cultural antiquity means that these characteristics of distinctiveness and homogeneity must be projected onto the past of the people and place, and as a result has a profound effect on the way that an archaeology embedded within state structures operates.

---

[6] Acklom, G., *A Forgotten Era in Archaeology: The Research Conducted by Early British Travellers in Palestine from c. 1670 to 1825*. Unpublished PhD, Department of Classics and Archaeology, University of Melbourne, 1995, 34.

[7] Cf. Brassey, Mrs. *Sunshine and Storm in the East or Cruises to Cyprus and Constantinople* (New York, Henry Holt and Company, 1880) and Haggard, H.R. *A Winter Pilgrimage, Being an Account of Travels through Palestine, Italy, and the Island of Cyprus, Accomplished in the Year 1900* (London; Longmans, Green and Co., 1901).

[8] There have been a number of recent studies which examine the relationship between nationalism and archaeology, and nationalism's use of the past. Chief amongst them are Kohl and Fawcett (1995), Diaz-Andreu and Champion (1996), Atkinson, Banks, et al. (1996) and Graves-Brown, Jones, et al. (1996).

[9] Cf. Graham et al. (2000), Gellner (1987) and Mouliou (1996).

The collective memory of the group is stimulated through symbols and commemorative events such as flags, national anthems and memorial days aimed at enhancing a sense of community. Collective memory, however, is not entirely fluid and adaptable as it is constrained to some degree by the actual historical past, i.e. the past can be 'selectively exploited' for ideological purposes but not entirely constructed.[10] Thus, Benedict Andersen's 'imagined community' of the nation can only be imagined because some real commonalities already existed; it is rarely, if ever, invented from scratch, as 'imagined' implies.

The key issue here is the transference of values, such as territoriality, nationality and continuity, from the nation-state to archaeology through the mechanisms of their shared institutional bodies and as expressed in antiquities laws.[11] Archaeology as a discipline could conceivably question the material evidence for the state's values of continuity and territoriality but is unlikely to do so when operating within state institutions;[12] to question the prior existence of such values is to question the legitimacy of the state itself.

These values are of such importance because, frequently, the international acceptance of the territorial and political integrity of a state is strengthened with the common acceptance of the ethnic or cultural unity of the group, traceable temporally in a given geographical territory. As a result, archaeology, history and the past in general are invested with special significance by the state as the tools which can best provide the necessary evidence of homogeneity and continuity in culture and identity through time. Archaeology and the past are thus ideally placed for the provision and shaping of the narratives and symbols which will henceforth identify and represent the nation-state.[13] Group collective memory and sense of community is then 'activated and articulated' by and through these narratives and symbols.[14]

This archaeological underpinning of ideological national narratives characterises in particular the relationship between the nation-state and the archaeology in the early days of the state, or in states where continued pressure on territorial borders from outside powers demands strong internal unity and solidarity. It has been my argument that in states that are well established and lack such urgency for internal cohesion, these ideological functions are often superseded, or at least matched on another level by financial imperatives with an equally potent impact on local archaeology. In this situation, archaeology, and archaeological heritage, now managed by state-controlled agencies, becomes central to the economic prosperity of the state by virtue of the important role played by the 'heritage industry' in modern tourism.[15] For many

[10] Zerubavel, Y. *Recovered Roots, Collective Memory and the Making of Israeli National Tradition* (Chicago; University of Chicago Press, 1995), 5.

[11] Firth. A, "Ghosts in the Machine." in: Cooper, M. A., Firth, A., Carman, J., and D. Wheatley, eds. *Managing Archaeology* (London; Routledge, 1995) 51–67.

[12] Ibid, 52.

[13] Knapp, B. and S. Antoniadou "Archaeology, Politics and the Cultural Heritage of Cyprus." in: Meskell, L. ed. *Archaeology Under Fire: Nationalism, Politics and Heritage in the Eastern Mediterranean and Middle East* (London; Routledge, 1998), 13–43, 14.

[14] Liakos, A. "The Construction of National Time: the Making of the Modern Greek Historical Imagination." *Mediterranean Historical Review* 16:1 (2001) 27–42, 28.

[15] Urry, J. *The Tourist Gaze: Leisure and Travel in Contemporary Societies* (London; Sage Publications, 1990).

nations, both developing and developed, economic solvency is as immediate a concern as internal unity (often positively affected by economic buoyancy) or the need to prove the legitimacy of territorial and political claims. Thus, simultaneous use is made of both the ideological and economic benefits of archaeology. Tourism provides the heritage industry, and thus the state, with a sizable domestic as well as international audience, while archaeology provides an effective means of transmitting ideologically generated, authoritative narratives to that audience through its provision of powerful and evocative symbols of national identity.

As noted, for many countries, especially those in the developing world, tourism plays a vital role in economic prosperity and in raising the international profile of the host country in both political and economic terms. This is a potentially crucial benefit for smaller, weaker countries which may otherwise lack such a voice. Within this context, whereby countries must compete for the attention of a frequently fickle tourism market, the development of a unique 'signature' which is easily marketed and memorable is essential. As highlighted in the discussion on nationalism, the archaeological heritage of a region is viewed as one of the key expressions of the unique individuality and personality of that region, which, in a market driven by the quest for an experience of the novel, yet authentic and the exotic, is a key selling point. This heritage is thus perfectly suited as a tool in the fashioning of a concise and attractive 'national signature'. The natural attractions of the country in question, in terms of landscape, scenery and so on may be incorporated into this signature, thereby presenting both nature and culture as the naturally occurring, inherent twin pillars linking people and place.

These, then, are the ideological and infrastructural factors, which have determined the shape of archaeological practice and management in Israel and the Republic of Cyprus. Despite many similarities in the history, structure and problems faced by archaeology in the two places, differences also exist in the ways that both countries address these issues and challenges. I will turn now to give an overview of how these particular factors have played out in Israel and to the kinds of ethical questions posed by this analysis for archaeological professionals working in this area.

Archaeology in Israel: Jerusalem Archaeological Park and Caesarea

The modern Israeli nation-state shares much in common with the nearby island of Cyprus, from pre-history to the present day. Similar groups have occupied both territories over centuries and in the modern period Ottoman rule was replaced by first British, and later, self-rule. Israel differs, however, in that the modern Israeli state is one based predominantly on *aliyah* — the return to Israel of Jews from the Diaspora. The contested nature of the territory between Israelis and Palestinians, and the need to create tangible links to the land for Israel's new citizens, means that the country's past, particularly those elements which pertain to previous Jewish presence in the land, becomes vitally important. The question of ethnogenesis, as in Cyprus, assumes the role of a forceful principle in archaeological investigation. Yet, as in Cyprus, this quest is not informed simply by national needs, but by the methodological and cognitive frameworks previously established in the colonial period.

As noted earlier, modern concerns and interests, particularly those of a political nature, frequently set the agenda for, and influence the results of, historical research. The discipline of archaeology is enmeshed, at both an intellectual and an institutional level, with the most potent political force in our age, nationalism. Archaeology, as a discipline and as an activity, operates almost exclusively within the framework of the nation-state, to the extent that its management structure is embedded within that of the state. Almost all modern nations exercise their sovereignty over the archaeological record (and thus over the representation of the past) through the establishment and running of state departments of antiquities, national museums, national parks and heritage sites, university archaeological departments, history curricula in schools, through the inclusion of the above in town and city planning and through the celebration of elements of the past in various patriotic commemorative events and festivals.[16] In this way, one dominant and frequently linear narrative of the past or mode of knowledge can be both presented and preserved.[17]

The notion of continuity in culture and identity is promoted through this supposed historical linearity, thus marginalising and silencing the complexities and nuances of cultural development through time. Israel is no different from other modern nations who thus seek to control, manage and own the remains of the past located within their borders. By investigating the manner in which archaeological sites are managed and presented to the public, we learn much regarding the concerns of Israeli society. From a purely archaeological point of view, questions are raised about the effectiveness of such approaches for the conservation of archaeological remains, and about the intellectual and ethical integrity of the narratives thereby constructed.

Fieldwork and Methodology

My Israeli fieldwork was conducted in April and May 2005, with some preliminary work carried out in the summer of 2004. I examined the interfaces between archaeology and the public and the impact of both nationalistic and economic agenda (primarily via the tourist industry), on the conservation and presentation of archaeological remains and the narratives created around and through them. Sites were selected for study based on their prominence in the managed heritage landscape. The nature of tourism in Israel, which is geared towards the organised group tour rather than the individual tourist, means that within the context of the heritage

---

[16] Cf. Abu el Haj (1998) and Fowler (1992).
[17] Cf. Graham et al., 2000; 19, 32, 37.

industry, the vast majority of tourist interest in archaeological remains is directed at a comparatively small number of archaeological sites. Because foreign, rather than domestic visitors, generate the bulk of revenue at archaeological attractions in Israel (as anecdotally, may be the case in many other countries also), it is those sites which attract the largest numbers of foreign tourists that receive the greatest financial investment in terms of site preservation and presentation to the public. These sites are thus prominently placed to transmit messages to both a domestic and a foreign public. In light of Urry's claim that an investigation of how societies construct their 'tourist gaze' is a good way of exposing the concerns of society at large,[18] an investigation into the types of sites chosen for such intense promotion should prove revealing of Israeli society and the building blocks with which Israeli group identity is being constructed. As a result, I chose to examine a select number of sites and museums prominent in the Israeli cultural landscape and conducted an in-depth study of their presentation to the public and also of the history of presentation at, and management of, these sites. Many of these sites and museums were located in and around Jerusalem, while the other major sites selected for study were Akko, Beth She'an, Caesarea and Masada, as well as the city of Jaffa.

The 'archaeological tour' has been constructing 'Israel' in the public imagination since the nineteenth century, when Cook's 'Eastern Tours' helped to create a new kind of pilgrimage to the Holy Land, providing Europeans with tangible support for their creed. The tours helped those of various persuasions to find a Catholic, Presbyterian or Lutheran Palestine, according to their individual needs. These tours are important in the construction of the imagined community of Israel today, spatially, diachronically and perhaps more importantly, in terms of modern cultural identity. In the course of these 'touring holidays', the Israeli landscape is dissected and choice elements are separated and isolated, to be presented to the tourist for consumption. A similar process occurs in the individual tours of archaeological sites, so that a specific Jewish or Judeo-Christian past can be created for the visitor, to the exclusion of the other groups and cultures who occupied this time and space. In addition, the monument or archaeological site has been presented since colonial times as the key destination for the visitor, and consequently, the socio-economic environment in which this monument is set has no bearing for the tourist whose aim is only to 'capture' this monument on film and bring his/her trophy home.[19] As will be discussed shortly, this is evident in the cases of the Jerusalem Archaeological Park and Caesarea, both sites with non-Judeo-Christian remains and located amidst Israeli Arab communities, though little or no reference to either is made in the tourist literature available on-site.

Because tourism in Israel is still geared towards the organised group tour rather than the individual tourist, the vast majority of tourist interest in archaeological remains is directed at a comparatively small number of archaeological sites. This interest frequently comes from a tourist audience who already have an expectation of the significance of such sites. And because foreign visitors generate the bulk of

---

[18] Urry, *The Tourist Gaze*, 2.

[19] Cf. Urry, *The Tourist Gaze*.

revenue at archaeological attractions in Israel, it is specifically those sites that receive the greatest financial investment in terms of site preservation and presentation to the public. Tours to these sites are the main point of contact between the public and archaeology and both the sites selected for touring itineraries and the nature of information provided, prove revealing, not only in terms of archaeological practice and academic interests in Israel, but of the concerns, at least at an official level, of Israeli society. These sites are prominently placed to transmit messages to both a domestic and a foreign public and the experience created for the visitor through these tours is a function of official state narratives and are a window into how Israeli group identity is being constructed and presented. To demonstrate the nature and content of archaeological site tours in Israel and their role in constructing Israel in the public imagination, I will provide evidence from two multi-period sites, both of which appear regularly on touring itineraries: the Jerusalem Archaeological Park and Caesarea.

Jerusalem Archaeological Park

The Jerusalem Archaeological Park is managed by the East Jerusalem Development Co. Ltd., founded in 1966, with the aim of 'the development and operation' of tourist sites in Eastern Jerusalem and the greater Jerusalem'.[20] The company is in the overall charge of the Prime Minister and the Minister of Education. The company also manages the Ophel Archaeological Garden and the Davidson Exhibition and Virtual Reconstruction Centre, both of which are located within the Jerusalem Archaeological Park.[21]

The Archaeological Park encompasses part of the Western wall of the Temple, Robinson's Arch, a Herodian Street, a complex of buildings from the Roman and Byzantine periods, remains of Umayyad Palaces and a Fatimad tower renovated by the Crusaders, the Ayyubids and the Mameluks. Some areas of the Park are highly manicured with garden and courtyard spaces, while others are left overgrown. There are limited information plaques, so if a visitor does not pay the inflated price for a guide (NIS 160, about €29), it would be impossible to decipher the complex jumble of archaeological remains. The official tour of the site begins in the Davidson Centre, which is located in rooms that were part of the basement of the seventh to eighth century Umayyad Palace, though information about the palace is not provided. This placement of the Centre erases the significance of the palace as a historic monument, and in a deliberate way eclipses its original importance. The Centre comprises a number of colour-coded displays outlining the chronological development of the city. A select number of artefacts, as well as reconstruction drawings, are used to illustrate the narrative. As elsewhere in Israel, information is provided only in Hebrew and English and not Arabic, one of the country's official languages, spoken by approximately 18% of the country's inhabitants. Guided tours are unavailable in Arabic, although advertised and provided in English. Limited

---

[20] Pami.co.il "Governmental Firm – Works under the Conditions of the Authority of Governmental Firms." Internet. Available from: <http://www.pami.co.il/eng/> [Accessed 19 September 2005].
[21] Images of these sites can be viewed in the accompanying podcast of this presentation.

Arabic is to be found on the few plaques in the site itself. Visitors are also presented with an informative and detailed video on the history of the excavations which provided us with information on the artefacts, as well as the information already presented in the displays. The overall focus of the Centre, however, is the evocation of the Second Temple Period (516 BCE–70 CE) and drawings of the Temple and its associated activities are to be found on the walls throughout the exhibition. The culmination of a visit to the Centre is a virtual reality film, narrated by the tour guide. The film is about Second Temple Period Jerusalem and specifically the Temple and its compound, and aims at presenting a picture of what a visit to the Temple would have entailed at that time. In effect, the visitor is presented with a virtual reality depiction of the remains about to be viewed outside and site photos of the actual remains can be seen on one side of the screen.

The tour of the site itself takes in only a very small number of the remains in the park – in essence, the Second Temple Period archaeology. Shades and information panels are provided at these 'important' points. The Roman and Umayyad remains (testimony to the historical 'other') are ignored entirely, although our guide, who informed me later that he had a personal interest in presenting a more multi-vocal narrative, made a point of indicating and giving a brief summary of these structures. The Umayyad Palaces themselves were removed by the excavators, though the tour ends where Palace One would have stood. Although some beautifully preserved mosaics and plastered walls survive from the Byzantine period residential area, they also do not form part of the tour. The Ophel Archaeological Garden, which forms part of the Jerusalem Archaeological Park, is also largely ignored by the tour. The garden, which comprises a multi-period site incorporating mostly residential remains, is located at the foot of the southern wall of the Temple Mount. It includes the steps of the Hulda Gates which led to the Temple in the Second Temple Period. The garden is fenced off from the road from whence the site can be viewed. Indeed, the only information plaques detailing the complex maze of multi-period remains in the garden are located along this fence on the roadside. These plaques are quite old and as a result of graffiti as well as weathering many are illegible. Those which can still be read, bear diagrams of a select number of remains. The garden is highly overgrown and in places, trees and bushes grow inside archaeological complexes. The site can be accessed through the Park, but few visitors incorporate the garden in their activities (although often they will include the steps of the Hulda Gate), as it does not form part of the official tour of the site and is too overgrown and ill-provided with information to be of interest to many.

The entire complex is an odd mix of high-tech, innovative and attractive presentation techniques combined with neglect, disinterest and occasional brief acknowledgement of non-Jewish Second Temple remains. At this site, the shame of such measures is more potent than elsewhere, for given the contentious location (at the perimeters of the contested holy location for Jews and Muslims, at the heart of the divided city of Jerusalem, amidst a large and mostly impoverished Palestinian community), a genuine acknowledgement in conservation and presentation terms, by the Israeli establishment of the multi-cultural past and present of the country at this site might well go a long way to creating a feeling of inclusion among Israel's non-Jewish citizens.

Caesarea

A similar picture is painted at the archaeological site at Caesarea. This multi-period monumental site is managed by the Israel Nature and National Parks Protection Authority. Within the Park, the Caesarea Edmond Benjamin de Rothschild Corporation operates *Caesarea Harbour*, a visitor centre with multi-media displays on the history of the site. The National Park extends from the Roman theatre in the south to the Crusader city to the north. Many, though not all, of the archaeological remains within the park have been prepared for public presentation and these include: the Byzantine square, the Herodian amphitheatre, the promontory palace, a bathhouse and a network of streets. In 1968, the Crusader city and the theatre became a national park. The Israel Antiquities Authority and Haifa University have been conducting extensive excavations since the early 1990s as part of the development of the site for tourist purposes within the framework of the Master Plan for Tourism in Caesarea.

As in the case of the Jerusalem Archaeological Park, the archaeological remains at the site are in varying states of preservation. Conservation attention has most obviously been paid to the theatre (which has undergone reconstruction work and is used as a venue for modern productions), the bathhouse complex (which houses a number of mosaics) and the hippodrome. By contrast, many other less illustrious remains are overgrown and ramshackle and many mosaics are left exposed to the hazards of the elements and visitors' feet, despite the lessons observed with the deterioration, and in some cases obliteration, of parts of the three mosaics discovered in the promontory palace at Caesarea in 1978.

Information panels at Caesarea are limited in number but instructive when provided. Again, they appear in greater quantity in the areas most readied for public presentation, but conversely would be most useful in the less manicured areas of the site. The remains of a nineteenth century Bosnian village, including a mosque located on the site, have been converted into a visitor centre. As in the case of the Umayyad Palace in the Jerusalem Archaeological Park, the original historic significance of these remains, and the populations who built them, is thereby erased. Indeed, the entire site has undergone extensive commercialisation. As can be seen from the figures, craft and souvenir shops have even been built into and underneath the archaeological remains. Again, the result is a diminishing of the significance of the actual archaeological remains. As the Rothschild Corporation phrases it:

> *Your visit to Caesarea Harbor will be an enchanting adventure filled with an abundance of captivating activities and presentations, a variety of restaurants and cafés, art and craft galleries that allow you to take part in the creative process, authentic boutiques and modern beach conveniences.*[22]

---

[22] caesarea.org.il "Welcome to Caesarea Harbor." Available from: <http://www.caesarea.org.il/namal/template_e/default.asp?catid = 61> [Accessed 19 September 2005].

A significant element of any visit to the site now is the multi-media presentation on the history of the site at Caesarea Harbour. Although tickets must be bought separately for this part of the site, they are heavily promoted at the site entrance and by the ticket sales staff. The presentation includes an interactive encounter with individuals from the past of the site, as well as digitised computer–aided visual presentations on the city and its history. In the words of the site's brochure:

> *The internationally renowned English company Past Forward, in conjunction with Atat Ltd., which transforms archaeological sites into tourist attractions through the use of advanced technology, rebuilds the city on an enormous screen, providing a thrilling encounter with history through an exciting, interactive journey.*[23]

The presentations are offered in Hebrew, English, French, Spanish and Russian, but notably as in the case of the Jerusalem Archaeological Park, not Arabic, one of the official languages of the country. The *Caesarea Experience* is completed with an introduction to 12 historical figures prominent in the history of the site. This interactive programme presents three-dimensional figures with a list of set questions and answers from which the visitor can choose to learn about the history of Caesarea. This programme divides the history of the site into four broad historical periods and introduces the visitor to three characters from each: the Early Roman period with King Herod, Pontius Pilate and Saint Paul; the Late Roman period with Rabbi Akiva, Rabbi Abbahu and Empress Helena; the Crusader period with Saladin, King Louis IX and Sultan Baybars; and finally, the twentieth century with Baron Edmond de Rothschild (who bought Caesarea and developed it), Hannah Senesh (the Jewish Resistance poet sentenced to death by the Nazis) and her mother Katrina Senesh (who made *aliya* to Israel to the kibbutz at Caesarea). This final section on the twentieth century deals with the anti-Semitism faced by Jews in Europe from the perspective of the young Jewish poet, Hannah Senesh, and the resulting importance of Zionism. Hannah was killed by the Nazis, but her family survived and came to Israel and settled on the land purchased by de Rothschild and his efforts in the area of the resettlement of Jews in Israel also feature in the programme. This display entirely ignores large elements in the past of Caesarea, choosing instead to focus on the Jewish and Christian past of the site (invariably appealing to the site's dominant clientele), while the few Arab or Muslim characters given a mention are presented (both physically and in their words) as demonic barbarians. Shavit argues in response that:

> *A visitor to Masada, for example, may be 'nationalistically' inspired, whereas a visitor to Caesarea, Beit Shean, or even Gamla will be impressed primarily by the 'archaeological merits' of the sites. In other words, we must distinguish between the function of archaeological sites or monuments as ideological agents, on the one hand, and the non-tendentious history that archaeology helps tell or retell on the other.*[24]

---

[23] Caesarea Harbor Brochure (2005).

[24] Cf. Shavit, Y. "Archaeology, Political Culture, and Culture in Israel." in: Silberman, N.A. and D.B. Small eds. *The Archaeology of Israel; Constructing the Past, Interpreting the Present* (Sheffield; Academic Press,1997) 237, 52–53.

Here, he ignores the point that regardless of what motivates a visit to a site, the potential for that site to tell multiple narratives, including nationalist ones, is still there as at Caesarea, as demonstrated in the de-Arabisation of Caesarea and the restoration of the Crusader remains, as borne out in the *Caesarea Experience*. In the Israeli context, it seems preferable to immortalise those who exterminated the Jewish communities of Europe (in the late eleventh and early twelfth centuries) and murdered the Jews of Jerusalem in 1099 than to preserve relics of the local Arab civilisation with whom today's Israelis must supposedly coexist. Crusader structures, both authentic and fabricated, lend a European romantic character to the country's landscape, whereas Arab buildings spoil the myth of an occupied land under foreign rule, awaiting liberation at the hands of the Jews returning to their homeland. And if it is impossible to erase the physical remains, it is at least possible to ascribe them to someone else: 'Crusaders, Mamluks or Ottomans'. In addition, by focusing on the harsh, war-faring characteristics of those 'Others' who occupied this territory in the past, Israel is playing to the national narrative of a tiny beleaguered state surrounded by barbaric enemies but prevailing against all odds.

The visitor to Caesarea is left in no doubt as to the message of Jewish redemption through reclamation of the land and of the perpetual brutal and brutish nature of the Arab East. At Caesarea, the tourist is encouraged to conduct his/her own tour, from a choice of four pre-designed routes printed on maps, all of which incorporate substantial time in the tri-partite visitor centre, viewing the technologically sophisticated displays. These displays take up the vast majority of tour time and the result is that the archaeological remains (which in this case provide testimony to the multi-cultural, turbulent nature of the site and Israel as a whole) become secondary to the narrative being promoted at the site through the displays. The archaeology thus becomes a redundant, if aesthetically pleasing aside to ideologically and economically driven narratives and concerns.

While guided tours are not available at all sites in Israel, they are available at the vast majority of those sites appearing regularly on touring itineraries or could be arranged in advance for such groups. It was my experience, however, that the information provided by a number of tour guides was inaccurate and almost always tended towards a strong Jewish bias in the presentation of information both historical and modern about a site and its environment. Narratives about sites and their surroundings relied heavily on the audience's ability to identify with Jewish customs and traditions. Guides also intermittently referred to ancient Israelites as Israelis and modern Israelis as Israelites, thereby conflating the two identities and linking them diachronically. Such conceptualisations of Israeli identity deny even the existence of any other than Jewish Israeli citizens. Indeed, as also noted by Abu el Haj, tour guides and information panels at sites and museums in Israel constantly make a distinction between a Jewish 'us' and an Other 'them', all narrated in the first-person plural 'we'.[25]

---

[25] Abu el Haj, N. "Translating Truths: the Practice of Archaeology, and the Remaking of the Past and Present in Contemporary Jerusalem." *American Ethnologist* (1998) 25:2, 166–88, 179.

Lessons to Be Learned from Case Studies

Landscape in Israel is understood on a vertical axis – the above ground and visible, with its ruins and monuments, and the equally vocal subterranean space, translated by archaeology.[26] The totality is a scientific (and hence irrefutable) expression of the cultural and ethnic identity of that landscape. Every rock, stone and even minor artefact becomes meaningful and important to the construction and expression of this identity. In Israel, however, through the selectivity introduced in part through archaeological tours, the kaleidoscope of cultural remainders are ignored or suppressed. This is not to say that the narratives presented to the public through tours and site displays are falsehoods or entirely new inventions, but merely that they highlight and elaborate on certain elements of the past while overlooking or ignoring others.

Problems arise when this monumental version of the nation's past silences vernacular or other minority or contested pasts in the same time and space. The anthropologist Roxani Caftanzoglu points out that the landscape can be an important symbolic resource and the archaeologist through his work with that landscape is a powerful agent in the construction and practice of national identity. Archaeologists and related professionals in the heritage industry therefore contribute to the creation of national narratives of inclusion and exclusion, and they may annihilate more inclusive narratives through the selectivity of their work, by isolating and excluding unwanted cultural forms.[27] The archaeological site tours, described in this chapter, are an expression of such exclusionary tendencies.

The archaeological profession (including heritage management) have an ethical obligation to represent all who have used the landscape and their respective narratives. We can do this by looking towards a more nuanced understanding of the role played by continuity, by shifting away from the view that sees continuity as a guiding principle and instead reading continuous discontinuity into the archaeological record. We must re-evaluate our understanding of such concepts as culture and ethnicity in light of their relationship to political idioms and concerns, and the way both of these relate to the archaeological record.

Equally, it is necessary to re-evaluate the nature of the relationship between archaeology and cultural heritage tourism. Not all the effects of tourism are negatives for archaeological sites and examples from Israel demonstrate both the positives and negatives of this relationship. The damage from wear and tear is evident at numerous sites in Israel; the building of visitor amenities such as car parks,

---

[26] Serghidou, A. "Imaginary Cyprus: Revisiting the Past and Redefining the Ancient Landscape." in: Tatton-Brown, V. ed. *Cyprus in the 19th Century AD: Fact, Fancy and Fiction* (Oxford; Oxbow Books, 2001) 21–31, 22.

[27] Caftanzoglu, R. "National Scholars and the Creation of National Landscapes: a Case of Exclusion." Paper presented at the International Conference Ancient Monuments and Modern Identities, the History of Archaeology in 19th and 20th Century Greece. Cambridge, 25th–27th March, 2002.

shops and restaurants causes irreparable damage to unexposed archaeological remains and may be aesthetically unpleasing.[28] This is equally true in the case of shades for visitors, archaeological shelters and modern entrances to the park. Such features, if ill-planned, can become obtrusive through their physical dominance at a site.

The commercialisation of some sites, such as Caesarea, can distract the visitor from the landscape, the archaeological remains themselves and from the historical significance of the site. Over-exposure of archaeological remains at sites such as Caesarea and the Archaeological Garden in Jerusalem results in the inevitable neglect of some remains at the cost of others and exposes all remains to unnecessary deterioration in the absence of long-term conservation plans and the necessary spreading of resources over a larger number of projects.

On the other hand, the complete neglect of a site once excavation has ceased will also lead to the deterioration of the archaeological remains, as the site becomes overgrown, exposed to vandalism, unmonitored visits from the public and environmental conditions.[29] In this case, not only are the archaeological remains themselves lost to the public and the scientific community, but so are the educational, spiritual or religious and aesthetic values attached to the site. It is the case that the development of a site also increases its educational value. Without tourism, many sites would remain mute, their history inaccessible to the public. Increased tourism to an area because of an archaeological site benefits the local economy and is a source of both pride and education to the public. The key then is to promote sustainable tourism, which takes the long-term preservation of archaeological remains into account.

Within this complex web of competing agenda and interests, the challenge to government officials, archaeologists, architects, conservators and the community in general is to instigate workable, long-term management and conservation plans for archaeological sites which have the interests of the archaeological remains at heart, for it is only through the conservation of the archaeology that the concerns of other interested parties can be protected also. The question is how is this to be done within the current parameters of the discipline, trapped, as it is, within the walls of the nation-state. I acknowledge that breaking free of those walls is no easy task, for while the conceptual and practical creation of a distinctive national heritage was the result of the creation of the nation-state, it is now difficult to conceive of any other organisation with the instruments capable of sponsoring and supporting even the current heritage remains, let alone the fruits of future research.[30] This, however, should not deter us from seeking to find other and better possibilities.

---

[28] Merhav, R. and A. Killebrew "Public Exposure: for Better and for Worse." *Museum International (UNESCO) (1998)* 50: 4, 15–20, 15.

[29] Ibid, 18.

[30] Cf. Graham et al. (2000), 184 and McIntosh and Togola (1996), 187.

Contested Archaeologies and Ethics

It was made clear through my fieldwork that the tensions between the interests and concerns of a government department and the preservation and presentation of archaeological material and knowledge can be overwhelming. Archaeologists produce the raw material for an industry which at the same time supports the archaeologists' endeavours. It seems to me now that this is a cycle from which it would be very difficult to extricate archaeology and so we must find ways to retain the beneficial elements for both parties whilst protecting each component from the negative impact they might have on the other. Modern technology and the demands of a global economy for progress and development have led to rapid economic growth in many countries. Internationally, destruction through excessively hurried change has occurred at a faster rate than an awareness of the needs of, and policies for preservation. As noted by Greene, economic growth moves faster than under-funded archaeology and its rewards are more immediately tangible than those of archaeology, which are often seen as irrelevant to the needs of daily life.[31]

The problem thus faced is the need to develop for the future whilst also preserving the past for that future. The lack of available time, money and personnel means that inevitably managers have to make difficult decisions about which sites to preserve and which to leave to destruction. Because they are not classified as developing countries, neither Cyprus nor Israel receives high levels of development aid that can sometimes be used for cultural resource protection. Both countries utilise the income borne of international interest in their past and the remains thereof to fund this endeavour. However, as demonstrated in the case studies discussed, a problem then arises when these archaeological remains become exploited to meet the needs of the all-consuming tourist industry, to the detriment of both current and future interests in their study and preservation.

Problems also arise when archaeological remains are used to uphold the needs and claims of certain ethnic voices and associated pasts whilst silencing others considered less palatable. This poses major problems for archaeological practice, site preservation and management. It raises important and difficult questions about the ownership of the past and its material remains. For example, if we argue that though modern Cypriots are not the 'direct' descendents of the Bronze or Iron Age inhabitants of the island in a literal sense, but that modern Cypriots' belief in their Hellenic identity, inherited from the Aegean settlers in the island during these pre-historic periods, is something that should be acknowledged and respected, how does this impact on the preservation of archaeological heritage?

---

[31] Cf. Greene, J.A. "Preserving which Past for Whose Future? The Dilemma of Cultural Resource Management in Case Studies from Tunisia, Cyprus and Jordan." *Conservation and Management of Archaeological Sites* (1999) 3, 43–4.

If we introduce the language of inheritance and ethnic association, do we imply that modern Cypriots are the 'owners' of some archaeological remains located on the island, and the 'caretakers' of those not pertaining to their self-identification as Hellenes and Christians?[32] In turn, does Turkey have 'rights' to archaeological remains in the Republic of Cyprus that pertain to the Turkish and Muslim past of the island? What implications does this have for the issue of the export of cultural remains or their repatriation from abroad? Silberman raises similar questions in relation to Israeli claims to archaeological remains lying in the Palestinian Territories:

Are the Israelis justified in mounting an effort to retrieve documents and artefacts of direct and demonstrable relevance to their culture and tradition? Even if those artefacts lay in disputed territory [the West Bank]? Do Palestinians, on the other hand, have a right to claim ownership of ancient Jewish artefacts in their part of the country, even if those artefacts are of relatively little significance to them? And if the antiquities of the country are to be partitioned by cultural association, do the Palestinians thereby have a right to custodianship of Muslim holy sites within Israel?[33]

While I do not profess to have the answers to these difficult questions, I suggest that part of the problem lies in the current focus on tracing ethnic groups temporally and misunderstandings of the role of continuity and change in cultural production and reproduction. Most modern theorists of ethnicity agree that ethnic identity, '...is based on shifting, situational, subjective identifications of self and others, which are rooted in ongoing daily practice and historical experience, but also subject to transformation and discontinuity'.[34]

Therefore, while maintaining a respect for people's ethnic self-definition, one should not necessarily encode this definition in legal standards (especially retrospective ones), given its proclivity to change. A more useful proposition might be to acknowledge discontinuities and changes wrought with time and enshrine custodial rather than ownership status over all archaeological monuments, landscapes and artefacts. This would not merely require changes in the relevant antiquities laws, but fundamental changes in attitude to the past and our relationship to it – viewing it as not merely as a resource to be selectively exploited for either economic or national or ethnic purposes, but as a valuable endangered species in our care.

---

[32] As demonstrated in this thesis, neither the Cypriot nor the Israeli administrations have been especially good caretakers to date of archaeological monuments and artefacts of periods of little interest or anathema to state definitions of self and self-interest.

[33] Silberman, N.A. "Operation Scroll." in: Vitelli K.D. ed. *Archaeological Ethics* (London; Altamira Press, 1996), 134–5.

[34] Jones, S. *The Archaeology of Ethnicity: Reconstructing Identities in the Past and Present* (London; Routledge, 1997), 13–14.

Bibliography

Abu el Haj N. "Translating Truths: the Practice of Archaeology, and the Remaking of the Past and Present in Contemporary Jerusalem". *Am Ethnol* 1998;25(2):166–88.

Acklom G. *A Forgotten Era in Archaeology: The Research Conducted by Early British Travellers in Palestine from c. 1670 to 1825.* University of Melbourne: Unpublished Ph. D, Department of Classics and Archaeology; 1995.

Atkinson J, Banks I, O'Sullivan J, editors. *Nationalism and Archaeology: Scottish Archaeological Forum.* Glasgow: Cruithne Press; 1996.

Bond GC, Gilliam A, editors. *Social Construction of the Past: Representation as Power.* London: Routledge; 1994.

Brassey A. *Sunshine and Storm in the East or Cruises to Cyprus and Constantinople.* New York, NY: Henry Holt and Company; 1880.

Caesarea.org.il "Welcome to Caesarea Harbor." Available from: <http://www.caesarea.org. il/namal/template_e/default.asp?catid = 61/> [accessed 19.09.05].

Caftanzoglu R.. "National Scholars and the Creation of National Landscapes: a Case of Exclusion." Paper presented at the International Conference Ancient Monuments and Modern Identities, the History of Archaeology in 19th and 20th Century Greece. Cambridge; 25–27 March, 2002.

Diaz-Andreu M, Champion T, editors. *Nationalism and Archaeology in Europe.* London: UCL Press; 1996.

Firth A. "Ghosts in the Machine". In: Cooper MA, Firth A, Carman J, Wheatley D, editors. *Managing Archaeology.* London: Routledge; 1995. p. 51–67.

Fowler P. *The Past in Contemporary Society Then, Now.* London/New York, NY: Routledge; 1992.

Gellner E. *Culture, Identity and Politics.* Cambridge: Cambridge University Press; 1987.

Gero J, Root D. "Public Presentations and Private Concerns: Archaeology in the Pages of National Geographic". In: Gathercole P, Lowenthal D, editors. *The Politics of the Past.* London: Routledge; 1994. p. 19–37.

Graham B, Ashworth GJ, Tunbridge JE. *A Geography of Heritage, Power Culture and Economy.* London: Arnold; 2000.

Graves-Brown P, Jones S, Gamble C, editors. *Cultural Identity and Archaeology: the Construction of European Communities.* London: Routledge; 1996.

Greene JA. "Preserving which Past for Whose Future? The Dilemma of Cultural Resource Management in Case Studies from Tunisia, Cyprus and Jordan". *Conserv Manage Archaeol Sites* 1999;3:43–60.

Haggard HR. *A Winter Pilgrimage, Being an Account of Travels Through Palestine, Italy, and the Island of Cyprus, Accomplished in the Year 1900.* London: Longmans, Green and Co.; 1901.

Jones S. *The Archaeology of Ethnicity: Reconstructing Identities in the Past and Present.* London: Routledge; 1997.

Knapp B, Antoniadou S. "Archaeology, Politics and the Cultural Heritage of Cyprus". In: Meskell L, editor. *Archaeology Under Fire: Nationalism, Politics and Heritage in the Eastern Mediterranean and Middle East.* London: Routledge; 1998. p. 13–43.

Kohl PL, Fawcett C, editors. *Nationalism, Politics and the Practice of Archaeology.* Cambridge: Cambridge University Press; 1995.

Liakos A. "The Construction of National Time: the Making of the Modern Greek Historical Imagination". *Mediterr Hist Rev* 2001;16(June):27–42.

Merhav R, Killebrew A. "Public Exposure: for Better and for Worse". *Mus Int (UNESCO)* 1998;50(4):15–20.

Mouliou M. "Ancient Greece, its Classical Heritage and the Modern Greeks, Aspects of Nationalism in Museum Exhibitions". In: Atkinson J, Banks I, O'Sullivan J, editors. *Nationalism and Archaeology/Scottish Archaeological Forum*. Glasgow: Cruithne Press; 1996. p. 174–99.

Pami.co.il "Governmental Firm – Works under the Conditions of the Authority of Governmental Firms." Available from: <http://www.pami.co.il/eng/> [accessed 19.09.05].

Serghidou A. "Imaginary Cyprus: Revisiting the Past and Redefining the Ancient Landscape". In: Tatton-Brown V, editor. *Cyprus in the 19th Century AD: Fact, Fancy and Fiction*. Oxford: Oxbow Books; 2001. p. 21–31.

Shavit Y. "Archaeology, Political Culture, and Culture in Israel". In: Silberman NA, Small DB, editors. *The Archaeology of Israel; Constructing the Past, Interpreting the Present*, vol. 237. Sheffield: Academic Press; 1997. p. 48–61.

Silberman NA. "Operation Scroll". In: Vitelli KD, editor. *Archaeological Ethics*. London: Altamira Press; 1996. p. 132–5.

Stritch, Deirdre. *Archaeology and the State: An Examination of Archaeological Practice and Official Interpretation of Archaeological Remains in Israel and the Republic of Cyprus*. Unpublished PhD thesis, Trinity College Dublin; 2007.

Urry J. *The Tourist Gaze: Leisure and Travel in Contemporary Societies*. London: Sage Publications; 1990.

Whitelam K. *The Invention of Ancient Israel: the Silencing of Palestinian History*. London: Routledge; 1996.

Zerubavel Y. *Recovered Roots, Collective Memory and the Making of Israeli National Tradition*. Chicago: University of Chicago Press; 1995.

11 Research Ethics in Divided and Violent Societies: Seizing the Ethical Opportunity

Gladys Ganiel

Irish School of Ecumenics (Belfast), Trinity College, Dublin, Ireland

Abstract

This chapter explores how to conduct social research in divided and violent societies by developing the concept of the 'ethical opportunity'. The 'ethical opportunity' is situated in a brief discussion of 'action' and feminist approaches to research. It argues that seizing the ethical opportunity requires researchers to: plan for their personal safety, plan for participants' personal safety and plan how they will communicate and disseminate their results. It draws on the author's personal experience researching in South Africa, Zimbabwe and Northern Ireland, concluding that it is in the communication and dissemination phase that researchers' hopes for 'making a difference' may be realised or dashed. It cautions would-be researchers to manage their own – and research participants' – expectations about what social research can achieve. Its effects may not often be as transforming and liberating as idealistic researchers hope for, but that should not dissuade them from striving towards those ends.

Key Words

Action research, feminist approach, divided society, violent society, informed consent, confidentiality, data protection, communication

Introduction

Many researchers decide to work in divided and violent societies because they want to 'make a difference'. They want their work to contribute to better social relations and to sustainable peace. This unabashedly normative position is not always accepted in the social sciences, but I consider myself part of this research tradition. I see research in divided and violent societies as an 'ethical opportunity' to promote

Ethics for Graduate Researchers. DOI: http://dx.doi.org/10.1016/B978-0-12-416049-1.00011-8

peace and justice. Attempting to seize this 'ethical opportunity' is at the heart of the type of research that I try to do, and which I encourage my students to undertake.

This chapter builds on an already extensive literature on conducting research in divided and violent societies.[1] In it, I develop my concept of the 'ethical opportunity', which flows out of other scholars' earlier work, drawing on 'action research' and feminist approaches. I begin this chapter by situating my conception of the 'ethical opportunity' in a brief discussion of these approaches. I then consider the three key ways in which social science researchers can seize the 'ethical opportunity' to promote peace and justice: by planning for their personal safety, planning for participants' personal safety and planning how they will communicate and disseminate their results. By way of illustration, I draw on my own research on South Africa, Zimbabwe and Northern Ireland, concluding that it is in the communication and dissemination phase that researchers' hopes for 'making a difference' may be realised or dashed. To that end, I caution would-be researchers to manage their own — and research participants' — expectations about what social research can achieve. Its effects may not often be as transforming and liberating as idealistic researchers hope for, but that should not dissuade them from striving towards those ends.

'Making a Difference?' — Seizing the Ethical Opportunity

I teach in Trinity College Dublin's master's programme in Conflict Resolution and Reconciliation, located in Belfast, Northern Ireland. I think our programme attracts a disproportionate number of students who want their research to 'make a difference' in the 'real world', and I do not want to discourage these students. As Smyth and Robinson have argued, it is difficult to justify research in situations where lives are being lost, if it cannot make some contribution to transforming the violence.[2] It is possible, just possible, that what researchers discover during the course of their work may help people to understand their social and political worlds better. And this in turn might encourage people to change their worlds in ways that will promote peace and justice.[3] Accordingly, I want — and I hope my students also

[1] Two of the best edited collections are Smyth, Marie and Robinson, Gillian (eds.) *Researching Violently Divided Societies: Ethical and Methodological Issues* (London: Pluto Press, 2001) and Lee, Raymond M. and Stanko, Elizabeth A. (eds.) *Researching Violence: Essays of Methodology and Measurement* (London: Routledge, 2003).
[2] Smyth and Robinson, "Introduction," in Smith and Robinson, (eds.) *Researching Violently Divided Societies*, 3–4.
[3] Of course, what constitutes 'peace' and 'justice' in particular contexts is always contested. Especially in divided societies, what seems like 'justice' for one 'side' may seem like 'injustice' for the 'other'. So researchers must always be careful to reflect on how their conceptions of peace and justice (or democracy or racial integration and so on) fit (or not) in the particular society or societies in which they are conducting research. It is best if researchers can articulate these conceptions and recognise their own subjectivity, including 'self-reflexive' analysis of their own identities, assumptions and possible biases. See Nason-Clark, Nancy and Neitz, Mary Jo (eds.) *Feminist Narratives in the Sociology of Religion* (Walnut Creek: Altamira Press, 2001) and Poloma, Margaret, *Main Street Mystics: The Toronto Blessing and Reviving Pentecostalism* (Walnut Creek: Altamira, 2003), 237–257.

want – to seize the 'ethical opportunity' to conduct research in such settings. My concept of 'ethical opportunity' is grounded in the idea that researchers in such settings have a moral responsibility to share the results of their work with those who have the means to use it to end division and violence. This includes policy makers and people who have participated in the research. As such, my concept of the 'ethical opportunity' builds on action and feminist approaches to research.

The action research tradition has developed precisely because researchers have wanted to work alongside research participants to facilitate social change. McNiff and Whitehead make this clear in their discussion of the 'underpinning assumptions of action research'. In contrast to the 'notionally value free' tradition of 'positivist' research, in which 'the researcher stays out of the research, so as not to "contaminate" it', action researchers are fully embedded in the worlds they are researching.[4] A full-blown action research project will involve participants in every stage of the research process, including framing the research questions, carrying out the work, writing up and disseminating the results. I have never personally conducted a full-blown action research project, although I have supervised master's students who have done so. To take one example, a master's student who worked for the North Belfast Interface Network used an action research approach in his dissertation, involving his colleagues and people in the local community in designing and carrying out a research project about what it might take to dismantle some of the area's notorious 'peace walls'.[5] Not every researcher will have the means or opportunity to gain that level of involvement with research participants – and not all research participants will want that level of involvement. After all, many participants in social research are already busy social activists whose top priority is not your research project! But researchers can still adopt some of the principles behind action research. For example, McNiff and Whitehead discuss the 'value laden' and 'morally committed' nature of action research demonstrating that its main goal is to have a 'social purpose'. This purpose can range from promoting democratic values, to improving the workplace or making the 'social order' more just.[6] In the case of divided or violent societies, I would add that the purpose of action research could include promoting better relationships between opposing groups, informing policy makers' approaches to overcoming division or challenging divisive social structures such as segregated education.

Similarly, feminist approaches to social research have emphasised that it can and should impact on the people who have participated in the study, and on society at large. Some feminist scholars have gone so far as to argue that the validity of research should be judged on the extent that it contributes to 'progressive' individual,

---

[4] McNiff, Jean and Whitehead, Jack, *All You Need to Know About Action Research* (London: Sage, 2011), 27. See also Costello, Patrick, *Effective Action Research: Developing Reflective Thinking and Practice* (London: Continuum, 2011).

[5] McCallum, Robert, "Living at the Interface: Research in Three Interface Areas of North Belfast," Dissertation submitted for the M.Phil. in Conflict Resolution and Reconciliation (Belfast and Dublin: the Irish School of Ecumenics, Trinity College Dublin, 2011).

[6] McNiff and Whitehead, *All You Need to Know About Action Research,* 38.

social or political change.[7] Cho and Trent call this 'transformational validity', explaining that this approach to research finds its worth in its 'ability to raise consciousness and thus provoke political action to remedy problems of oppressed peoples'.[8] This said, it is difficult to establish what (if any) are the core components of feminist approaches. In her discussion of feminist and post-colonial theory, Ali uses Campbell's term 'theoretical field' to refer to 'a diverse group of theorists and research projects that coalesce around shared political and theoretical investments'.[9] The concept of a theoretical field is intended to convey the sense that there is both unity and diversity in the theoretical and action-based approaches of scholars who identify with feminism, rather than a strict set of philosophies or practical guidelines to which they sign up. This also captures the contested nature of feminism and recognises the impossibility of defining *the* feminist approach. But it is worth sketching what the 'shared political and theoretical investments' of feminism might be. Ali identifies the following components[10]:

- a challenge to 'unproblematic understandings of rationality, objectivity and neutrality in research',
- the idea that 'all knowledge is partial and situated',
- the idea that 'all knowledge and its production are political',
- a concern to expose and challenge abuses of power, and
- a 'commitment to collective knowledge production'.

Watts (2006) chooses these criteria[11]:

- 'the power relations between researcher and participants,
- the foregrounding of participants' or subjects' viewpoints,
- a commitment to the group being researched,
- an aim of using the research to improve women's lives, and
- an awareness of the different relation to the production of knowledge between researcher and subjects.'

Neitz sketches the convergences between feminism and the 'cultural turn' in sociology, emphasising 'the movement away from binary categories [that] leads to a more relational conceptualization of the self', which has occurred alongside 'the

---

[7] Lather, Patti, "Issues of Validity in Openly Ideological Research," *Interchange* 17(4), (2006), 63–84, available at: http://web.media.mit.edu/∼kbrennan/mas790/06/Lather,%20Issues%20of%20validity%20in%20openly%20ideological%20research.pdf, accessed 22 December 2011; Wolcott, H.F., "On Seeking – and Rejecting – Validity in Qualitative Research," in Eisner and Peshkin, (eds.) *Qualitative Inquiry in Education: The Continuing Debate* (New York: Teachers College Press, 1990), 121–152.

[8] Cho, Jeasik and Trent, Allen, "Validity in Qualitative Research Revisited," *Qualitative Research* 6, (2006), 319–340, direct quote p 325.

[9] Ali, Suki, "Introduction: Feminist and Postcolonial: Challenging Knowledge," *Ethnic and Racial Studies Special Issue, Feminism and Postcolonialism: Knowledge/Politics* 30 (2007),191–212; Campbell, Kirsten, *Jacques Lacan and Feminist Epistemology* (London: Routledge, 2004), quoted in Ali, "Introduction," 193.

[10] Ali, Suki, "Racializing Research: Managing Power and Politics?" *Ethnic and Racial Studies* 29 (2006), 471–486, direct quote p 472.

[11] Watts, Jacqueline, "The Outsider Within: Dilemmas of Qualitative Feminist Research within a Culture of Resistance," *Qualitative Research* 6 (2006), 385–402, direct quote p 385–386.

political activism associated with what have come to be called the new social movements'.[12] Feminist approaches also include a renewed emphasis on analysing narrative, storytelling, rituals and practices, as well as consideration of how 'relational selves are constituted in performance and narrative'.[13]

In my work, I have found that action and feminist approaches provide the best foundations on which researchers who want to 'make a difference' can build. Although my conception of the 'ethical opportunity' is grounded in these approaches, a deeper analysis of their theoretical and philosophical assumptions is beyond the scope of this chapter. Now, I turn to my three key ways in which social researchers can seize the ethical opportunity when conducting fieldwork in divided and violent societies.

A Plan for Protection — Personal Safety

As a young post-doctoral researcher at the University of Cape Town, I was conducting interviews with people who attended a diverse, charismatic Christian congregation not far from campus. I usually arranged to meet participants at the church, or in their homes, and I rode a bicycle to our meetings. One afternoon, I arranged to meet a woman in her home in a neighbourhood with which I was not familiar. When I arrived at her home, an apartment block, I rang the outside bell corresponding to her flat number. There was no answer.

As I waited, I began to attract unwanted attention. I looked different from most of the people in the neighbourhood, and I had a bag slung over my shoulder that — while only containing papers and my relatively low-tech recording device — was designed to hold a laptop. Several elderly women walking by warned me that I should not be hanging around, but I did not want to break the appointment, so I rang again. Within minutes, a group of young men had surrounded me and one began to tug on my bag, and another knocked over my bicycle. Fortunately for me, at this point a man driving an SUV pulled over and startled the other men, causing them to disperse. The man in the SUV indicated I should jump in, with my bicycle, and while this also did not sound like a great idea (how many times had I been told not to accept a lift from a stranger?), at that point it seemed like my best alternative. The man drove me back to the neighbourhood where the church was located, and all was well.

The first lesson I learned from this experience is to listen to the wisdom of elderly women who warn you that you could be in danger. But I also learned that I had not adequately prepared myself for fieldwork in what is still a divided society, in which personal violence, as opposed to the violence of apartheid, is still common. I had not asked anyone about the particular neighbourhood I was going to

[12] Neitz, Mary Jo, "Gender and Culture: Challenges to the Sociology of Religion," *Sociology of Religion* 65 (2004), 391–402, direct quote p 391.
[13] Neitz, "Gender and Culture," 400.

and I had not told anyone else (housemates, friends, work colleagues) where I was going or when I expected to be back.

As I now know, researchers in divided or violent societies should have a better plan than I did on that day. From then on, I always asked people at the church about the neighbourhood I was travelling to for interviews, told my housemates where I was going and when I expected to be back, and on occasion, even asked them to ring my mobile phone during the time when I was conducting the interview so I could confirm that I was okay. (Yes, this meant briefly interrupting the interview, but I decided I would trade a moment of rudeness for my own peace of mind.) And while the incident described above happened during the day, I also decided I would not travel to interviews after dark on my bicycle – I would either hire a taxi or try to conduct interviews during daylight hours.

It is not uncommon for researchers to have to think on their feet to develop better strategies for their own and others' safety, as described in Belousov et al.'s article on their research on the enforcement of health and safety regulations in the shipping industry in Russia.[14] Shortly into their fieldwork, their key 'gatekeeper', the captain of the port who had agreed to facilitate their work, was assassinated. While Belousov et al. write that his murder did not seem to be linked to their research project, it did raise tensions at the port and make their ability to access research participants much more difficult. Unlike my individual, small-scale project in Cape Town, Belousov et al.'s project had significant funding and employed a research team. So the funders commissioned a professional security firm to undertake a risk assessment before their fieldwork would be allowed to resume after the murder. A list of fieldwork precautions was developed. While such precautions would not apply to every situation, I reproduce them here because I think they are useful for helping other researchers think through steps to take in their own difficult or dangerous contexts[15]:

* work in pairs during fieldwork;
* telephone checks: a phone call leading up to the interview, and after the interview (all field researchers should have mobile telephones);
* introductions: the researchers are employees of the Sociological Institute of the Russian Academy of Sciences, and the research is a confidential academic study and is not of an investigative character;
* during the ship inspections, the researchers must follow all of the instructions given by the inspecting officials;
* close attention should be given to guidance from the inspectors, regarding making your way through the port and ships;
* always have complete documentation on one's person (passes, passports, etc.);
* make clear that the research project is not being extensively advertised, and only a select number of people who are directly involved will have knowledge of it.

---

[14] Belousov, Konstantin, Horlick-Jones, Tom, Bloor, Michael, Gilinsky, Yakov, Golbert, Valentin, Kostikovsky, Yakov, Levi, Michael, and Pentsov, Dmitri, "Any Port in a Storm: Fieldwork Difficulties in Dangerous and Crisis-Ridden Settings," *Qualitative Research*, 7 (2007), 155–175.
[15] Belousov et al., "Any Port in a Storm," 167 (the last six points are quoted verbatim).

My purpose here is not to unduly alarm would-be researchers. On the contrary, I think most of the time researchers in divided and violent contexts are much safer and take far fewer risks than the people who they ask to participate in their projects. Nowadays, I jokingly tell would-be researchers that when conducting research in potentially dangerous settings, they should take the same precautions that they would take when going to see someone they met through an online dating site for the first time. A little common sense goes a long way when it comes to planning your personal safety.

A Plan for Protection – Participants' Safety

In 2007, I conducted fieldwork at a diverse, charismatic congregation in Harare, Zimbabwe. The political situation in Zimbabwe was (and remains) dangerous and precarious, and the country's economy had collapsed. My research concerns were not 'Political' with a capital 'P', in that I was not interested in whether people at this particular church supported the ruling ZANU-PF party and the country's long-time president, Robert Mugabe. Rather, I asked people about their personal faith, their relationships with other people in the congregation from different ethnic backgrounds and what their congregation was doing to respond to the economic collapse and the social and human problems that followed in its wake. Probably inevitably, when some people spoke about their congregation's response to Zimbabwe's deterioration, they spoke about 'politics', at least with a lowercase 'p'. No one named or criticised Mugabe or ZANU-PF directly, but they had views on why Zimbabwe was in the state it was in. I was deeply conscious that the political situation meant that people could be taking a risk by talking to me. I entered the field intending to make the name and location of the congregation anonymous – although the elders and others who participated in the research insisted that I use its name: Mount Pleasant Community Church.[16] They were excited about what their church was doing and they wanted others to know about it and perhaps learn some lessons from it, so this was understandable.

But at the level of individuals, I insisted on protecting people's confidentiality. In the West, we are usually required by our universities or funders to ask research participants to sign a consent form or disclaimer, indicating that the research has been explained to them and that by signing, they are indicating their willingness to take part in it. I did not want to use consent forms, because I knew that when I left Zimbabwe, I did not want a hard copy record of the people who had participated in the research. So, I relied on their verbal consent before beginning the interviews. I did record the interviews, but I made it a point to transcribe and erase the interviews almost immediately, so that a digital record of their voices and what they had said did not survive. When I finished the interview transcriptions (removing any obvious identifying characteristics), I sent an electronic copy to a colleague in

---

[16] The congregation has since changed its name.

Ireland, who stored them for me. I then erased the transcripts of all the interviews from my laptop, just in case this was examined or seized on my way out of Harare. As it happened, my departure from Zimbabwe was without incident. Some of my friends and research participants in Zimbabwe laughed when I described this process to them – they thought me paranoid. But I like to think that others were grateful for my cautiousness and that this helped them to speak more freely.

Most departments or schools within universities now have research ethics committees which must approve social scientific research with human subjects. The existence of such committees, and graduate researchers' awareness that they must submit their research proposals to them, should drive home the importance of having a plan to protect research participants during fieldwork, as I did in Zimbabwe.[17] This plan should include how participants will be protected during research activities such as participant observation and before and after conducting interviews. Ethics committees are especially stringent in evaluating research proposals that include fieldwork with children and vulnerable adults. Because almost all people living in divided and violent societies are taking a risk when they participate in social scientific research, especially if the research is related to the division or the violence itself, the same stringency should be applied to all research in these contexts. My brief description of my work in Zimbabwe illustrates some strategies for protecting the confidentiality of participants, including in the storage of data. Other areas researchers should be especially concerned about are gaining informed consent, preparing to interact with people who have experienced traumatic events and communicating with participants about the research.

To put it simply and bluntly, gaining informed consent means that you do not deceive people about your research subject and your intentions. That it is ethical – and good research practice – to be honest may seem so obvious as to hardly merit writing here. But researchers should be aware that they may be tempted to be vague about their research to gain favour with participants. For instance, it is possible to imagine researchers in Ireland who wish to interview Catholic priests about the impact of the child sexual abuse scandals, introducing their research as about the 'contemporary Irish Catholic Church', without mentioning that the main focus of their work is the scandals. Participants who start a research interview under such pretence could feel deceived when the interview turns out to focus mainly on this subject. The British Sociological Association provides a useful conceptualisation of informed consent in its Statement of Ethical Practice[18] :

> ... [Informed consent] implies a responsibility on the sociologist to explain in appropriate detail, and in terms meaningful to participants, what the research is about, who is undertaking and financing it, why it is being undertaken, and how it is to be disseminated and used.

---

[17] For more on having a plan, including what to do if your data is subpoenaed, see Israel, Mark and Hay, Iain, *Research Ethics for Social Scientists* (London: Sage, 2006).

[18] "Statement of Ethical Practice for the British Sociological Association," paragraphs 16 & 17, available at: http://www.britsoc.co.uk/equality/, accessed 21 December 2011.

*... Research participants should be made aware of their right to refuse partici-
pation whenever and for whatever reason they wish.*

Conducting research in divided and violent societies means that you may, more
often than not depending on the subject matter of your research, be interacting with
people who have experienced traumatic events.[19] Indeed, it is possible that your
research interview can stir up old traumas for people – even if your interview is
not necessarily about division or violence. For example, for a research project on
evangelicalism in Northern Ireland, I had a research assistant conducting interviews
with people who had left the evangelical faith. During one interview, a participant
began to weep as she recalled the traumatic events that had contributed to her leaving her church. In this case, the researcher had contact details available for a counselling hotline, which she provided for the participant.[20]

Research focused on the effect of violence on direct victims and survivors has
even greater potential to re-traumatise participants. Paul Connolly, in a document
titled 'Ethical Principles for Researching Vulnerable Groups,' which he prepared
for Northern Ireland's Office of the First Minister and Deputy First Minister,
recommends considering if people who have experienced severe traumas really
should be interviewed at all. If researchers make the decision that yes, this is the
case; they must devise a plan that includes support arrangements for participants
both during and after the research. Connolly summarises some of the options[21]:

> *The researcher therefore needs to explain their concerns with the participant and
> to discuss with them what arrangements they would like to be made in terms of
> possible support. This could include simply having a friend or relative present in
> the interview or waiting to meet them afterwards.*
>
> *However, it may also mean having suitably trained counsellors available to
> meet them either after the interview or at a later date. At the very least, it should
> include the researcher identifying appropriate support mechanisms and having
> details at hand to pass on to the participant. Overall, such issues need to be dis-
> cussed clearly with each potential participant and arrangements for support
> agreed and set in place before the research begins.*

Finally, researchers should remember it is not their stories that are being told in
the public domain – it is the stories of their participants and these should be treated

---

[19] For a brief discussion of the methodology used in a research project with victims and survivors in Northern
Ireland, see Templer, Sara and Radford, Katy, "Hearing the Voices: Sharing Perspectives in the Victim/
Survivor Sector" (Belfast: Community Relations Council, 2008), 14–15, available at: http://qub.academia.
edu/SaraTempler/Papers/935895/Hearing_the_voices_Sharing_perspectives_in_the_victim_survivor_sector,
accessed 23 December 2011.

[20] Mitchell, Claire and Ganiel, Gladys, *Evangelical Journeys: Choice and Change in a Northern Irish
Religious Subculture* (Dublin: UCD Press, 2011). The research assistant was Sara Templer.

[21] Connolly, Paul, "Ethical Principles for Researching Vulnerable Groups" (Belfast: Office of the First
Minister and Deputy First Minister, 2003) 25, available at: http://www.ofmdfmni.gov.uk/ethicalprinci-
ples.pdf, accessed 21 December 2011.

with respect. Assuming that researchers have built up an adequate level of trust during the research process,[22] when they share drafts of the work and/or publication plans with participants, they build on that trust. Participants should be satisfied that researchers are not simply 'using' them to publicise their research or advance their own careers.

A Plan for Communication and Dissemination

Seizing the ethical opportunity presented by researching in divided and violent societies hinges on researchers' ability to communicate with various audiences. The importance of communication has been noted by Smyth and Robinson[23]:

> *If research is to inform international organisations, policy makers and the public both outside and within divided societies, then the researcher must be able to communicate with integrity in several languages: as a specialist, as a generalist, as an academic, as a populist, as a public speaker, and as a journalist.*

Many researchers, such as Smyth and Darby, emphasise the importance of communicating with policy makers.[24] I agree that this is important, but I think that researchers' priority should be communicating with the participants themselves. After all, it is these people who have given the most of themselves throughout the research, and it is most likely they who have the most to gain and to lose from it. A plan for communication and dissemination with research participants also can guard against a breakdown of relationships with participants after leaving the field.[25] At a minimum, participants should have the opportunity to read and respond to any work based on their input that is going forward for publication, or that will be put in the hands of policy makers. At the risk of stating the obvious,

---

[22] On trust see Brewer, John. D. "Sensitivity as a Problem in Field Research: A Study of Routine Policing in Northern Ireland," in Renzetti, Claire M. and Lee, Raymond (eds.) *Researching Sensitive Topics* (London: Sage, 1993) 125–145; on how building trust relates to researchers managing their own identities in relation to others, see Ganiel, Gladys and Mitchell, Claire, "Turning the Categories Inside-Out: Complex Identifications and Multiple Interactions in Religious Ethnography," *Sociology of Religion* 67(1) (2006), 3–21.

[23] Smyth and Robinson, "Introduction," in Smith and Robinson, (eds.) *Researching Violently Divided Societies*, 6.

[24] Smyth, Marie and Darby, John "Does Research Make Any Difference? The Case of Northern Ireland," in Smyth and Robinson (eds.) *Researching Violently Divided Societies* (London: Pluto Press, 2001), 34–54; See also Schubotz, Dirk, "Beyond the Orange and the Green: The Diversification of the Qualitative Social Research Landscape in Northern Ireland," *Forum: Qualitative Social Research* 6(3) (2005), Art. 29, available at: http://www.qualitative-research.net/index.php/fqs/article/view/11, accessed 23 December 2011.

[25] For a classic ethnographic study with an excellent appendix describing how the researcher interacted with his participants throughout the research process all the way up to the publication of his book – in which the participants shared in the profits – see Duneier, Mitchell, *Sidewalk* (New York: Straus and Giroux, 1999).

when researchers commit to this level of involvement for participants, it takes more time. Researchers must wait for participants to 'get back to them', and may need to revise what they have written to incorporate participants' criticisms and insights. So some strategies for enhancing communication with research participants include:

• Presenting the research to participants at workshops, where they can offer oral feedback (this may not be possible in situations where it is necessary that participants' identities are kept anonymous from other participants).
• In-depth conversations with individual participants.
• Inviting some research participants to help in the 'writing up' of research (this may include shared authorship in newspaper or academic journal articles).
• Sending participants drafts of articles and other publications for comment.
• Agreeing to produce a report for participants that is written in a more accessible form than standard academic work.

Earlier in my career, when sharing research results with participants, I often emailed them only a draft of the academic paper on which I was working. As I quickly realised, people outside of academia do not usually want to read an 8000–10,000 word paper that includes a heavy theoretical section. Even so, in those earlier days, some research participants persisted in reading those papers and provided helpful feedback. In the case of my research on the charismatic congregation in Cape Town, the feedback provided by different participants was at times seemingly contradictory, as illustrated below by examples from two emails I received shortly after the research in 2006:

> *You encapsulated everything well and your conclusions were brilliant and should help our elders to put something in place in 2006 re: leaders training, etc. . . . I am so grateful to God for sending you to us and helping us to open the way for discussion again. Since you left I have been able to have four very meaningful discussions with [an elder] which has opened the way for us to pick up the 'storytelling' component which is so necessary that people from each race group tell their stories and are listened to without interruptions or explanations. Thereafter there needs to be workshops to talk through what we have heard. He is very open to this so I reckon that [our congregation] is now ready for the next, and deeper step, into reconciliation. I am chuffed about this!*

An email like this of course encouraged me, making me think that my results might somehow be used by the congregation to 'make a difference' – to further improve relationships between people of different ethnicities. But this email, from a participant who had left the congregation, cast doubt on that:

> *For me, probably the most important part of the document involves the last paragraph, which acts as a summation of all that was discussed before, and is effectively the 'take home' message. . . I must say that I am surprised at the upbeat tone of the summation. There are some reservations, admittedly, that are made – recognizing that reconciliation has not been 'completely realized' and encouraging*

dialogue, for instance, but it is undeniable that the message is a relatively enthusi-
astic one for the course chosen for the church in question. I am uncertain whether
this is a reflection of the analysis of your data or the push to find a positive mes-
sage in your research that can be exported to other contexts.

After the publication of three academic articles based on my research,[26] some
participants requested that I cease from further publication. Unlike the email above,
in which the participant said he thought my analysis of the congregation's work on
ethnic relations was too 'positive', they thought that it was inappropriate for me to
impose analytical, sociological categories on a Christian organisation. They also
thought I had given too much weight in the analysis to the views of people who
had left the congregation. Out of respect for these participants, I stopped using the
information I had gathered for academic publication. This was of course disappointing for me, especially given my own idealistic hopes that my results would, as
the first email respondent also hoped, be helpful for the congregation. I look back
on this example as a failure of communication on my part, both to explain how
their congregation might appear in an academic publication, and to explain that I
thought that the critiques of others, such as the participants who had left the congregation, could actually help the congregation to improve its (what I actually
thought were already quite good) practices. Balancing participants' expectations
with the analytical demands of academic publication was trickier than I thought it
would be – most social scientists who read my work on this congregation, such as
peer reviewers for journals, wondered if I had been too 'positive' about ethnic relations within it. Indeed, my research on that congregation has provided one of the
few relatively 'positive' examples of a multi-ethnic congregation in the wider literature on charismatic Christianity in Southern Africa.[27]

Since my research in Cape Town, I have refined my practices for communicating
with participants. Now, instead of sending people only an academic article, I also send
a summary of the article, written in more accessible language and without laborious
theoretical discussion. I also alert individuals to particular pages on which quotations
from their interviews are used. This allows people to grasp the content of what I have
written more quickly and easily. Below is a short example from correspondence I sent
to participants in Zimbabwe, in which I raised the issue of lowercase 'p' politics:

Social science research is almost always concerned with politics, but social scien-
tists tend to use a broader definition of politics than other people. When I was in

---

[26] The publications are: Ganiel, Gladys, "Is the Multiracial Congregation an Answer to the Problem of
Race? Comparative Perspectives from South Africa and the USA," *Journal of Religion in Africa* 38
(2008), 263–283; "Religion and Transformation in South Africa? Institutional and Discursive Change
in a Charismatic Congregation," *Transformation: Critical Perspectives on Southern Africa* 63 (2007),
1–22; "Race, Religion and Identity in South Africa: A Case Study of a Charismatic Congregation,"
Nationalism and Ethnic Politics 12(304) (2006), 555–576.

[27] I have written an overview of the literature, see Ganiel, Gladys, "Pentecostal and Charismatic
Christianity in South Africa and Zimbabwe: A Review," *Religion Compass*, 5 (2010), 130–143, available at: http://religion-compass.com/.

Zimbabwe, it seemed to me that people equated politics either with what the gov-ernment was doing, or with what people in opposition groups were doing (such as protesting). However, I think that introducing a broader conception of politics can be useful in helping people in congregations see how what their congregation is doing may have a wider impact. For example, in a context in which political agita-tion may be dangerous or unproductive, engaging in social activities that enable orphans, widows and other marginalized people to begin to feed and clothe them-selves, and become educated, can (eventually) have wider political consequences. Such activities, slowly but surely, address some of the social and economic pro-blems that keep Zimbabweans materially poor and politically marginalized. This is what I would like to emphasize to you from this discussion of politics: what your congregation is doing for widows, orphans, the poor — is important and may even-tually have broader consequences.

One response I received from a participant read:

I was reading your email with one of my 'politically active' friends who found the concept of feeding the poor and caring for widows as one of the most influential forms of being a political activist. I'm glad that you have noticed that in Zimbabwe our emphasis with regards to political issues centres around what the government is or is not doing. ...It is inspiring to note that the little we are doing to impact the lives of the less privileged in our community, is in itself a major contribution to the political process. Lives are changed, poverty datum lines redefined, people realize God's love for them through other people... What an amazing eventuality it can be.

Social Science research on congregations is crucial, we would not have seen some of the things we are doing as good had you not taken your time to research on us.

Again, while I was encouraged by this email, I am not claiming (because I do not have the empirical evidence for it) that this or any other research I have done has made a major difference; either for how the various organisations, con-gregations or individuals think about themselves, or for how they practice their lowercase 'p' politics. In fact, I would say that some of the 'action research' projects my students have taken on for their dissertations have had more direct impacts on the organisations they were working with.[28] But in some of the feed-back that I have received, I find evidence that a small 'difference' has been made, at least for some individuals. As a researcher, it is these glimmers of feedback that give me hope, while at the same time reminding me to manage my own expectations about what social research in divided and violent contexts can actually achieve.

---

[28] Takashima, Keita, "Extending the Effects of Intergroup Contact: An Action Research with Peaceplayers International Northern Ireland," Dissertation submitted for the M.Phil. in Conflict Resolution and Reconciliation (Belfast and Dublin: the Irish School of Ecumenics, Trinity College Dublin, 2011) McCallum, "Living at the Interface."

Conclusion

If researchers want to seize what I have called the 'ethical opportunity' for their research to contribute to peace, justice or socio-political change, they must have a plan — before beginning fieldwork — for protecting participants and themselves. They must remember that individual participants' safety and right to confidentiality are always more important than the findings of a particular project or the advancement of one's career. The rights of individual participants should even trump researchers' desire to get out the message that they, probably rather naïvely, think could 'change the world'. So, I urge would-be researchers to take particular care in planning how they will disseminate and communicate about their research, especially with policy makers and participants. But do not neglect participants at the expense of policy makers. Seizing the 'ethical opportunity' means helping your research participants understand how they themselves can make the changes that can transform the divided and violent societies in which they live.

Bibliography

Ali S. "Introduction: Feminist and Postcolonial: Challenging Knowledge". *Ethnic Racial Stud Spec Issue, Fem Postcolonialism: Knowl Polit* 2007;30:191−212.

Ali S. "Racializing Research: Managing Power and Politics?" *Ethnic Racial Stud* 2006;29:471−86 [direct quote p. 472].

Belousov K, Horlick-Jones T, Bloor M, Gilinsky Y, Golbert V, Kostikovsky Y, et al. "Any Port in a Storm: Fieldwork Difficulties in Dangerous and Crisis-Ridden Settings". *Qual Res* 2007;7:155−75.

Brewer JD. "Sensitivity as a Problem in Field Research: A Study of Routine Policing in Northern Ireland". In: Renzetti CM, Lee R, editors. *Researching Sensitive Topics*. London: Sage; 1993. p. 125−45.

Cho J, Trent A. "Validity in Qualitative Research Revisited". *Qual Res* 2006;6:319−40 [direct quote p. 325].

Costello P. *Effective Action Research: Developing Reflective Thinking and Practice*. London: Continuum; 2011.

Ganiel G, Mitchell C. "Turning the Categories Inside-Out: Complex Identifications and Multiple Interactions in Religious Ethnography". *Sociol Relig* 2006;67(1):3−21.

Ganiel G. "Is the Multiracial Congregation an Answer to the Problem of Race? Comparative Perspectives from South Africa and the USA". *J Relig Afr* 2008;38:263−83.

Ganiel G. "Religion and Transformation in South Africa? Institutional and Discursive Change in a Charismatic Congregation". *Transform Crit Perspect South Afr* 2007;63:1−22.

Ganiel G. "Race, Religion and Identity in South Africa: A Case Study of a Charismatic Congregation". *Natl Ethnic Polit* 2006;12(304):555−76.

Ganiel G. "Pentecostal and Charismatic Christianity in South Africa and Zimbabwe: A Review". *Relig Compass* 2010;5:130−43 <http://religion-compass.com/>.

Israel M, Hay I. *Research Ethics for Social Scientists*. London: Sage; 2006.

Lather P. "Issues of Validity in Openly Ideological Research". *Interchange* 2006;17 (4):63−84 <http://web.media.mit.edu/~kbrennan/mas790/06/Lather,%20Issues%20of %20validity%20in%20openly%20ideological%20research.pdf/>; [accessed 22.12.11].

Lee RM, Stanko EA, editors. *Researching Violence: Essays of Methodology and Measurement.* London: Routledge; 2003.

McCallum R "Living at the Interface: Research in Three Interface Areas of North Belfast." Dissertation submitted for the M.Phil. in Conflict Resolution and Reconciliation. Belfast and Dublin: the Irish School of Ecumenics, Trinity College Dublin; 2011.

McNiff J, Whitehead J. *All You Need to Know About Action Research.* London: Sage; 2011.

Nason-Clark N, Neitz MJ, editors. *Feminist Narratives in the Sociology of Religion.* Walnut Creek: Altamira Press; 2001.

Neitz MJ. "Gender and Culture: Challenges to the Sociology of Religion". *Sociol Relig* 2004;65:391−402 [direct quote p. 391].

Poloma M. *Main Street Mystics: The Toronto Blessing and Reviving Pentecostalism.* Walnut Creek: Altamira Press; 2003. p. 237−57.

Schubotz D. "Beyond the Orange and the Green: The Diversification of the Qualitative Social Research Landscape in Northern Ireland". *Forum: Qual Soc Res* 2005;6(3): Art. 29, <http://www.qualitative-research.net/index.php/fqs/article/view/11/>; [accessed 23.12.11].

Smyth M, Robinson G, editors. *Researching Violently Divided Societies: Ethical and Methodological Issues.* London: Pluto Press; 2001.

Smyth Marie, Darby J. "Does Research Make Any Difference? The Case of Northern Ireland". In: Smyth, Robinson, editors. *Researching Violently Divided Societies.* London: Pluto Press; 2001. p. 34−54.

"Statement of Ethical Practice for the British Sociological Association." Available at: <http://www.britsoc.co.uk/equality/>; [accessed 21.12.11].

Takashima K "Extending the Effects of Intergroup Contact: An Action Research with Peaceplayers International Northern Ireland." Dissertation submitted for the M.Phil. in Conflict Resolution and Reconciliation. Belfast and Dublin: the Irish School of Ecumenics, Trinity College Dublin; 2011.

Templer S, Radford K. *Hearing the Voices: Sharing Perspectives in the Victim/Survivor Sector.* Belfast: Community Relations Council; 2008. p. 14−15, <http://qub.academia. edu/SaraTempler/Papers/935895/ Hearing_the_voices_Sharing_perspectives_in_the_victim_survivor_sector/>, [accessed 23.12.11].

Watts J. "The Outsider Within: Dilemmas of Qualitative Feminist Research within a Culture of Resistance". *Qual Res* 2006;6:385−402 [direct quote p. 385−86].

12 Ethics of Oral Interviews with Children

Elizabeth Nixon

School of Psychology and Children's Research Centre, Trinity College, Dublin, Ireland

Abstract

Changing theoretical conceptions of children and childhood have resulted in a shift in the research agenda towards understanding what it means to be a child. Qualitative interview methods are highly compatible with the research endeavour aimed at understanding unknown aspects of children's worlds, and their role as social actors in their world. The ethical issues associated with conducting interviews with children centre around balancing children's rights to participation and rights to protection from harm and exploitation. Central to balancing these rights is an understanding of the different – not inferior – competencies of children, and of the disparities in power status between children and adults which permeate structures in society and which may be duplicated in the research process. These distinctions form the backdrop to reflecting upon key ethical issues including: how children can be enabled to give informed consent to participate in research, how power dynamics between researchers and young participants may be redressed in the interview setting and how children's well-being and safety can be protected in the interview process.

Key Words

Children, childhood, interviews, children's rights, participation, consent, power dynamics, empowerment, protection, confidentiality

> *The child is familiar to us and yet strange, she/he inhabits our world and yet seems to answer to another, she/he is essentially of ourselves and yet appears to display a different order of being. [1]*

In recent times, there has been increasing recognition of the importance of taking account of children's perspectives on various aspects of their lives. This stands in contrast to the long tradition of research which has been 'about' children rather than

Ethics for Graduate Researchers. DOI: http://dx.doi.org/10.1016/B978-0-12-416049-1.00012-X

'with' children. The increased involvement of children as informants in research has been underpinned by shifts in how childhood and children are conceptualised within psychology, sociology and other disciplines concerned with children's lives, as well as a growing recognition of children's rights to be heard and participate in decisions that affect their lives. Coinciding with these conceptual shifts, researchers' relationships with their child participants and the methods they use to elicit children's experiences have come under increasing scrutiny and like any research with human participants are subject to ethical consideration. This chapter considers the ethical issues involved in conducting research with children. This chapter focuses specifically on the oral interview method, although many of the issues covered equally apply to an array of methods and methodological approaches for conducting research with children.

Changing Conceptions of Children and Childhood

Beginning early in the twentieth century, the scientific study of children and their development became an established field, guided by the work of psychological theorists such as Gesell, Kohlberg and Erikson [2]. Alongside this, sociological and anthropological accounts [3,4] emphasised how cultural and social institutions such as family and school moulded children into socialised beings [5]. These early approaches shared assumptions of the child as an 'object' to be socialised and consequently little attention was paid to children's subjectivity and agency.

Early popular research methodologies for understanding child development included systematic observation and testing, often under controlled laboratory conditions [6]. The agenda behind this was to delineate universal and 'normal' patterns of development and to strip away confounding influences of the environment, thereby exposing the true nature of 'the child'. The use of controlled procedures and standardised measures, where children's performance was often compared to a standard or norm, often based upon a dominant societal group (such as white middle-class Americans) was related to inherent assumptions that childhood is context-free, the essence of the child is isolable and that development is a universal process [7,8]. Developmental researchers adopted an objective stance, whereby their subject of enquiry – the child – was transformed into a de-contextualised and somewhat de-personalised object who is in a state of 'not yet being' [9] as they progressed towards adulthood. Hogan [8] has suggested that an implication arising from this conceptualization of the unformed child as a 'becoming' rather than a 'being'[10] was that children's subjective experiences were deemed to be irrelevant and children were considered as unreliable informants in research. She went on to state:

If childhood is a highly regulated and universal experience, unrelated to historical time and to social contexts, then adults, with their superior capacity for objectivity and more sophisticated understanding, who themselves have been children, can claim to possess expertise on the experiences of any given child. Children's personal experience of events, relationships and everyday life receive little attention, with the result that knowledge about what it is to be a child can scarcely be described within the literature.

Together, these assumptions validated the status of 'expert' adults and endorsed the marginalisation of children's own perspectives in research. The marginalised position of children's views in research is not unique to the research arena, but reflects the broader positioning of children in society. Qvortrup [11] has suggested that children can be characterised as a minority group in relation to adults, while Mayall [12] has argued that children are a distinct social group because they lack adulthood, a lack which is variously characterised in terms of dependency, disadvantage, deficiency and oppression. For example, within families, children have been assigned a position as dependents, under the moral and economic responsibility of their parents [13]. Children are on the receiving end of family values and are seen to belong to their parents, not as autonomous actors, but rather as an extension of their family, reflecting their parents' social status, set of values and models of conduct [14,15]. Children in industrial societies are increasingly served by age-segregated institutions, such as day-care centres, schools, extracurricular activities, paediatric health care services and juvenile courts, such that every age now has its own set of contexts and professionals [16,17]. According to Gillis [16], age segregation is underpinned by assumptions about the innocence and vulnerability of children, which justifies the prescription of special services and contexts for childhood.

Critiques of the developmental paradigm have paralleled the emergence of social studies of childhood or childhood studies. Central to this discipline is the notion that childhood is no longer seen as a natural or universal stage in the life course but rather as a social context of children's lives. The notion of childhood as a social phenomenon is not wholly novel, having been previously written about within pedagogy, philosophy and anthropology [18–21]. Nor has developmental theory and research been devoid of mention of the contextualised child [22,23]. However, the importance of considering the various contexts and historical periods within which development occurs is now deeply entrenched in developmental science. For example, the strategic plan of the Society for Research in Child Development, a professional association with almost 6000 members representative of the various disciplines and professions that contribute to the knowledge of child development, commits to the principle that 'a full understanding of development requires inclusion of cultural, racial, ethnic, national or other contexts as influences on individuals and the families and communities in which they live' [24]. Thus, it is acknowledged that behaviour, which is constructed as 'normal' and reflective of natural and appropriate development, is simply that which corresponds to certain norms and mores of a particular society [25]. Developmental theorists Vygotsky and Bronfenbrenner were particularly significant opponents of the decontextualisation of children and proponents of the view that children must be studied in their own context [7]. Paralleling these developments, sociologists proposed that a view of childhood as a specific and cultural component of many societies, rather than as a natural or universal feature of human groups, represented a central component of an emergent paradigm for the sociology of childhood [26]. In this view, childhood is understood as a social construction [27]:

> There is not one childhood, but many, formed at the intersection of different cultural, social and economic systems, natural and man-made physical environments. Different positions in society produce different experiences.

This tenet emphasises that there is no 'universal child', as traditional models suggested, but rather that childhood is a reality constructed by children as they engage with their social and cultural world.

Related to this is the perspective that children should be viewed as social actors, who play a role in constructing and determining their own social lives, and the lives of those around them, rather than just being passive recipients of adult teaching and influence. This shift to recognising the child as an active agent is well exemplified in the parenting literature. Early approaches to understanding parenting were concerned with the study of parental 'traits', such as warmth, responsiveness and power-assertion and their associations with children's outcomes. This social mould framework [28] was a top-down unidirectional formulation, in which parenting was seen as something that was 'done' to children, as parents 'shaped' their children towards socially and culturally desired outcomes. Little attention was paid to the intervening interaction processes between parent and child whereby this shaping was assumed to happen [29]. Mothers' parenting behaviour in particular was assigned causal responsibility for children's problems as evidenced by the dominant mother-blaming discourse in major clinical journals during the 1970s [30]. Increasingly, however, empirical findings necessitated the generation of new theoretical approaches for understanding parenting. Parent-effect models were expanded to account for child effects on parenting processes, thereby giving rise to a bi-directional conceptualisation of parenting as parents and children interacting as intentional and active agents [31]. Conceptualising children as agents in the functioning of families has opened up new understandings of how co-operation, compliance, discipline, monitoring and conflict are interpreted and negotiated by children and parents [32,33].

These shifts illustrate that notions of childhood as a social construction and of children as agents in the construction and determination of their own lives have been embraced by various academic disciplines concerned with understanding the lives and development of children. Shifting conceptualisations of childhood and children within various academic disciplines are also reflected in policy discourses and within this context, the United Nations (UN) Convention on the Rights of the Child, ratified almost universally, is of major significance. According to Freeman [34], the treaty has been significant because the child is constructed as a subject in his/her own right, rather than as a concern or object of intervention. Particularly relevant to research with children is Article 12, which refers to children's right to express an opinion and to have that opinion taken into account, in any matter or procedure affecting them, in accordance with their age and maturity. Freeman has further suggested that the treaty sets forth expectations that can legitimise policy and programmes and contribute to changing attitudes and actions relating to children's participation in society and in research. Children are now seen as worthy of study in their own right and in relation to matters affecting their everyday lives, and not just in respect of what they will become as adults. These changing assumptions about the nature of childhood and children (known as ontological assumptions) have implications for the research questions that we ask and the methodologies that we adopt to address those questions.

Methods in Research with Children

With childhood conceptualised as socially and culturally constructed and children as agents in the production of their everyday life, the research lens has been somewhat re-directed to reflect a new epistemological agenda. Thus, where in the traditional paradigm research was conducted *on* children, the new paradigm proposes research with children [35], or involving children as research partners [7]. Rather than dealing with children as objects of concern, children become more engaged as active participants in the research process [36]. In this sense, adults attempt to enter into children's worlds to try to understand what it means to be a child and how children experience the world. A central tenet of this approach is the rejection of a long-standing practice where researchers have preferred to ask adult respondents, such as parents or teachers, to report on children's lives, rather than to ask children themselves. Put another way, the best people to provide information on children's perspectives, understandings and experiences are children themselves [37].

A trend towards qualitative approaches to research with children has become increasingly evident. Such open-ended approaches enable researchers to engage with children as competent research participants and collaborative research partners [5]. This is perhaps not surprising as such open-ended approaches are compatible with the goal of understanding how children themselves construe and negotiate their worlds (more so than, e.g. the use of standardized tools, which are typically developed by adults) [38]. There has also been an upsurge in the development of creative and participative methodologies for conducting research with children [36,39,40]. The rationale behind the use of participative approaches is to empower children and young people to generate knowledge about their lives (as opposed to the researcher trying to extract knowledge), while creative approaches employ methods that draw upon imagination and inventive processes, such as drawing, play, storytelling and drama [41].

However, these are by no means the only methods by which we can truly gain access to and understand children's socially and culturally located lives. As Christensen and James [42] have argued, '...to carry out research with children does not necessarily entail adopting different or particular methods'. Ultimately, the choice about what methods to use should be guided by the specific research question to be addressed [38].

Qualitative Interviews as a Window into Children's Lives

The qualitative research interview has become one of the most widely used methods in the new social studies of childhood. Such qualitative research has yielded important insights into an array of topics, including family relationships and family transitions [14,43], experiences of poverty [44] and life at school [45,46]. However, this should not be taken to mean that interviews had never been used in research with children before the emergence of social studies of childhood. Examples of research that have utilised interviews (often of the clinical or structured kind) to uncover some underlying developmental processes are common in developmental psychology. Perhaps one of the most famous interviewers of children was Piaget [47], who derived his groundbreaking theory on children's thinking on the basis of interviews and observation of children at play and engaged in logical and scientific tasks. As Woodhead and Faulkner [6] have described, Piaget's innovative use of the clinical interview method enabled children to freely express themselves as they worked through various problems, thereby revealing their thinking processes to the researcher.

Another important area of research that has relied heavily upon the interview method with children is that of eyewitness memory and investigative interviewing [48]. This research was primarily concerned with ascertaining children's ability to recall events that happened to them (most often abuse) and more specifically the reliability of their reports. This research was implicitly underpinned by a model of the child as an unreliable informant. The findings of these studies are instructive to researchers who use interviews in their research with children. Bruck, Ceci and Hembrooke [49] concluded that children are competent in providing accurate, detailed and valid accounts of events provided they are not influenced by suggestive interviewing techniques. Young children are more susceptible to suggestibility when interviewed by an adult than by a peer, and are more likely to be swayed when interviewed by an authority figure or adult with high prestige [50,51]. Bruck and colleagues [49] suggested that within the context of disclosure of child abuse, children are competent witnesses with the potential to provide important evidence so long as they are interviewed under appropriate circumstances.

Thus, while it is acknowledged that children may have different competencies to adults, this does not mean that their knowledge and competencies should be considered inferior to adults' [52]. Findings on children's eyewitness memory challenge the idea that children provide unreliable accounts of events or their own experiences, and importantly, bolster the argument that children have important contributions to make to research. Moreover, a series of studies by Waterman and colleagues in which children were asked nonsensical closed and open questions has indicated the type of questions that may work best when interviewing children. They found that children were more likely to answer closed nonsensical questions (requiring a yes/no response) (e.g. Is a jumpier angrier than a tree?) than open questions (e.g. What do feet have for breakfast?). If the nonsensical question required the children to generate their own response (an open question), the majority of the children indicated that they did not understand. In the case of closed nonsensical questions, however, most children gave a yes or no response rather than indicating uncertainty. But when children were asked to elaborate upon the reason for their yes or no response, the researchers discovered that many children had used the no response to indicate that they thought the question was silly or that they were unable to answer it. The authors concluded that question format may have a strong effect on children's tendency to admit when they cannot answer the question and cautioned that interviewers should use open questions whenever possible [53]. The implications of this research for those interviewing children are clear: it is incumbent upon us to closely attend to our style of questioning to take account of children's suggestibility, language use and conceptual meanings to enable them to generate a narrative that adequately captures their own concerns and experiences.

Ethical Considerations for Conducting Interviews with Children

The ethics of conducting interviews with children are centred on balancing the child's right to protection from exploitation (enshrined in Article 19 of UNCRC) with the child's right to participation and right to freedom of expression (enshrined in Articles 12 and 13 of the UNCRC). Of course, how researchers balance these rights is inherent to all research processes, regardless of the age or developmental status of participants. Furthermore, ethical principles underpin all stages of the research process, not just at the point of contact with potential participants [54]. Alderson and Morrow [55] proposed that 'ethical questions are woven through every aspect of the research, shaping the methods and findings'. Here, I consider ethical issues pertaining to interviewing children as part of the data collection phase of the research, though they may equally apply to stages of choosing a research topic, design, data analysis and dissemination of findings.

While there are pitfalls in over-emphasising distinctions between children and adults (indeed, previously this resulted in the marginalisation of children's voices from research altogether), an acknowledgement of how children and adults differ is vital to ensuring their rights are protected [56]. In addition to distinctions from adults, 'children' themselves are highly a differentiated group (as are 'adults'). They vary widely in their cognitive, linguistic, emotional competencies, attention span and life experiences. Other characteristics that differentiate children may include gender, age, ethnicity, social class and presence of illness/disability. Depending upon these competencies and other characteristics, children's understanding of what research is, what their participation in the research will entail and what will happen with the information that is generated in the course of the research is likely to vary. This variation has important implications for researchers trying to secure informed consent.

A second important distinction between adults and children relates to children's status within the institutions where they typically participate in research (and within society more generally). Relative to adults, children have less power, and their sub-ordinate position is accentuated by the hierarchical and adult-led organisation of the majority of institutions within which children are researched (such as childcare, education or health care settings). Even within the family, the distribution of power is asymmetrical [31]. Punch [57, p. 324] suggests that 'children are used to having much of their lives dominated by adults, they tend to expect adults' power over them and they are not used to being treated as equals by adults'. So what are the implications of this for the adult researcher going into a school setting to interview children? Will children perceive the researcher to be like any other adult they encounter in the school setting — one vested with authority and who they should respect and obey? And is it possible for the researcher to overcome this so that researcher and participant are on an equal footing? Do children have any power and how might they exercise this power? At the very least, this differential power status needs to be acknowledged so that efforts to address the imbalance can begin.

Together assumptions of differential competencies and diminished power status mean that children are perceived as vulnerable and in need of special protection in the research process. This is also true of many 'disempowered' groups, such as individuals with disabilities, mental health problems or literacy difficulties, refugees, and asylum seekers and so on. These distinctions in terms of competencies and status form the backdrop to reflecting upon the ethics of conducting interviews with children. Central to these ethical reflections are questions of consent and choice, power dynamics and protection from harm in the interview setting.

Consent and Choice

Concern about enabling child participants to make an informed choice about whether to participate has predominated discussion about the ethics of doing research with children and much of what has been written about consent relates to consent about medical treatment [54,55]. Some guidelines refer to assent, rather than consent, where it is assumed that children cannot give legally valid consent until they are aged 18. According to Alderson and Morrow [55], assent refers to agreement by children who understand some but not all of the issues required for consent. These authors question whether a decision based on partial understanding counts as a decision at all. Instead, they suggest that children who are 'Gillick competent' to make decisions are giving consent/refusing consent, rather than assent. 'Gillick competence' (so named after a landmark case in England) is used to decide whether a child 16 years or younger is able to consent to his or her own medical treatment, without the need for parental permission or knowledge.

Researching children's experiences necessarily involves negotiating the nature (e.g. location, duration and activity) of the researcher—child contact with adult gatekeepers, as well as with children themselves. Researchers need the informed consent of a parent or guardian of a child before the child can be invited to partici-pate in research. This may give rise to tensions, in the event of parents refusing consent for their children despite their children's desire to participate. Alternatively, parents may pressurise children to participate, when children themselves have no real motivation or interest [40]. The following are the questions that need to be answered, in order for potential participants and adult gatekeepers to give informed consent.

- What is the research about?
- What will taking part entail – what is being asked of them in terms of time and effort required?
- What will happen to the information that is collected – Who will have access to it? Who will know that they contributed information to the research? Will their data be anonymous?
- Will they be told anything about the results?
- Will the information they provide be confidential, and if not, what information will be shared and under what circumstances?
- If they decide to take part, can they later change their mind and withdraw their consent?
- If they decide not to take part, do they understand that this will not impact upon services that they receive?
- Will participants receive payment/gift for their participation?
- Do participants have information which will enable them to follow up with the research team afterwards, if they wish to comment, question, complain or seek support around any issues that emerged?

The manner in which this information is communicated to children and young people is central – unless the information is accessible, efforts to secure consent are meaningless. The use of convoluted and technical research terms should be carefully considered, if not abandoned altogether, not only because such terms may be incomprehensible to potential participants but also because they may exacerbate existing power differentials between researchers and participants. Children's rights to confidentiality and the limits to those rights must be clearly communicated as part of the consent process. Boundaries to confidentiality have received particular attention due to the potential that children may reveal something that indicates their safety or well-being is at risk in some way [58]. Furthermore, the nature of the qualitative interview setting may render such disclosures more probable [59]. It is generally agreed that necessary follow-up on any revelations deemed to constitute abuse or risk of harm should be discussed with the child before any action is taken [55,56].

Consent is also an ongoing process, not just something to be 'gotten out of the way' at the beginning. New and unanticipated questions in relation to the research may emerge at any time. As a result, the researcher needs to consider consent as a contract between the participant and the researcher, and as such something that is open to renewal, termination or negotiation throughout. A freely given 'no' may trouble a researcher, but could also be interpreted as a sign that the processes of providing information and seeking informed consent have been effective. Finally, a child may consent to be interviewed, but then be non-communicative in the interview as a means of withdrawing their consent to participate [56].

Alderson and Morrow [55] proposed that researchers working with children should move to a conceptualisation of consent as a process based on enabling children's understanding through a two-way exchange of information, rather than a view of consent as an event, based on testing children's static knowledge through a one-way communication of 'facts'. Furthermore, this process must accommodate to the needs of children, especially those with learning, reading or sensory disabilities, or who use another first language.

Power Dynamics in the Interview Setting

The disparities in power status between children and adults which permeate structures in society are also replicated in the researcher relationship [60]. What actions can the researcher take to diminish this differential power status? Is it possible to ever diminish one's status as an adult, and is it even desirable? Mandell [61] has advocated adopting the least adult role which focuses on minimising differences between children and adults, and entails casting aside all adult-like characteristics except physical size. Similarly, in her research with children in schools, Thorne [62] described the adoption of the least adult role, where she attempted to blend into their social world by occupying a position somewhere between their adult authority figures (teachers) and the children she was observing. James, Jenks and Prout [63] have argued that 'it is not possible for adults to pass unnoticed in the company of children – age, size and authority always intervene... However friendly we are or however small, we can only ever have a semi-participatory role in children's lives'. They also suggested that facing up to these inevitable differences between adults and children may enable the researcher to adopt the 'middle ground of semi-participant or friend'. However, one must also question whether it is desirable or ethical to adopt a friend-like relationship with participants. After all, friendship is based on a relationship between equals, and it may be disingenuous to suggest that the relationship between researcher and research participants is equal. James et al. [63, p. 189–190] themselves concede this point:

> To be friends with children – the role adopted by many researchers – is from the children's point of view a potentially uncertain and disruptive action. It leaves many questions unanswered. Who is this woman? What does she want and why does she want it from us? What book is she writing and why can't our names be in it? Children may be rightly suspicious or cautious.

Children may feel uneasy with any attempt by a strange adult to befriend them – after all, babies are adaptively and instinctively programmed to exhibit stranger anxiety, and children are instructed from a young age to be wary and not talk to friendly strangers. It behoves us then to reflect upon how we as 'strange adults' may be perceived by our child participants. Small actions on the part of the researcher may go some way towards empowering a young person to say 'no' to participating in research or to opt out of responding to particular questions in an interview setting. These may include actions such as dressing informally (to distinguish oneself from other adult figures in the setting), avoiding titles such as Dr., Ms. or Mr., sitting at eye level, not too close and not too distant, and generally displaying a friendly and approachable demeanour. Another mechanism by which the power imbalance between child participant and adult researcher could be redressed might involve allowing the child greater control to set the agenda. This might include enabling the child to decide where and when the interview takes place, or who else might be present. Practically, however, these factors may have to be determined by or negotiated with gatekeepers.

Notwithstanding these efforts to minimise power differentials, the interview setting may pose additional challenges in terms of establishing a less vertical power hierarchy. It could be argued that this is more so the case with interviews than with other methods, such as naturalistic observation where the researcher watches and takes note as children's naturally occurring activities unfold. Interviews often proceed in a question-and-answer exchange of information, although interviews do vary considerably in the extent to which they are structured by the researcher [64]. Most common are semi-structured interviews, in which set questions and prompts around specific topics are used, while at the same time, giving space for participants to generate their own narratives and develop their ideas. The structure of interviews generally militates against equal statuses, as adults usually set the agenda. Also, when children are typically questioned by non-parental adults, they are under conditions of examination (such as at school or when they see a health professional). As a result, children may draw upon these experiences to guide their behaviour in the interview setting. They may say what they think the researcher wants to hear, or may fear giving what is perceived as an 'incorrect' response. Reassurances such as 'this is not a test' and 'I am only interested in your ideas, and there are no right or wrong answers', and expressing genuine interest in what they have to say may go some way towards challenging children's preconceptions about question-and-answer exchanges with adults. Lewis [65] has similarly suggested that the researcher could stress to the child that he/she knows more about the issue/event than the researcher does, to counter the child's assumption that the adult already knows the answer. In this way, the child is positioned as an expert. Further suggestions from Lewis and drawing upon some of the literature previously alluded to include encouraging 'don't know' responses and requests for clarification. Avoiding repeat questions is also suggested as children may interpret a repeated question as one that was incorrectly responded to the first time. Closed questions (those that demand a yes/no response) may also give rise to responses even when children do not understand the question or do not know a response to a question [65].

Often methods that are used to redress the power imbalance are considered under the label 'rapport building'. Punch [57] has suggested that it is a mistake to assume that all adults have the skills to build rapport with children, and some researchers may feel uncomfortable with establishing camaraderie with young participants. Some authors endorse the use of activities and props, such as drawing, puppets/dolls, photographs, diaries and worksheets, to supplement the interview and help put the child at ease [42,66]. The assumptions underpinning the use of these approaches are worth considering: children find these methods fun and inter- esting, they sustain children's attention and children may be more accustomed to using visual and written techniques for communication, rather than relying solely upon verbal exchanges. These methods may draw upon children's competencies and customary tools for communicating ideas. Furthermore, the attention of researcher and participant may be centred on the tool, rather than on each other, thus alleviating some of the power imbalance inherent in the research- er–participant relationship. But do these methods always work in the manner that is expected and do they yield useful data? As highlighted by Punch [57, p. 330]:

> ...These task-based methods can enable children to feel more comfortable with an adult researcher. The problem with using innovative techniques is that the benefits and drawbacks of using them are not always scrutinized. A reflexive and critical approach is needed to recognize their disadvantages and limits, as well as the rea- sons for using them.

Not all children will feel comfortable with these tools, and their use may inhibit rather than encourage expression, and may undermine efforts to address power imbalances. As previously highlighted, children are not homogeneous and the abil- ity to be flexible and adapt to the needs of different children and different contexts is an important skill for the researcher. Furthermore, we should be cautious in assuming that age or developmental status is the only difference between an adult researcher and a child participant. Other differences, such as gender, ethnicity or where one comes from may also be significant sources of power disparities [60].

Interviewing children in a group format may be another way to impact upon the power imbalance inherent in the individual interview setting. Children may feel more comfortable in the presence of their peers, and may not feel pressure to respond to every question. On the other hand, interviewing in a group setting gives rise to questions about how the confidentiality of the participants' perspectives and experiences can be respected. Hennessy and Heary [67] have highlighted two ethi- cal issues specific to focus group methods. The first is concerned with the height- ened risk of disclosure of individual's personal information outside the group setting. To address this, children may be requested not to disclose the content of the group discussion to non-participants, although this should not preclude children from seeking support with a trusted adult after the focus group, if necessary. In advance of the group, participants should also be advised of the possibility that the content of the focus group discussion might be disclosed to non-participants [68]. The second issue is concerned with how children may be emotionally affected by the opinions or disclosures of other individuals in the group. Thus, it is incumbent upon the researcher to monitor stress levels of participants and to intervene when necessary. Overall, while group interviews may go some way towards redressing the vertical adult–child power dynamic, they may not be appropriate for all research questions, specifically research that requires participants to disclose sensi- tive information.

Protection from Harm

Assessment and declaration of the possible risks which may arise as a result of being interviewed is a central ethical consideration. The risks most commonly associated with interviews involve risk of distress, anxiety, loss of self-esteem or embarrassment [55]. It may not be possible to determine all risks beforehand or to anticipate what might cause distress or who might become distressed – what is innocuous to one person or in one context may not be to another person or in another context. These possibilities highlight the need to be alert and sensitive to participants' emotional responses during the interview process and to gauge the appropriateness of pursuing particular lines of enquiry.

Children can also be protected from potential harm within the research process through opening up the private space of the interview to other individuals. This may result in interviews being conducted in a group setting, as opposed to individuals, as discussed in the previous section. Parents or other gatekeepers may also request to sit in during the interview with the child, and for some children, the presence of a trusted adult may make them feel more comfortable in the interview setting. Parents may supplement their children's replies and help their children develop their narratives, yielding a richer account of their experiences. However, children may also feel more constrained in what they say, or may become compliant or prone to suggestibility in their responses. Thus, while protection is important, over-protection can lead to children's voices being silenced within the research. Their right to protection must be balanced with their right to privacy and right to participate and express their opinion freely. The following example from a colleague's research on children's experiences of parental separation illustrates the potential impact of parental presence in an interview [69]. In this extract, the interviewer is talking to a 9-year-old girl about the frequency with which she sees her non-resident father.

> *Researcher:* Do you see other people in the family? Like your dad?
> *Child:* Yes, I see me dad ... they (siblings) don't see him but I see me da.
> *Researcher:* How often would you see him?
> *Child:* How often do I see him, ma? *[Defers to mother]*
> *Mother:* Once a month, every six weeks.
> *Child:* Every six ... no...every, every week.
> *Mother:* [Child's name] that's telling a lie. You don't see your daddy every week. How long is it since you seen him? ... when he came back from Spain and that was in October.
> *Child:* Yes... October.
> *Mother:* ... she sees him about every six weeks ...if she's lucky.
> *[Researcher note: Child becomes quiet for a while after this exchange...]*

In this exchange, the mother's reprimand of the child's response may have resulted in the child feeling that she was not responding in a 'correct' manner to the researcher's questions and she may have felt disempowered within the interview process. The presence of the parent in this example interfered with the child's right to speak autonomously about her experiences.

Conclusion

The ethics of interviewing children requires a careful balance between enabling children's meaningful participation while at the same time ensuring that their well-being is protected within the research process. Somewhat paradoxically, the conceptualisation of children as competent social actors across many disciplines, which has given a welcome rise to children's participation in research, is not always reflected in the research process. A protectionist discourse continues to pervade, where children are positioned as vulnerable and as occupying a subordinate power position within the research process. While protection is of paramount importance, over-protection can lead to the exclusion of children from research, or within research, the silencing of their voices. Children's vulnerabilities and subordinate power position are not insurmountable barriers to children's participation. Appropriate participation is possible and worthwhile, through a reflexive, sensitive and flexible engagement among the research community, children and young people, and adult gatekeepers.

References

[1] Jenks C. *The Sociology of Childhood. Essential Reading.* London: Batsford; 1982.
[2] Woodhead M. "Child Development and the Development of Childhood". In: Qvortrup J, Corsaro W, Honig MS, editors. *The Palgrave Handbook of Childhood Studies.* London: Palgrave Macmillan; 2009. p. 46–61.
[3] Denzin N. *Childhood Socialization.* San Francisco, CA: Jossey-Bass; 1977.
[4] Whiting J, Child I. *Child Training and Personality: A Cross-Cultural Study.* New Haven, CT: Yale University Press; 1953.
[5] Christensen P, Prout A. "Anthropological and Sociological Perspectives on the Study of Children". In: Greene S, Hogan D, editors. *Researching Children's Experience.* London: Sage; 2005. p. 42–60.
[6] Woodhead M, Faulkner D. "Subjects, Objects or Participants? Dilemmas of Psychological Research with Children". In: Christensen P, James A, editors. *Research with Children. Perspectives and Practices.* London: Falmer; 2000. p. 9–35.
[7] Hogan D. "Valuing the Child in Research: Historical and Current Influences on Research Methodology with Children". In: Hogan D, Gilligan R, editors. *Researching Children's Experiences: Qualitative Approaches.* Dublin: The Children's Research Centre; 1998. p. 1–9.
[8] Hogan D. "Researching the 'Child' in Developmental Psychology". In: Greene S, Hogan D, editors. *Researching Children's Experience.* London: Sage; 2005. p. 22–41.
[9] Verhellen E. *Convention on the Rights of the Child.* Leuven: Garant Publishers; 1997.
[10] Morss J. *Growing Critical: Alternatives to Developmental Psychology.* London: Routledge; 1996.
[11] Qvortrup J. "Introduction". In: Qvortrup J, Bardy M, Sgritt G, Wintersberger H, editors. *Childhood Matters: Social Theory, Practice and Politics.* Aldershow: Averbury; 1994. p. 1–23.
[12] Mayall B. *Children's Childhoods: Observed and Experienced.* London: Falmer; 1994.

[13] Brannen J. "Reconsidering Children and Childhood: Sociological and Policy Perspectives". In: Silva E, Smart C, editors. *The New Family?* London: Sage; 1999. p. 143–58.

[14] Smart C, Neale B, Wade A. *The Changing Experience of Childhood. Families and Divorce.* Oxford: Polity; 2001.

[15] Makrinioti D. "Conceptualisation of Childhood in a Welfare State: A Critical Re-Appraisal". In: Qvortrup J, Bardy M, Sgritta G, Wintersberger H, editors. *Childhood Matters: Social Theory, Practice and Politics.* Aldershot: Avebury; 1994. p. 267–83.

[16] Gillis J. "Transitions to Modernity". In: Qvortrup J, Corsaro W, Honig MS, editors. *The Palgrave Handbook of Childhood Studies.* London: Palgrave Macmillan; 2009. p. 114–26.

[17] Zeiher H. "Institutionalization as a Secular Trend". In: Qvortrup J, Corsaro W, Honig MS, editors. *The Palgrave Handbook of Childhood Studies.* London: Palgrave Macmillan; 2009. p. 127–39.

[18] Ariès P. *Centuries of Childhood.* London: Jonathan Cape; 1962.

[19] Hardman C. "Can there be an Anthropology of Children?" *J Anthropol Soc Oxf* 1973;4:85–99.

[20] Mead M. *Culture and Commitment: The New Relationships between the Generations in the 1970s.* New York, NY: Columbia University Press; 1978.

[21] Zelizer V. *Pricing the Priceless Child. The Changing Social Value of Children.* New York, NY: Basic Books; 1985.

[22] Bronfenbrenner U. *The Ecology of Human Development: Experiments by Nature and Design.* Cambridge, MA: Harvard University Press; 1979.

[23] Kessen W. "The American Child and Other Cultural Inventions". *Am Psychol* 1979;34:810–5.

[24] Society for Research in Child Development. "The Society for Research on Child Development Strategic Plan," <www.srcd.org/>; 2005.

[25] Greene S. *The Psychological Development of Girls and Women. Rethinking Change in Time.* London: Routledge; 2003.

[26] Prout Alan, Allison J. "A New Paradigm for the Sociology of Childhood? Provenance, Promise and Problems". In: James A, Prout A, editors. *Constructing and Reconstructing Childhood.* 2nd ed. London: Falmer; 1997. p. 7–33.

[27] Frønes I. "Changing Childhood". *Childhood* 1993;1:1.

[28] Hartup W. "Perspectives on Child and Family Interaction: Past, Present and Future". In: Lerner R, Spanier G, editors. *Child Influences on Marital and Family Interaction: A Life-Span Perspective.* New York, NY: Academic Press; 1978. p. 23–45.

[29] Maccoby E. "Dynamic Viewpoints on Parent–Child Relations – their Implications for Socialization Processes". In: Kuczynski L, editor. *Handbook of Dynamics in Parent–Child Relations.* Thousand Oaks, CA: Sage; 2003. p. 439–52.

[30] Caplan P, Hall-McCorquodale I. "Mother Blaming in Major Clinical Journals". *Am J Orthopsychiatry* 1985;55:345–53.

[31] Kuczynski L. "Beyond Bidirectionality. Bilateral Conceptual Frameworks for Understanding Dynamics in Parent–Child Relations". In: Kuczynski L, editor. *Handbook of Dynamics in Parent–Child Relations.* Thousand Oaks, CA: Sage; 2003. p. 3–24.

[32] Stattin H, Kerr M. "Parental Monitoring: A Reinterpretation". *Child Dev* 2000;71:1072–85.

[33] Kuczynski Leon, Kochanska G. "The Development of Children's Non-Compliance Strategies from Toddlerhood to Age 5". *Dev Psychol* 1990;26:398–408.

[34] Freeman M. "Children's Rights as Human Rights: Reading the UNCRC". In: Qvortrup J, Corsaro W, Honig MS, editors. *The Palgrave Handbook of Childhood Studies*. London: Palgrave Macmillan; 2009. p. 377−93.

[35] Mayall B. "Conversations with Children: Working with Generational Issues". In: Christensen P, James A, editors. *Research with Children. Perspectives and Practices*. London: Falmer; 2000. p. 120−35.

[36] O'Kane C. "The Development of Participatory Techniques: Facilitating Children's Views about Decisions which Affect them". In: Christensen P, James A, editors. *Research with Children. Perspectives and Practices*. London: Falmer; 2000. p. 136−59.

[37] Scott J. "Children as Respondents: the Challenge for Quantitative Methods". In: Christensen P, James A, editors. *Research with Children. Perspectives and Practices*. London: Falmer; 2000. p. 99−119.

[38] Greene S, Hill M. "Researching children's experience: Methods and methodological issues". In: Greene S, Hogan D, editors. *Researching Children's Experience*. London: Sage; 2005. p. 1−21.

[39] Alderson P. "Research by Children". *Int J Soc Res Methodol* 2001;4:139−53.

[40] Kellett M. "Children as Active Researchers: A New Paradigm for the 21st Century?" *National Centre for Research Methods Review Papers/003* 2005;: <eprints.ncrm.ac. uk/87/1/MethodsReviewPaperNCRM-003.pdf>.

[41] Veale A. "Creative Methodologies in Participatory Research with Children". In: Greene S, Hogan D, editors. *Researching Children's Experience*. London: Sage; 2005. p. 253−72.

[42] Christensen P, Allison J. *Research with children: perspectives and practices*. London: Falmer Press; 2000.

[43] Nixon E, Greene S, Hogan D. "Negotiating Relationships in Single-Parent Households: Children's and Mothers' Perspectives". *Fam Relat* 2012;61:142−56.

[44] Ridge T. "The Everyday Costs of Poverty in Childhood: A Review of Qualitative Research Exploring the Lives and Experiences of Low-Income Children in the UK". *Child Soc* 2011;25:73−84.

[45] Christensen P, Allison J. "What are Schools for? The Temporal Experience of Children's Learning in Northern England". In: Alanen L, Mayall B, editors. *Conceptualizing Child−Adult Relations*. London: Falmer Press; 2001. p. 70−85.

[46] Mayall B. "Understanding Childhoods: a London Study". In: Alanen L, Mayall B, editors. *Conceptualizing Child−Adult Relations*. London: Falmer; 2001. p. 114−28.

[47] Piaget J. *The Moral Judgement of the Child*. London: Routledge and Kegan Paul; 1975.

[48] Westcott H, Davies G, Bull R. *Children's Testimony: A Handbook of Psychological Research and Forensic Practice*. Chichester: Wiley; 2002.

[49] Bruck M, Ceci S, Hembrooke H. "Reliability and Credibility of Young Children's Reports". *Am Psychol* 1998;53:136−51.

[50] Ceci S, Ross D, Toglia M. "Age Differences in Suggestibility: Psycholegal Implications". *J Exp Psychol [Gen]* 1987;117:38−49.

[51] Tobey A. "Children's Eyewitness Memory: Effects of Participation and Forensic Context". *Child Abuse Neglect* 1992;16:779−96.

[52] Solberg A. "The Challenge in Child research from 'Being' to 'Doing'". In: Branner J, O'Brien M, editors. *Children in Families: Research and Policy*. London: Falmer; 1996. p. 53−65.

[53] Waterman A, Blades M, Spencer C. "Is a Jumper Angrier than a Tree?" *Psychologist* 2001;14:474−7.

[54] Morrow V, Richards M. "The Ethics of Social Research with Children: An Overview". *Child Soc* 1996;10:90−105.

[55] Alderson P, Morrow V. *The Ethics of Research with Children and Young People.* London: Sage; 2011.

[56] Hill M. "Ethical Considerations in Researching Children's Experiences". In: Greene S, Hogan D, editors. *Researching Children's Experience.* London: Sage; 2005. p. 61−81.

[57] Punch S. "Research with Children: The Same or Different from Research with Adults?" *Childhood* 2002;9:321−41.

[58] Kirk S. "Methodological and Ethical Issues in Conducting Qualitative Research with Children and Young People: A Literature Review". *Int J Nurs Stud* 2007;44:1250−60.

[59] Duncan R, Drew S, Hodgson J, Sawyer S. "Is my Mum Going to Hear This? Methodological and Ethical Challenges in Qualitative Health Research with Young People". *Soc Sci Med* 2009;69:1691−999.

[60] Harden J, Scott S, Backett-Millburn K, Jackson S. "Can't Talk, Won't Talk? Methodological Issues in Researching Children." In: Sociol Res Online 5, <socresonline.org.uk/5/2/harden.html/>.

[61] Mandell N. "The Least Adult Role in Studying Children". In: Waksler F, editor. *Studying the Social Worlds of Children.* Basingstoke: Falmer; 1991. p. 38−59.

[62] Thorne B. *Gender Play: Girls and Boys in School.* Buckingham: Open University Press; 1993.

[63] James A, Jenks C, Prout A. *Theorizing Childhood.* Cambridge, MA: Polity Press; 1998.

[64] Grieg A, Taylor J, MacKay T. *Doing Research with Children.* 2nd ed. London: Sage; 2007.

[65] Lewis A. "'And when did you last see your Father?' Exploring the View of Children with Learning Difficulties/Disabilities". *Br J Spec Educ* 2004;31:3−9.

[66] Westcott H, Littleton K. "Exploring Meaning in Interviews with Children". In: Greene S, Hogan D, editors. *Researching Children's Experience.* London: Sage; 2005. p. 141−57.

[67] Hennessy E, Heary C. "Exploring Children's Views through Focus Groups". In: Greene S, Hogan D, editors. *Researching Children's Experience.* London: Sage; 2005. p. 236−51.

[68] Smith M. "Ethics in Focus Groups: A Few Concerns". *Qual Health Res* 1995;5:478−86.

[69] Halpenny AM. "Children's Perceptions of Closeness and Security in Relationships with Parents Following Parental Separation," PhD dissertation, Trinity College Dublin; 2005.

Section 4

Emerging Debates and Future Prospects

Linda Hogan

University of Dublin, Trinity College, Dublin, Ireland

plus ça change, plus c'est la même chose

Abstract

Section 4 reflects on the manner in which research ethics is constantly changing. It discusses the influence of the social, cultural and scientific context in which research is pursued. It ends with a discussion of the deliberative and pluralist context in which ethical reflection occurs.

Key Words

Social justice, distributive justice, deliberative democracy, public reason, pluralism

As one reflects on the emerging debates in research ethics, one can recognise the wisdom of the adage that the more things change, the more things stay the same. Research is an inherently dynamic activity, and its successes are critical to the economic, social and political well-being of individuals and communities worldwide. Yet, even as major innovations in research continue to be announced, especially in science and technology, many of the fundamental ethical issues persist. Historically, the major issues of concern have revolved around three main themes: the nature and purpose of research, with a specific concern for the balancing of benefits and harm; the status and treatment of research subjects, including the nature of consent required and the treatment of vulnerable subjects; and the conduct of research, including the ownership and use of research outcomes, as well as issues of confidentiality and privacy. More recently, two further themes have emerged in research ethics. The first relates to issues of social justice and the

Ethics for Graduate Researchers. DOI: http://dx.doi.org/10.1016/B978-0-12-416049-1.00033-7

distribution of the benefits of research, and often arises in relation to whether research participants are in a position to gain from the outcomes of the research to which they have contributed. It is a particular issue of concern for researchers involved in clinical trials in vulnerable populations.[1] The second relates to the role of research in a globalised society, and specifically whether and how social responsibility and accountability can be achieved.

New developments in science and technology also give rise to what appear to be new ethical dilemmas involving new questions and new subjects. The fields of nanoscience and information technology are especially likely to throw up ethical questions with which we have heretofore not had to contend. Recent debates in reproductive technology, genetics and nanotechnology provide multiple examples of the ways in which technological advancements are raising fundamental questions about how human beings understand themselves and their world. In this section, Hille Haker's chapter on synthetic biology provides a careful analysis of some of the emerging issues in this field, and discusses some of the concerns for the governance of such research in the European context. Of course, many of these fundamental issues are not new, but rather appear in more acute forms, with these new technologies. For example, embryonic stem-cell research and therapies such as germ-line gene therapy raise again the fundamental and much debated issue of the moral status of the embryo[2] and of the ethical limits of enhancement.[3] In recent years, disability advocates have added their voices to this debate, with many arguing against what they regard as an emerging perfectionism in society, driven by scientific advancement, and which ultimately further disadvantages those whose 'disabilities' cannot be overcome through such interventions.[4] These new technologies have also re-opened the debate about the problematic of consent in research ethics, because with many of the new interventions, the subjects most affected by the technology, namely unborn siblings or future generations, have no voice in the process of seeking consent.[5] Beyond these specific issues, moreover, are more fundamental questions about the role of science in society and the extent to which its practices can and should be governed.

In addition to the ethical issues that arise from the research itself, new methodologies and new modes of working also have an impact on the emerging issues in

---

[1] See Farmer, Paul, *Pathologies of Power: Health, Human Rights and the New War on the Poor* (Berkeley, University of California Press, 2005) and World Health Organisation (WHO), UNAIDS, UNICEF *Towards Universal Access: Scaling up Priority HIV/AIDS Interventions in the Health Sector; Progress Report 2009* (Geneva, WHO, 2009) for a comprehensive discussion of the issue in the context of HIV/AIDS research.

[2] Status of the embryo.

[3] See Habermas, Jürgen, *The Future of Human Nature* (Cambridge, Polity, 2003).

[4] See Savulescu, Julian and Kahane, Guy, "The Moral Obligation to Create Children with the Best Chance of the Best Possible Life," *Bioethics* 23, no. 5 (2009) 274–290, and, from a theological perspective Junker-Kenny, Maureen "Genetic Perfection, or Fulfilment of Creation in Christ?" in Deane-Drummond, C. and Manley Scott, P., (eds.) *Future Perfect? God, Medicine and Human Identity* (London–New York, NY, T & T Clark 2006), 155–167.

[5] Different interventions impact on future generations in different ways. Particularly acute moral issues arise with some therapies, such as germ-line therapies, that produce viable eggs and spermatozoa.

research ethics. In this regard, Cathriona Russell's chapter on environmental considerations in research highlights the importance of the natural sciences and economics when the ethical dimensions of new food biotechnologies are being developed and promoted. Russell's chapter admirably demonstrates that the fundamental ethical questions inherent in such developments cannot be considered without a thorough engagement with the scientific, philosophical and social–scientific assumptions which underpin both the technologies themselves and the policies that promote their use. Researchers today are aware, as never before, of the limits of their own disciplinary perspectives and of the consequent need to engage in interdisciplinary conversations. Russell's chapter makes this abundantly clear. Such conversations can be vital in generating new insights about the unforeseen impacts of research, or creating enhanced awareness of particular blind spots that may be embedded in inherited disciplinary norms and practices. The benefit of such interdisciplinary reflection is also discussed by Amy Daughton in 'Lessons from Teaching Research Ethics Across the Disciplines'. In her chapter, Daughton argues that all researchers must develop a framework through which they can reflect, in a critical manner, on the ethical challenges that arise in their research and that, importantly, researchers must also be able to communicate the principles that guide this ethical reflection to research supervisors, to peers and to research participants. Daughton's case studies, based at Trinity College Dublin, highlight the challenges that researchers encounter as they clarify and refine their language and as they develop their ethical argumentation. However, notwithstanding the diversity of ethical frameworks and the disagreements about particular norms and principles, her conclusion confirms that such conversations are indispensible for the graduate researcher as he/she develops his/her research programme.

Ethical Reflection and the Social Context of Research

Much of the graduate researcher's effort is focused on acquiring the technical competencies of his/her discipline, as well as on delivering particular outcomes from his/her research project. This is as it should be. However, recent trends in graduate education have highlighted the importance of other skills, including those associated with competency in ethical reflection, with the development of such skills now regarded as an essential part of research training. Graduate researchers are increasingly expected, not only to conduct research, but also to reflect on the purpose of that research and on how that research is conducted. Of course, there are limits to the extent to which graduate researchers can influence the programmes of research on which they work. This is particularly true in the scientific disciplines where graduate researchers typically join large research groups comprising PIs, post-doctoral and graduate researchers. In this context, many of the most significant ethical questions may not be visible to the graduate researcher, as the fundamental issues about the purpose of the research, the status of the biological materials used or the recruitment of vulnerable populations are likely to have been already decided at the design phase of a research programme. Notwithstanding these limitations, however, the graduate researcher can nonetheless have a critical input into the ethical discussions about the nature, purpose and conduct of their research.

In her chapter 'Synthetic Biology — An Emerging Debate in European Ethics', Haker argues that, 'in the context of research, the task of ethics is to address and analyse the personal values and social norms underlying different claims, to address their inter-relation and to work on the normative claims that enable us to identify and prioritise rights and obligations'. As the graduate researcher encounters different views as to the appropriateness of particular research objectives or practices, he/she is expected to engage critically with the various perspectives, to come to a determination as to the appropriateness of a particular course of action. In the research context, graduates can often be expected to implement decisions that have been decided at a more senior level, or to undertake pre-determined programmes of investigation. However, this does not negate the duty that all researchers have, including those who are still in training, to ensure that the research in which they are engaged is conducted according to the highest ethical standards. It is essential therefore that graduates develop an understanding of the nature of ethical decision-making and its critical role in research ethics. As both Haker and Daughton argue, this is a deliberative process which depends on graduate researchers developing an appreciation of the different theories and principles that underpin ethical reflection. Indeed, as will become clear to the graduate researcher, many of the most fundamental conflicts in research ethics are the direct result of differing views about the relative importance of consequences or duties or rights in the determination of the right course of action. Graduate researchers will undoubtedly have their own personal views about the relative significance of these dimensions of decision-making and are likely to favour either consequentialist, deontological or communitarian frameworks in their own ethical reflection. The process of ethical reflection, however, requires that graduate researchers interrogate their own assumptions about the relative importance of these dimensions of ethical decision-making, consider their applicability in relation to their particular research projects, engage with contrary points of view and defend or revise their ethical assessments of their research projects. Of course, such ethical reflection does not occur in a vacuum. As many of the chapters in this book make clear, there is now a body of law, including international codes governing research, which provide the baseline for the ethical evaluation of research. It is vital therefore that graduate researchers are aware of these regulations, especially as they relate to their own fields of research, and that they have a full appreciation of the scandals and abuses that have occasioned such regulation. However, as such regulation is typically concerned with minimum standards, it should be regarded as the first rather than the last word in research ethics.

Even when the primary focus remains on the individual as moral decision-maker, however, one cannot neglect the significance of the broader context in which such decisions are made. Indeed, this issue of the nature of moral reasoning and its relationship with the intellectual and social contexts from which it emerges is one of the most contested debates in ethics today. Most theories of ethics have recalibrated their universalist claims and no longer seek to defend forms of abstract reasoning which have little or no connection with the social matrices in which such reasoning is exercised. There is, rather, a growing recognition that the norms of rationality are enmeshed in lived traditions of enquiry and that the normative principles that individuals defend are intimately linked to the cultural, historical and religious contexts in which they have been articulated. Moreover, it is gradually coming to be acknowledged that 'the objective standards of reason' are themselves the result of socially embedded assumptions about what is reasonable, logical, coherent and self-evident. We are creatures of tradition and history. Our expressions of value, our accounts of the good life, our apprehension of the virtues, our practical reasoning about how to live a dignified life, these and all our other deeply held convictions emerge from the communities we inhabit and become our own through the worldviews we encounter, and through the narratives we construct and re-construct. This contingent character of our understanding, especially of our moral understanding, is at the heart of how we now think about ethics, including the ethics of research.

As the graduate researcher becomes more attentive to the importance of context in ethics, she/he will inevitably need to think about the nature of his/her truth-claims and specifically about the issue of relativism. Many ethicists worry that if the contingency of moral knowledge is conceded, there will be no firm ground on which to stand and from whence the truth of ethical claims can be established. Although understandable, however, this reveals a basic misunderstanding about the nature of truth and justification in ethics. One can acknowledge that rationality is contingent and that justification is contextual without also endorsing a relativist position in respect to truth. Indeed, Paul Ricoeur's ethical framework upon which Daughton draws is one such example of a moral theory that is simultaneously realist in respect to truth, and contextualist in respect of justification.[6] At the core of such an ethical framework is the recognition that as we adjudicate amongst the ethical claims we make and as we justify our positions to one another, we must do so in a way that allows for a degree of durability to be attributed to such processes, while at the same time allowing for the recognition that these conclusions are ultimately provisional and therefore must be open to change. Notwithstanding the fact that our ethical judgements are inevitably shaped by the historical and cultural contexts of our moral formation; however, we can nonetheless strive to embody the virtues and excellences that we have come to believe reflect the best to which we can aspire, in research, as in life.

Research Ethics in a Deliberative Democracy

Whether conducted in privately funded institutions or in publicly funded universities, the objectives, conduct and outputs of research are matters of major social concern. Scientific research has an impact on some of the most fundamental

---

[6] See Ricoeur, Paul, *Oneself as Another* (Chicago University Press, Chicago 1996). See also, for example, Stout, Jeffrey, Democracy and Tradition, (Princeton NJ: Princeton University Press, 2004), Brandom, Robert, *Making it Explicit: Reasoning, Representing and Discursive Commitment* (Cambridge, MA, Harvard University Press, 1994) and Fergusson, David, *Community, Liberalism and Christian Ethics* (Cambridge, Cambridge University Press, 1998).

aspects of human biological life, including the prospects for future generations. Moreover, given the level of economic investment in scientific research globally, the issues of accountability for its responsible use, and of the just distribution of the benefits of that research, are quite reasonably matters of social interest. These issues are complex and wide-ranging and have the potential to impact on a significant proportion of the world's population, often in direct and enduring ways. They often also have impacts on future generations about which we can know very little, but about which we ought to be concerned. Society therefore has a collective interest in the objectives, conduct and outcomes of research and has an important role in determining the nature and scope of the research that it permits, and which it often funds. Its interest is legitimately in the common good and is based on a society's responsibility to ensure the welfare and protection of its members, and especially of its most vulnerable members. Research is ultimately supported by society for the benefit of that society and its members. The challenge therefore is to ensure that research is supported within an environment that balances innovation and scientific progress with social accountability and equity.

Ethics is a deliberative process which, when pursued in the research context, requires that the researcher be prepared not only to interrogate his/her own ethical values and principles, but also to defend or modify these normative claims in the context of his/her reflection on the research process. It is important to note moreover that this ethical deliberation now occurs in a social and political context that is unambiguously pluralist, and that the fact of this pluralism has a profound effect on how we view the moral frameworks and ethical principles of others. In *A Secular Age*,[7] Charles Taylor analyses the nature of modern pluralism, insisting that we moderns live in situation that is qualitatively different than any other preceding age, namely in a condition 'where we cannot help but be aware that there are a number of different construals, views which intelligent, reasonably undeluded people, of good will, can and do disagree on'.[8] He argues that in the late modern period there has been a dramatic change in what it means to believe so that we are no longer troubled or challenged by the fact of moral pluralism. Rather we accept that our global context 'contains different millieux, within each of which the default option may be different from others, although the dwellers within each are very aware of the options favoured by the others, and cannot just dismiss them as an inexplicable exotic error'.[9] Pluralism therefore is the condition of modernity, it frames all aspects of our ethical deliberation, determines how we treat the normative claims of others and shapes whether and how we expect to achieve ethical agreement on matters of serious social and political concern.

It is inevitable that differences of moral judgement will emerge in the research context, and that these differences may be based either on deep disagreements about fundamental values, or on more culturally or historically based variations of norms and practices. Either way, such ethical disagreement requires that we

---

[7] Taylor, Charles, *A Secular Age* (Cambridge, MA, Belknap Press of Harvard University Press, 2007).
[8] Ibid., 11.
[9] Ibid., 21.

consider how and on what basis we can adjudicate amongst deeply held principles and their applications, particularly in matters of public interest in research. When considering the problematic of how fundamental disagreements in research ethics can be managed, it is worth turning to the work of the political philosopher John Rawls, who has been concerned with the broader question of how to handle moral pluralism in democratic societies. Rawls argues that the state has an obligation to manage the reasonable pluralism that inevitably occurs in democratic societies, and that it ought to do so in a manner that supports 'the underlying ideas of citizens as free and equal persons and of society as a fair system of cooperation over time'.[10] He recognises that it is to be expected that citizens, who are generally motivated by different philosophical worldviews, will hold diverse views on the values by which individuals ought to live their lives and on the nature of the human goods by which a society ought to order itself. Rawls argues that a society must allow for 'the plurality of conflicting, and indeed incommensurable, conceptions of the meaning, value and purpose of human life (or what [he calls] for short "conceptions of the good") affirmed by citizens of democratic societies'.[11] Moreover, given what he calls 'the political fact of the incommensurability' and given that he believes that there is no political basis on which citizens can adjudicate among these diverse views of the good, he believes that a well-ordered society must develop a political conception of justice (namely justice as fairness) independent of and free from any consideration of the good. Indeed, according to Rawls, it is on this basis that 'an overlapping consensus' on fundamental matters among people with diverse commitments can be forged. The means by which this overlapping consensus can be achieved, according to Rawls, is by public reason, namely a process by which citizens replace their comprehensive doctrines of truth or right with an idea of the politically reasonable addressed to citizens as citizens.[12] More explicitly, public reason is the form of reasoning that citizens ought to adopt when they deliberate on matters of basic justice, and it is based on the conviction that when citizens make their case for the exercise of coercive political power (as e.g. in the research context) they should only do so when they 'sincerely believe that the reasons we offer for our political action may reasonably be accepted by other citizens as a justification of those actions'.[13] Citizens must therefore be prepared to translate their distinctive religious our philosophical claims into shared political values as they seek to persuade other citizens about the merits of their respective ethical positions.

The concept of public reason has generated significant debate in the last two decades, much of it focused on the extent to which citizens can or ought to translate their distinctive ethical claims into shared political principles. Jürgen Habermas is critical of the Rawlsian approach and argues instead that we need to develop a form of deliberative politics in which citizens are not expected to reserve

---

[10] John Rawls "The Idea of Public Reason," reprinted in *The Law of Peoples*, (Cambridge, MA, Harvard University Press, 1999) 141.
[11] John Rawls "The Idea of an Overlapping Consensus," *Oxford Journal of Legal Studies* 7, no. 1, 4.
[12] Idem. 132.
[13] "The Idea of Public Reason," 135.

their systematic doctrines but rather to explain and translate them. Thus, for Rawls, researchers should not invoke their religiously based convictions about, for example, the status of the embryo to resist or support particular forms of biomedical research, but rather should seek to justify their resistance or support for research on embryos according to principles that may reasonably be accepted by other citizens as a justification of those actions. For Habermas, in contrast, there is no such expectation. Rather, according to Habermas, 'citizens of a democratic community owe one another good reasons' for their respective positions, and therefore 'the requirement of translation must be conceived as a cooperative task'[14] in which citizens seek to forge reasonable consensus on matters of fundamental ethical significance.

The debate about the precise nature of the language through which we debate matters of moral significance is likely to continue, although there is an emerging consensus that fruitful conversation does not necessarily require a common language, nor shared concepts nor public reason. Rather, our public discourse on research ethics, as on other matters of moral significance should facilitate 'contextually sensitive, dialectical, improvisational, candid conversation between genuinely different points of view'.[15] It is essential that researchers, including graduate researchers, contribute to the fundamental societal debates about the nature and purpose of their research and about the values and principles according to which it ought to be conducted. Indeed, such debates flourish in democratic societies and are essential to its functioning. Moreover, as research continues to push the boundaries of knowledge, it becomes ever more important for those who are at the forefront of such scientific development to be engaged in such public debate.

Captions and links for PODCAST files for this section.

Hille Haker

1. Cultural, social and ethical reflection in addition to ELSA: synthetic biology.
2. Role of the European Group in Ethics.
3. Being a moral agent in an open society.

These can be found at http://booksite.elsevier.com/9780124160491

---

[14] Habermas, Jürgen, "Religion in the Public Sphere," *European Journal of Philosophy* 14:1 pp. 1−25, at 11.
[15] Nigel Biggar, "Against Translation: Theology in Public Debate About Euthanasia," in Biggar, Nigel and Hogan, Linda, *Religious Voices in Public Places* (Oxford, Oxford University Press, 2009) 151−193 at 192.

13 Environmental Perspectives in Research Ethics

Cathriona Russell

Department of Religions & Theology, Trinity College, Dublin, and
All Hallows College, Dublin City University, Ireland

Abstract

Sustainability is a key concept in environmental research ethics and policy formation. In this chapter, I will outline three ethical principles for modelling sustainability: autonomy, stewardship and subsidiarity. Autonomy champions human freedom
and communicative participation as both the end and the means of development.
Stewardship, as a resource-management model, argues for the market as a necessary but not sufficient route to sustainable development and lastly subsidiarity is
the principle that mediates between networks to integrate the local, the national and
the global.

In the second part of the paper I briefly present a case study to show how these
three principles work in practice. The case study examines no-till agriculture from
the perspective of John van Buren's four criteria in environmental hermeneutics –
the biophysical, the historical, the technical and the ethical–political. No-till agriculture represents a quiet but influential revolution in that it replaces the plough –
the pivotal technology that gave us modern agriculture – with a cropping model
that minimises soil disturbance, reducing erosion and soil-carbon loss while protecting soil macropores that allow drainage and aeration. I investigate the scope
and limits of no-till agriculture as a sustainable practice applying these three principles and four criteria. They provide a framework for any ethical evaluation of the
life cycle of new technologies – including products and processes – that are to be
applied in agriculture or released into the open environment.

Key Words

Productionism, agricultural ethics, environmental ethics, hermeneutics, no-till agriculture, autonomy, sustainability, subsidiarity, stewardship

Ethics for Graduate Researchers. DOI: http://dx.doi.org/10.1016/B978-0-12-416049-1.00013-1

Sustainability and Productionism

Research in the natural sciences, apart perhaps from some trajectories in the environmental sciences, is often argued for and presented in the language and value-framework of productionism, as if human culture maximises production as the highest good.[1] Productionism conflicts with the goals of sustainability in that it tends to externalise its full environmental costs. The productionist paradigm is, on the one hand, the driving force to which sustainability is a response and, on the other hand, the deeply implicit value system at work in research in industrial agriculture and economics that acts as a barrier to any substantial shift to more sustainable systems.

Thompson defines production as 'the intentional transformation of materials from a less valued to a more valued state'.[2] This implies that any meaningful conception of production already must carry with it an accompanying theory of value. Production ethics therefore (and research ethics by implication) needs a companion ethic of the environment, since the raw materials for production and research are ultimately rooted in finite biophysical resources and processes. This is nowhere more visible than in relation to agriculture, because field 'crops and animal grazing are ... easily the most spatially extensive human activities having impact upon land masses' and many current 'and emerging environmental controversies continue to involve agriculture'.

If agriculture and agricultural research are about production, productionism is the 'philosophy that emerges when production is taken to be the sole norm for ethically evaluating agriculture' and where the productionist criterion amounts to a principle that 'more production is always better'.[3] Productionism is an ideology and in fact immediately recognisable as a straw man; maximising production is not the longed-for goal of human existence, and farmers, producers and consumers cannot be reduced to rational maximisers. As Thompson puts it:

> *Productionism is an absurd philosophical position. It is contradicted by the oldest of old saws: man does not live by bread alone. There are no sophisticated philosophical defences of productionism. Arguably, no individual has ever believed in it.*[4]

Yet, it has been found in sloganeering; in industrial agriculture, for example, in the maxim 'get big or get out'; in the inappropriate transfer of technology to developing economies; and in research and extension initiatives in industrialised countries; even if politicians, economists and farmers alike know that 'at some point production costs are bound to exceed the value of additional commodities

---

[1] Cf. Hardin G. "The Tragedy of the Commons" *Science* 1968, 162:1243–1248 http://www.sciencemag.org/cgi/reprint/162/3859/1243.pdf.

[2] Thompson P. *The Spirit of the Soil: Agriculture and Environmental Ethics.* (London: Routledge, 1995), 11.

[3] Ibid., 48.

[4] Thompson, *The Spirit of the Soil*, 48.

produced'.[5] As an ideology, it has also been found implicitly in 'social policies, human organisation and cultural norms and has come to dominate agriculture in developed countries since World War II'.[6] Thompson argues that we need to understand this ideology of productionism in agriculture as 'a precondition for envisioning an environmentally responsible agriculture'.[7] If this is true for agriculture, then it also applies to agricultural research – including food biotechnology and synthetic biotechnology – especially insofar as the products of that research are irreversibly applied or 'released' into the farm environment itself.

In addition, although productionist underpinnings are philosophically untenable, they are nonetheless alive and well in the popular culture of research students in the natural sciences. Thompson suggests indeed that for natural 'scientists, productionist beliefs attain implicit, uncritical acceptance though the continuing influence of two discredited dogmas: positivist science and naïve economic Utilitarianism'.[8] And this continues to lead, however unintentionally, to the ongoing generation of scientists and policy makers who uncritically 'rationalise the construction of public organisations, private enterprises and government policies that effectively institutionalised productionist beliefs'. In agricultural ethics, we find carefully innocuous statements like this: 'Using the Utilitarian calculus, the productivity enhancements that characterise modern agriculture have been good for farmers and non-farmers alike'; rapidly followed by this: 'By any Utilitarian calculus, the impacts of these changes on people are dramatically positive. For those who remained in farming, incomes rose in relative as well as absolute terms'.[9] Paarlberg does mention that the regrettable historical displacement of a majority to the cities (or indeed slums) was the price paid for these economies of scale. What is regrettable for us is that he also appears to be advocating such clearances as a present model for modernising agriculture in developing countries without being aware that there are other styles of production that may in fact be a better fit. Paarlberg concludes that although he admits that 'the ethics of modern farming are mixed', he bemoans the fact that among citizens in modern prosperous societies, where few people know farming first hand, misunderstandings of the science and economics of agriculture proliferate. He is blind to his own somewhat patronising affirmation of the Utilitarian calculus. It is not agricultural science or appropriate technology transfer that is at issue, but productionism itself.

The basis of the productionist paradigm is a world view that interprets science as value-free, and which is characterised by total confidence in technologies that increase production.[10] So although it is considered philosophically and environmentally naïve at best in the early twenty-first century, it has cemented a value-framework still being propagated. It is alive and well in the current vision document from the Irish Department of Agriculture, Food and the Marine, *Food*

[5] Ibid., 48.
[6] Ibid., 49.
[7] Ibid., 50.
[8] Ibid., 60.
[9] Paarlberg, R. "The Ethics of Modern Agriculture" *Soc* (2009) 46: 4–8.
[10] Thompson, *The Spirit of the Soil*, 60.

Harvest 2020.[11] This re-discovery of productionism at departmental level may well owe more to bureaucrats than farmers or consumers, and demands greater scrutiny.

Thompson argues that ironically, any 'statement that science is and must be value-free is amusingly self-contradictory, since it stipulates a norm for scientists at the same time that it denies the validity of norms'.[12] And he rightly adds that agricultural science, much like medicine, has never been value-free. They are both always already applied and have an implicit 'mission of public utility' (food and fibre production) not universally demanded of scientific research in general.[13] Often agricultural scientists regard their work to be successful only and exactly when it is widely adopted and usually because it increases productivity through the creation of a production-increasing technology.[14]

This productionist paradigm only comes under pressure with the practical realisation that it can be self-defeating, because it tends towards the undersupply of public goods, or non-market goods on which production itself depends – soil functions, clean air and water, and the ability of non-renewable resources to persist over time. The early environmental movement was focused on these concerns. It may be no coincidence that this movement grew up in North America in response to the excesses of productionism, and so only truly makes sense in that context. Early environmentalism was not concerned with agriculture, but was more interested in the conservation of the so-called wildernesses and defending an intrinsic value for nature that resisted all forms of commodification. The rhetoric of the environmental movement did entail a critique of production but it did not, in its early manifestation at least, engender an ethic of production,[15] let alone a concern for food security or entitlement with which environmental philosophy and economics are deeply concerned today. Yet, it is clear that if agriculture and production need an environmental ethic, then environmental ethics must also consider a food production and distribution ethic.[16] Environmental theories of value likewise, in expressing the interdependence in the planetary earth system, cannot confine their effort to the articulation of the intrinsic value of natural areas in an untransformed state.[17] Rather, they need to turn their attention to agriculture and production, as these need to be as much a concern for environmental ethics as they are for environmental studies in the natural sciences.[18] If agricultural production is to become truly sensitive to environmental quality, then 'it will require conceptual sources not

---

[11] Department of Agriculture, Food and the Marine *Food Harvast 2020: a vision for Irish agri-food and fisheries* (2010). Cf. http://www.agriculture.gov.ie/media/migration/agri-foodindustry/foodharvest2020/2020FoodHarvestEng240810.pdf.
[12] Thompson, *The Spirit of the Soil*, 61.
[13] Ibid., 62.
[14] Ibid., 68.
[15] Ibid., 11.
[16] Ibid., 13.
[17] Ibid., 11.
[18] Ibid., 5.

present in the productionist ethic'.[19] Otherwise, we are once more left pitching 'free-market exchange value' against 'the deepest ecology of human extinction'.[20]

The concept of sustainability offers an alternative to the overplayed dichotomy between ecosystem preservation and human development. Looking at sustainability provides an opportunity to map the points of divergence between production and conservation and to examine the possibilities for reintegrating these goals in the interests of human development and sustainability.

Sustainability as a Concept of Convergence

The concept of sustainability offers an alternative to the dichotomy between wise-use advocates and those who would champion intrinsic value for earth systems, pitching ecosystem preservation against humanity.[21] Here I outline three ethical criteria for modelling sustainability: autonomy, stewardship and subsidiarity. Autonomy can be translated literally as 'self-rule' or 'self-legislation'. There are several schools of thought as to its meaning and application. However, in international human rights law and conventions, it is related to the dignity and the integrity of each human person and that is how it will be applied here. Autonomy defends human freedom and communicative participation as not just the end but also the means to development.

Traditionally, stewardship is interpreted as human creativity in the service of human needs, society and – for those who would include a divinity – God. Humanity stewards natural resources for the public or common good of society applying the tools of creative management. Stewardship here stands for the idea that the market is a necessary but not a sufficient route to sustainable development. Lastly, subsidiarity is a principle that helps to mediate between levels of activities to integrate the local, the national and the global.

Modelling Sustainability

Environmental sustainability, understood as the ability of non-renewable resources to persist over time, at first glance seems to have little to do with ethics. In the environmental sciences it is involved with carrying-capacities, critical limits and regulating consumption – but not with ethics. Devising sustainable systems is therefore a technical question better left to the natural scientists (and perhaps the economists). Sustainability, however, is not just about resources, it is also about people. The landmark Brundtland definition, despite much critique and refinement, captures this aspect of sustainability well. Development is sustainable where it 'meets the needs

---

[19] Ibid., 71.

[20] Ibid., 11.

[21] These concepts are also discussed in Russell, C. "Burden-sharing in a Changing Climate: Which Principles and Practices can Theologians Endorse?" *Studies in Christian Ethics* 2011, 24: 67–76, doi:10.1177/0953946810389119 and Russell, C. *Autonomy and Food Biotechnology in Theological Ethics* (Oxford: Peter Lang, 2009).

of the present without compromising the ability of future generations to meet their own needs'.[22] As a concept in environmental ethics, it is the bearer of at least two essential ideas: the dangers of growth[23] through the destruction of non-renewables, and at the same time, the rights of current and future generations in relation to those same resources. As a descriptive concept, sustainability is firmly based in the sciences (and economics). As a normative principle, however, it requires social and ethical foundations.

In environmental and agricultural ethics, sustainability is a word that is applied to systems, and systems do not have 'natural' borders, rather they are constructed in relation to the problem that a systems-analysis is expected to resolve.[24] The choices of borders and performance criteria are open to debate. As Thompson remarks, this 'means that knowing about the sustainability of the system apart from knowing how borders and performance criteria are selected means one knows very little'.[25] And this is not just an issue of more and more sophisticated modelling. Aiming at completeness is not the problem, the problem is that of confusing functionality with truth.[26]

The role of the natural sciences therefore in environmental sustainability is to describe the possibilities open to policy makers within the capacity of the biosphere; the role for ethics is to make clear the normative aspects of any claim that a system is sustainable. It may be possible, for example, to have a sustainable slave society (or indeed a slave society that is not sustainable) in the descriptive sense, as Thompson argues. So we could propose coercion for the control of human populations, as Garret Hardin among others would advocate, but with no evidence of an environmental dividend. Additionally, it might be that we could find that our systems will not be descriptively sustainable unless and until they are also committed to distributive justice, as the economist Amartya Sen argues. Poor countries, for example, may not be in a position to forgo development opportunities that consume natural resources, such as forestry or biodiversity, without international cooperation to close the incentive gap.[27] It is important therefore not to just define or advocate sustainability, but to make the philosophical assumptions in our understanding of natural and human systems explicit.[28] Three ethical principles are particularly relevant to models for sustainability: autonomy, stewardship and subsidiarity, and it is to these that I will now turn.

---

[22] Sen, A. "Why We Should Preserve the Spotted Owl" *London Review of Books* 2004 26: 3, 10–11.

[23] That is, the dangers of growth, not growth *per-se*, in addition a distinction needs to be made between efficiency and effectiveness cf. McDonough, W and Braungart, M *Cradle to Cradle: Remaking the Way We Make Things* (New York; North Point Press, 2002).

[24] Ibid., 156.

[25] Thompson, *The Spirit of the Soil*, 156.

[26] Ibid., 157.

[27] Kaul I., Grunberg I. and Stern M. *Global Public Goods: International Cooperation in the 21st Century* (Oxford: University Press, 1999), xxiv.

[28] Thompson, *The Spirit of the Soil*, 167.

Sustainability and Autonomy

The first principle, autonomy or freedom, argues for participation not coercion in environmental decision-making as the means and end of sustainable development. An autonomy approach resists the coercion and instrumentalisation of the human person, found, ironically, in the excesses of both the free-market approach and some environmental discourse. The dignity, uniqueness and irreplaceability of the human person (along with other principles such as the common good, social solidarity and distributive justice) are already widely defended in principle and law. But they are under pressure from market forces that commodify the human person or that conceptualise them as maximisers of their own self-interest. Such tendencies are also found in the unexamined value judgements in environmental discourse. We see them, for example, in Garret Hardin's 'Tragedy of the Commons,' in the misanthropy of Paul Erlich, and in the 'Fortress Conservation' approach of Holmes Rolston III.[29] They continue to re-appear in many guises: most usually under the rubric of over-population. Either we need to accelerate the productionist paradigm or we need to coerce human populations (usually those other than our own) to live sacrificially for the sake of the planet.

This has left environmentalists open to charges of misanthropy and often serves the agenda of neo-conservatives who have more interest in markets than morality. Deep ecology and ecocentrism, although worthy correctives to instrumentalism, continue to carry this ambiguity and are in danger of undermining hard-won protections for the human person. Ironically, they can do so without ensuring any pathway to an 'environmental dividend'.[30] An autonomy approach defends the dignity and integrity of the human person and therefore resists instrumentalising the person in the call for environmental justice. That does not mean that such an approach is not interested in how a vision of human development intersects with the question of economic sustainability. There may be an environmental cost in defending human dignity and human rights, or it may be the case that this is the shortest route to environmental sustainability.

Sustainability and Economics: Stewardship Revisited

The second principle relocates economics within the scope of moral frameworks and envisages market mechanisms and production as necessary if not sufficient routes to sustainability. Stewardship has become part of the discourse of environmental management. If markets are to be one tool in the delivery of human development and economic sustainability, they need to prioritise those ends in exchange relationships. Sen observes that the impact of environmental degradation falls disproportionately on the poor. What he is innovative in doing is arguing that because environmental issues are an inescapable part of the battle against poverty, weenvironmental sustainability will be delivered only with, and not in spite of, human

---

[29] Siuruna, H. "Nature Above People: Rolston and 'Fortress' Conservation in the South" *Ethics and Environment*, 2006 11:1. pp. 71–96.

[30] Sen, A. *Development as Freedom* (Oxford: University Press, 1999).

development. This is especially the case where development is understood foundationally as an expansion of human freedoms rather than the expansion of 'inanimate objects of convenience' such as increased Gross Domestic Product (GDP).[31] There can therefore be an instrumental justification for poverty alleviation,[32] as a means to protect the environment, an argument that should appeal even to the most economistic policy makers.[33] Development is simply tied not only to wealth creation but also (beyond a certain level of wealth) to other 'freedoms' that people have reason to value. For Sen, developing countries should not wait to develop basic education and health care until after a certain level of opulence has been achieved. Rather it is these 'public goods' that are themselves both the means and the end of development. Sen has shown, both theoretically and empirically, that human development and environmental sustainability are not necessarily in conflict, most especially in his critique of the use of coercion in population control.

Sen does, however, take issue with the use of the term 'needs' in the Bruntland definition of sustainability. Economics usually treats agents inadequately as with motives reduced to a rational core – maximising self-interest in accordance with the principle of utility. He argues instead that if economics is concerned with real people it is hard to believe that real people would 'stick exclusively to the rudimentary hard-headedness attributed to them by modern economweics'.[34] He removes the strait-jacket of self-interest as it leaves us unable to give a greater concreteness to the conception of needs. Sen in contrast talks not of needs but of capabilities. We require this broader view of human persons, as 'agents whose freedoms matter' and who live 'lives they have reason to value' and who are 'more than their living standards'.[35]

Sen also argues that if economic growth is effective as a means to sustainable development, its success is contingent on many other factors: it is certainly not unique as a means. Market mechanisms have their blind spots; they cannot take account on their own of the distribution of benefits or burdens, or long-term consequences or the active participation of all. The market is a necessary but not a sufficient mechanism for human development and environmental sustainability.[36]

He defends economics as a tool while also pointing out that the problems of environmental sustainability do not lie only in economic analysis but in political action. Most significantly, there is a lack of incentive (mechanisms and structures) to do the right thing for the environment: society and economy have us act on

---

[31] Sen, A. *The Idea of Justice* (London: Penguin, 2009), 225.

[32] Anand S and Sen A. Human Development and Economic Sustainability. *World Development* 2000 28 (12) 2029–2049.

[33] Cf. Sen, A. *Development as Freedom* (Oxford: University Press, 1999).

[34] Sen, A. *On Ethics and Economics* (Oxford: Blackwell, 1988), 1.

[35] Sen, *Why we should preserve the spotted owl*, 11.

[36] For example, the higher the average income of a country the more likely it is to have a higher life expectancy, lower infant mortality rate, higher score on the 'human development index'. But income difference only explains some of that variation, for example China, Kerala score higher that would be expected given their Gross National Product. Cf. Sen, S *Development as Freedom* Chapter 9.

different sets of priorities.[37] If stewardship is the key link between economy and ecology that produces sustainable development[38] then we need to find ways of matching sustainable development as a societal goal with economic policies and instruments that work to achieve it. The Forest Stewardship Council is one such initiative, notwithstanding its shortcomings.[39]

Admittedly, stewardship is not without its critics. For some environmentalists, management under the rubric of stewardship is too little too late, it is a default word and not a considered concept. It is merely 'an unconscious synonym for the unavoidable interactions between us as living beings and... the environment that surrounds us'.[40] It is instrumentalist and human centred and therefore cannot deliver sustainability. There is something utterly correct in this critique. The reason the market works is exactly because it depends on things outside of itself that are beyond market value; beauty, truth and goodness. We cannot be insensitive to Ricoeur's lament that history 'showcases the ever increasing defeat of what is without price, driven back by the advances of commercial society'.[41] That which is without price includes moral dignity, the integrity of the human body and the splendour of the natural landscape. There is something both disorienting and reorienting in the recognition of the integrity and splendour of the world, and in the spontaneity that we encounter, rather than create. It is exactly that which environmentalists continue to both try to express and also to defend against the absolute tyranny of productionism.[42]

Notwithstanding that critique, stewardship can help uncover the economic frameworks and mechanisms (market, social and other) that could deliver on the sharing of the benefits and burdens of resource use. It points to the need to develop national, regional and international institutions, applying the principle of subsidiarity to which I will shortly turn to explore the role of citizenship and participation, and of regulations and incentives in the interests of human development and economic sustainability.

Sustainability and Subsidiarity: Integrating the Local and the Global

The third principle, subsidiarity, acts as a test for how well local and regional action can be integrated in the interests of benefit- and burden-sharing in the life we hold in common :

> The principal advantage of subsidiarity as a structural principle... is that it integrates international, domestic, and subnational levels of social order on the basis

[37] Sen A. "Environment and Poverty: One World or Two?" *International Conference on Energy, Environment and Development: Analysing opportunities for reducing poverty.* Bangalore, India, 2006. http://www.institut.veolia.org/ive/ressources/documents/1/166,Amartya-Sen.pdf.
[38] Berry RJ, (ed). *Environmental Stewardship* (London: T&T Clark, 2006).
[39] Cf. http://www.fsc.org/.
[40] Berry, *Environmental Stewardship*, 1.
[41] Ricoeur, P. *The Course of Recognition* (Cambridge: Harvard University Press, 2005), 235.
[42] Cf. Feehan, J. *The Singing Heart of the World* (Dublin: Columba, 2010).

of a substantive vision of human dignity and freedom, while encouraging and protecting pluralism among them.[43]

It is a principle rooted in the common good tradition, which also includes sociability and solidarity, for discovering ways to integrate the good life for the individual with the social good. This principle has the effect of safeguarding the mediation between institutions of civil society and between the state and the individual.[44] Subsidiarity defends the freedom of the human person on two fronts: by arguing that it is wrong, first, to take from individuals that which they can accomplish by their own initiative, and second, it is also a distortion of society to assign to a greater or higher association what lesser and subordinate organisations can do.

Subsidiarity is the principle that seeks to reconcile the universal goals of sustainable development with the plurality of forms of good practice at local and regional level.[45] Less attention has been given in environmental ethics to the mechanisms by which local systems for sustainability interface and integrate with regional systems. Global eco-governance often deals in abstractions that can fail to account for the difficulties of contextualising wider goals at the local level. Local systems of action are frequently too partial to offer sufficient guarantees for sustainability. The concern to offset global climate change through biofuel production, for example, must be integrated with the concern to protect food security – both globally and locally. Biofuel mandates, from governments in the European Union (EU) and in North America, appear to have had the effect of increasing world food prices and increasing food deprivation.[46] A recent bulletin from the European Environmental Agency's scientific committee recommended a new comprehensive study on the environmental risks and benefits of biofuels and a suspension of the EU target to increase the share of biofuels used in transport to 10% by 2020.[47] The lesson for research is that institutions need to be reflexive and that societal commitments to research need to be revisable in the interests of these higher-level principles. Biofuels cannot be specified narrowly under technical definitions, they represent a technological trajectory, and as such, their adoption is a political question that needs to be debated widely and democratically.[48]

---

[43] Carozza, P. "Subsidiarity as a Structural Principle of International Human Rights Law" *The American Journal of International Law* 2003 97: 38 pp. 38–79.

[44] Grasso, K., G. Bradley, and R. Hunt, eds. *Catholicism, Liberalism and Communitarianism* (Lanhan: Rowman and Littlefield, 1995), 98.

[45] Integrating freedom of the press with the individuals, right to privacy, for example.

[46] Matthews, A. Professor for Agricultural Policy in the Department of Economics, and the Director of the Institute for International Integration Studies, Trinity College Dublin. "EU agricultural policy and developing countries: what do we know?" Public Lecture Series May 5th 2010. Available as a pod cast with slides http://www.tcd.ie/iiis/publications/podcasts.php.

[47] European Environmental Agency, Opinion of the EEA scientific committee on the environmental impacts of biofuel utilisation in the EU (2012) http://www.eea.europa.eu/highlights/suspend-10-percent-biofuels-target-says-eeas-scientific-advisory-body.

[48] Thompson, P. "The Agricultural Ethics of Biofuels" *Journal of Agricultural and Environmental Ethics* 2008 21: 183–198, 189.

In the next Section entitled 'No-Till Agriculture: A Case Study in Environmental Hermeneutics', the adoption of no-till agriculture is examined using John van Buren's four criteria; the biophysical, the historical, the technical and the ethical–political.

No-Till Agriculture: A Case Study in Environmental Hermeneutics

Environmental hermeneutics is an emerging aspect of environmental philosophy and can be defined as the philosophical study of interpretation; it is predicated on the idea that all human experience is mediated though language, which in turn always needs to be interpreted.[49] A critical environmental hermeneutics, in whatever way we narrate our understanding and approach to the environment, 'considers the conditions within which we interpret the environment while at the same time seeks to uncover distortions in interpretation' as well as communication.[50] Van Buren suggests that one of the more practical tasks of hermeneutics is to address 'conflicts of interpretation' in the world, and he outlines four criteria that might assist in assessing our interpretation of the environment to that end; the biophysical, the historical, the technological and the ethical–political.[51] I would like to outline and apply these four criteria to assess the claim that no-till farming is a sustainable model for agriculture, that it integrates agricultural production and the conservation of non-renewable resources.

Agriculture is a human activity aimed at producing usable food and fibre from land-based renewable natural resources.[52] Ploughing is used to kill competing weeds, bury surface fibrous organic matter and create a warmed seedbed for crops. It has also been revealed as a leading cause of farmland degradation through soil erosion and loss of soil organic matter.[53] No-till agriculture, in contrast to ploughing, seeks to minimise soil disruption, and to contribute to a more sustainable agriculture. This move away from ploughing is described as a quiet revolution in farming in response to particular conditions and contexts and is considered an intrinsic element in conservation agriculture. Conservation tillage is a term applied to 'any method that retains enough of the previous crop residues such that at least 30 per cent of the soil surface is covered after planting'.[54] Crop rotation and cover crops are essential elements of conservation agriculture, which in turn is based on

---

[49] Utsler, D. "Paul Ricoeur's Hermeneutics as a Model for Environmental Philosophy" *Philosophy Today* 2009 173–178.

[50] Utsler, *Paul Ricoeur's*, 177.

[51] van Buren, John "Critical Environmental Hermeneutics" *Environmental Ethics* 1995 17:259–275.

[52] Thompson, *The Spirit of the Soil*, 47.

[53] Huggins, David "No-Till: the Quiet Revolution" *Scientific American* 2008 299: 1 pp. 70–77, 1.

[54] Huggins, *No-Till*, 4.

three principles: continuous minimal mechanical disturbance, permanent organic cover and diversification of crops grown in sequence or association.[55]

Retaining continuous cover can increase water filtration and reduce run-off and evaporation, encourage biodiversity and good soil structure, and carbon sequestration as well as offering economic advantages to the farmer in reducing the number of passes to establish and harvest the crop, reducing time and fuel use. It may also allow the expansion of agriculture to marginal soils.[56] Given the advantages that are claimed for it in contrast to intensively tilled systems, in terms of soil conservation and conditioning and its contribution to carbon sequestration, we could ask the question then what are the barriers that have stalled its adoption globally. There are four common barriers outlined by Derpsch: know-how, tradition, inadequate structural supports and the unavailability of suitable herbicides to facilitate weed management.[57] No-till agriculture depends on intensive herbicide use and this is one of its great drawbacks from an environmental perspective. Although advocates of no-till agriculture would argue that there is more to no-till agriculture than the 'herbicides-only' approach, in its current manifestations, weed-control in no-till systems relies heavily on herbicides as an alternative to the plough.[58] Notwithstanding that drawback, agricultural researchers assume that once there is a wide recognition that no-till farming is a truly sustainable system, its use will spread to areas where adoption is low 'as soon as the barriers to its adoption have been overcome'.[59] I test this assumption about technology transfer using van Buren's four criteria and in the light of the three preceding principles.

Biophysical Fit of No-Till Agriculture

The first question we can ask is under what conditions no-till farming can be considered to be more sustainable than intensive tillage. Borrowing from the hermeneutics of Ricoeur, van Buren argues that the first criterion, the 'biophysical criterion stipulates only that interpretations must be "fitting" to the bioregion, that they must fit the biophysical world to which they belong'.[60] A new technology must adequately correspond to the context in which it is being applied. No-till agriculture is not just seeding without tillage, but involves a switch in a whole set of factors: seeding techniques, timing, weed and pest management and crop varieties.[61] It requires investment in new machinery, new management know-how and the risk of initial failures as the farmer develops new skills. Permanent continuous

---

[55] Derpsch, R, Friedrich, T, Kassam, A and Hongwen, L. "Current status of adoption of no-till farming in the world and some of its main benefits" *International Journal of Agricultural and Biological Engineering* 2010 3(1) pp. 1–25, 4 Open Access at http://www.ijabe.org.

[56] Derpsch et al., *Current status*, 3.

[57] Ibid., 3.

[58] Goddard,T., Zoebisch, M. Gan, Y. Ellis, W. Watson, A. and Sombatpanit, S. (eds) *No-Till Farming Systems* (Thailand: World Association of Soil and Water Conservation, 2008).

[59] Derpsch et al., *Current status*, 3.

[60] van Buren, *Critical environmental hermeneutics*, 269.

[61] Derpsch et al., *Current status*, 4.

no-till cover is aimed at, rather than occasional tilling. It grew up in the plains of North America. The United States now has the highest area under no-till in the world followed by Brazil, Argentina, Canada and Australia.[62] It may also come as no surprise that it is not extensively practised in Europe, which is interpreted as 'a developing continent in terms of the adoption of Conservation Agriculture'.[63] European farmers are not fully convinced that it meets the requirements of environmentally friendly farming, lower production costs and consumer demand, as Derpsch et al. point out. Adoption rates are low too in Africa and much of Asia because farmers in developing countries already use crop residues for fuel, fodder and bedding and work on very different models of land holding, tenure and labour resources. No-till agriculture is an alternative to or refinement of industrial large-scale farming which is currently already dependent on tillage and herbicide use on soils that are prone to erosion and loss of soil condition.

Historical Origins and Implications of No-Till Agriculture

The historical is the second criterion for deciding the fittingness of interpretations, and much like that of biophysical fit, it also involves a version of 'the coherence theory of truth because it calls for examination of how an interpretation coheres or fits in with historical traditions'.[64] Agriculture on the Great Plains has a relatively short history. Until the invention of the modern plough (such as the John Deere in 1837), the tall-grass prairie of the Midwestern United States had resisted widespread farming because the thick sticky sod was a barrier to cultivation; this land is now home to one of the most agriculturally productive areas of the world.[65] However, this new tillage practice was not without its costs. The Dust Bowl era (1931–1939) exposed the vulnerability of plough-based agriculture as wind blew soil from the plains in times of drought. Soil conservation became a new concern, and conservation agriculture became a movement that challenged the necessity of ploughing itself.

New interpretations of farming can and have led to cultural displacement, alienation and homelessness for traditional users. International agreements on climate change that hope to manage mitigation and adaptation are hedging against just such alienation and culture shock. However, tradition as a barrier to adoption cannot just be interpreted in terms of the risks and hazards of adopting new farming styles. Indigenous forms of production may already be a good 'biophysical' fit and not in need of the remedy that no-till agriculture is offering. Historical analysis can help trace these different technological trajectories in local styles of agriculture.[66] One-model-fits-all approaches to farming styles can under-determine and alienate the embedded skills-base that best fits a locality.

[62] Huggins, *No-Till*, 5.
[63] Derpsch et al., *Current status*, 5.
[64] van Buren, *Critical environmental hermeneutics*, 270.
[65] Huggins, *No-Till*, 3.
[66] van Buren, *Critical environmental hermeneutics*, 271.

We should not return by another route to the 'fallacies of misplaced Utilitarianism' and productionism. Even in the historical context in which it grew up, the conservation movement has been interpreted as 'just another instance' of the validity of productionism.[67] Conservation agriculture, as represented by no-till, is therefore only one trajectory in a larger vision for sustainable agriculture, which needs to be more diverse,[68] taking on successful practices from other systems for best biophysical and historical fit.

The Technical Criterion and Sustainability

The third criterion for assessment is the technical, meaning that form of knowledge that lies in the domain of instrumental reason. This criterion borrows from the idea that what is good and true corresponds to what works in practice. It is concerned solely with efficiency of use and the manipulation of the world to achieve desired ends. In that way, it helps 'to decide which are the better means for a given end' but it is not sufficient in itself, it 'cannot choose between alternative ends themselves and rationally legitimate this choice'.[69] The danger in this approach, as van Buren points out, is that this technical ability becomes concentrated in an elite of experts or technicians and agency falls under the sway of 'technocracy' or 'expertocracy', and finally becomes a kind of unfreedom, or authoritarian rule.[70]

In the case of no-till agriculture, it is clear that changing from tillage-based agriculture is not easy, it demands a change in management at all levels, not just a reduction in ploughing.[71] As a style in farming, it has established itself through farmers' own effort.[72] Farmers are not passive recipients of agricultural research, but rather, they develop new indigenous systems that are a product of their own effort and social networking. They do not copy new models or styles of farming, but reconstruct them.[73] This is both an example of subsidiarity in action and a lesson in technology transfer. First, producers are not, in practice, induced to innovate nor are they simply passive recipients of expert knowledge; rather, they reconstruct innovations to meet pragmatic goals that integrate loosely coupled technologies into practices that fit their own farms, abilities, resources and markets. Second, there is always the danger that in missing this aspect, agricultural 'researchers were "not even close" to predicting farmer's conservation behaviour from their personal characteristics, the characteristics of their farms, or their linkages to institutions and information sources'.[74] Farming styles are internally coherent and externally

---

[67] Thompson, *The Spirit of the Soil*, 67.
[68] Huggins, *No-Till*, 7.
[69] van Buren, *Critical environmental hermeneutics*, 271.
[70] Ibid., 271.
[71] Huggins, *No-Till*, 6.
[72] Derpsch et al., *Current status*, 1.
[73] Milton Coughenour, C "Innovating Conservation Agriculture: The Case of No-Till Cropping" *Rural Sociology* 2003 68 (2), pp. 278–304.
[74] Milton Coughenour, *Innovating*, 279.

distinctive modes of ordering farm systems.[75] No-till farming represents one technological shift, among a plurality, towards a more sustainable agriculture.

Communicative Ethical—Political Sustainability

What in the ancient world was called 'practical reason' — which was concerned with the ends of human action worked out in rational discourse between free citizens in the public or political sphere — has come to be called communicative reason in contemporary thought, according to van Buren.[76] Communicative action implies a procedural approach, which is concerned with not so much what is being talked about, but how it is being talked about.[77] Applying van Buren's approach to intensive till versus no-till agriculture, for example, we could ask to what extent either approach falsely universalises itself as being the whole truth about agricultural production. No-till may not be the best biophysical fit in all instances; it may truncate other historical trajectories in faming styles or under-determine the agency of farmers and producers.

To take a final example, conservation agriculture is championed because it has the potential to mitigate climate change by sequestering more carbon in the soil than intensive tillage systems.[78] As a relative argument that can be true, it does mitigate agricultural emissions. Globally, however, mitigation is better effected agriculturally by halting tropical and sub-tropical deforestation (and the burning of fossil fuel).[79] It would be a step in the wrong direction to argue, at the global level, that these forests could be sustainably replaced with conservation agriculture in the interests of reducing carbon emissions. Alternative models of farming, such as agroforestry, may be a better biophysical fit, less likely to alienate indigenous practices and more appropriate technologically. Conservation agriculture may be a step closer to sustainable production in the Midwestern Corn Belt and in other places in the world that farm industrially on soils that are easily eroded, but may only represent a minor element under different biophysical, historical or political conditions. Success in agricultural research needs to be decoupled from the 'one-size-fits-all' model implicit in productionism.

Implications for Research Ethics

In this chapter, I have presented three background principles (autonomy, stewardship and subsidiarity) that set an ethical framework for the concept of subsidiarity,

---

[75] Garstenauer, R. Langthaler, E and Tod, S. "Get Big or Get Out? Farm Development in the PostWar 'Agricultural Revolution' in Austria, 1945—1980" Paper to the international conference Quantitative Agricultural and Natural Resources History in Zaragoza/E, June 2—4, 2011 http://estructuraehistoria. unizar.es/gihea/documents/Zaragoza_Garstenauer-Langthaler-Tod.pdf.

[76] van Buren, *Critical environmental hermeneutics*, 272.

[77] Ibid., 272.

[78] Smith, P., Powlson, D., Glendenning, M and Smith, J. "Preliminary estimates of the potential for carbon mitigation in European Soils through no-till farming" *Global Change Biology* (1998) 4, 679—685.

[79] Ibid.

and four foreground criteria (biophysical, historical, technical, ethical–political) that can be used to begin to assess the environmental impact of production innovations. Autonomy implies participation, not coercion, in environmental decision-making as the means and the end of sustainable development; farmers, e.g. as adopters of agricultural research, are not passive recipients but active agents in reconstructing new loosely bound technologies to 'fit'. Stewardship relocates economics within the scope of moral frameworks and it validates a production ethic and varieties of instrumental reason when it comes to valuing nature. It is not productionism, however, that can be characterised as a self-defeating naïve Utilitarianism. Markets are a necessary but partial mechanism for the sustainable management of systems. Lastly, subsidiarity tests how well local and regional action can be integrated in the interests of benefit- and burden-sharing. As a structural principle, it has not reached its potential for integration in the effort to secure the 'needs' of the current generation without compromising the ability of future generations to meet theirs. We can clearly see it at work, however, in the recent reappraisal of the biofuel targets for transport in the EU in the interests of food security.

No-till agriculture does appear to deliver a more sustainable agriculture within the limits of its biophysical, historical and technological fit, it is an improvement on the intensive tillage system it replaces. However, it is by no means established that it is as universally applicable as its advocates suggest or that it can be taken as a fully developed model of sustainability in its own right. The three background principles of autonomy, stewardship and subsidiarity map the environmental ethics landscape, while the four criteria locate innovations in practice. They can be used as a reference point in any environmental ethical assessment of research in food and fibre production.

Acknowledgements

Thanks to Thomas Cummins, UCD, for reading a draft of this paper and for his helpful comments and critique.

Bibliography

Anand S, Sen A. "Human Development and Economic Sustainability". *World Dev* 2000;28 (12):2029–49.

Berry RJ, editor. *Environmental Stewardship*. London: T&T Clark; 2006.

Carozza P. "Subsidiarity as a Structural Principle of International Human Rights Law". *Am J Int Law* 2003;97:38–79.

Department of Agriculture, Fisheries and Food. *Food Harvest 2020: a vision for Irish agri-food and fisheries*; 2010. Cf. <http://www.agriculture.gov.ie/media/migration/agri-foodindustry/foodharvest2020/2020FoodHarvestEng240810.pdf/>.

Derpsch R, Friedrich T, Kassam A, Hongwen L. "Current status of adoption of no-till farming in the world and some of its main benefits". *Int J Agric Biol Eng* 2010;3(1):1–25 Open Access at: <http://www.ijabe.org/>.

European Environmental Agency. Opinion of the EEA scientific committee on the environmental impacts of biofuel utilisation in the EU; 2012. <http://www.eea.europa.eu/highlights/suspend-10-percent-biofuels-target-says-eeas-scientific-advisory-body/>.

Feehan J. *The Singing Heart of the World*. Dublin: Columba; 2010.

Forest Stewardship Council. <http://www.fsc.org/>.

Garstenauer R, Langthaler E, Tod S. "Get Big or Get Out? Farm Development in the Postwar 'Agricultural Revolution in Austria' 1945−1980." Paper to the international conference Quantitative Agricultural and Natural Resources History in Zaragoza/E; June 2−4, 2011. <http://estructuraehistoria.unizar.es/gihea/documents/Zaragoza_Garstenauer-Langthaler-Tod.pdf/>.

Goddard T, Zoebisch M, Gan Y, Ellis W, Watson A, Sombatpanit S, editors. *No-Till Farming Systems*. Thailand: World Association of Soil and Water Conservation; 2008.

Grasso K, Bradley G, Hunt R, editors. *Catholicism, Liberalism and Communitarianism*. Lanhan: Rowman and Littlefield; 1995.

Hardin G. "The Tragedy of the Commons". *Science* 1968;162:1243−8 <http://www.sciencemag.org/cgi/reprint/162/3859/1243.pdf/>.

Huggins D. "No-Till: the Quiet Revolution". *Sci Am* 2008;299(1):70−7.

Kaul I, Grunberg I, Stern M. *Global Public Goods: International Cooperation in the 21st Century*. Oxford: University Press; 1999, xxiv.

Matthews A. Professor for Agricultural Policy in the Department Of Economics, and the Director of the Institute for International Integration Studies, Trinity College Dublin. "EU agricultural policy and developing countries: what do we know?" Public Lecture Series; May 5 2010. Available at: <http://www.tcd.ie/iiis/publications/podcasts.php/.

McDonough W, Braungart M. *Cradle to Cradle: remaking the way we make things*. New York, NY: North Point Press; 2002.

Milton Coughenour C. "Innovating Conservation Agriculture: The Case of No-Till Cropping". *Rural Sociol* 2003;68(2):278−304.

Paarlberg R. "The Ethics of Modern Agriculture". *Society* 2009;46:4−8.

Ricoeur P. *The Course of Recognition*. Cambridge: Harvard University Press; 2005.

Russell C. *Autonomy and Food Biotechnology in Theological Ethics*. Oxford: Peter Lang; 2009.

Russell C. "Burden-sharing in a Changing Climate: Which Principles and Practices can Theologians Endorse?" *Stud Christ Ethics* 2011;24:67−76. doi:10.1177/0953946810389119.

Sen A. *The Idea of Justice*. London: Penguin; 2009.

Sen A. Environment and Poverty: One World or Two? *International Conference on Energy, Environment and Development: Analysing opportunities for reducing poverty*. Bangalore, India; 2006. <http://www.institut.veolia.org/ive/ressources/documents/1/166,Amartya-Sen.pdf/>.

Sen A. "Why We Should Preserve the Spotted Owl". *Lond Rev Books* 2004;26(3):10−1.

Sen A. *Development as Freedom*. Oxford: Oxford University Press; 1999.

Sen A. *On Ethics and Economics*. Oxford: Blackwell; 1988.

Siuruna H. "Nature Above People: Rolston and 'Fortress' Conservation in the South". *Ethics Environ* 2006;11(1):71−96.

Smith P, Powlson D, Glendenning M, Smith J. "Preliminary estimates of the potential for carbon mitigation in European Soils through no-till farming". *Glob Change Biol* 1998;4:679−85.

Thompson P. "The Agricultural Ethics of Biofuels". *J Agric Environ Ethics* 2008;21:183−98.

Thompson P. *The Spirit of the Soil: Agriculture and Environmental Ethics.* London: Routledge; 1995. p. 11.

Utsler D. "Paul Ricoeur's Hermeneutics as a Model for Environmental Philosophy". *Philos Today* 2009;:173−8.

van Buren J. "Critical Environmental Hermeneutics". *Environ Ethics* 1995;17:259−75.

14 Synthetic Biology – An Emerging Debate in European Ethics – Part Two

Hille Haker

Theology Department, Loyola University Chicago, Chicago, IL

Abstract

In this chapter, I ask what the role of ethics is or could be with respect to science and new technologies, turning particularly to synthetic biology. Following up on the first part of this chapter, which focused on nanotechnology, I argue that the so-called ethical, legal, social aspect (ELSA) methodology needs to be complemented by a distinct social–ethical methodology that enables ethics to address new technologies as social practices whose categories, goals and means are open to philosophical and societal deliberation. I demonstrate that a normative approach founded on human rights enables ethics to reverse the perspective of ethical analysis; which instead of assessing a technology using ELSA, rather regards science and technologies as social practices that need to be justified in light of the normative framework. I then turn to the emerging debate on synthetic biology and present the conclusions of the Opinion that was issued by the European Group on Ethics in 2009.

Key Words

Ethics, bioethics, synthetic biology, European Group on Ethics

Modern sciences analyse more and more the constitutive elements of human nature and nature as such. The life sciences have shown that nature is no longer the normative limit of human intervention, but rather it is the raw material science takes as the occasion for potentially infinite interventions. In this process, the concept of 'life' may radically change. As shown in Chapter 6, the transition from therapeutic to 'enhancing' interventions is already easily blurred in genetics and nanomedicine. This trend is further deepened when the new developments in synthetic biology are taken into consideration. What is and hence should be considered as the normative limit of human intervention, and what is open to changes by the sciences, is not

Ethics for Graduate Researchers. DOI: http://dx.doi.org/10.1016/B978-0-12-416049-1.00014-3

easily to be determined. The normative concept of life and nature that could be used as the moral framework for the deliberation on humanity's relationship towards nature has long been questioned; with the new developments, however, nature seems to lose all normative force.[1]

The transition from the genetic modification to the genetic engineering of organisms via synthetic biology is subtle, and where exactly 'synthetic biology' over against the modification of existing organisms begins is contested among scientists. However, synthetic biology embraces the engineering of biological components and systems that do not exist in nature, and the re-engineering of existing biological elements. It therefore seems to be reasonable to suggest that the use of non-natural DNA sequences is the dividing line between genetic engineering and synthetic biology. Synthetic biology involves three related aspects: the design of minimal cells or minimal organisms, the identification and use of existing biological elements to create new organisms and the construction of biological systems that may, one day, be completely artificial.

'We have got to the point in human history where we simply do not have to accept what nature has given us',[2] comments researcher Keasling. He works on one of the most prominent projects in synthetic biology, producing artemisinin, the biological material that is needed to produce the main anti-malaria drug. The aim of synthetic biology is to understand life processes, and to construct biological 'material' or organisms to develop renewable energy, anti-toxic and anti-pollutant bacteria, diagnostic and therapeutic tools, new cosmetics, agricultural products or new textiles. These applications sound familiar when compared to the nanosciences which work in exactly the same fields; this stresses the point I made earlier, namely that the new technologies cannot be considered separately but rather need to be seen as 'converging' technologies which may increase trends in the different fields of research.

The European Union is now bound by the Lisbon Treaty and the Charter of Fundamental Rights of the European Union.[3] These documents state that dignity and human rights, together with the values of solidarity, subsidiarity and tolerance, are the main moral pillars that should guide social practices, including scientific and technological innovation. I will quote from the beginning of the Treaty. It states that the contract partners establish the European Union

DRAWING INSPIRATION from the cultural, religious and humanist inheritance of Europe, from which have developed the universal values of the inviolable and inalienable rights of the human person, freedom, democracy, equality and the rule of law,

---

[1] Cahill, L., Haker, Hille "Natural law. a controversy." *Concilium* 2010, 46 (3).

[2] Keasling, J. "A Life of Its Own." In The New Yorker (2009). Cf. online: http://www.newyorker.com/reporting/2009/09/28/090928fa_fact_specter.3. And European Group on Ethics in Science and New Technologies, *Opinion 25: Ethics of Synthetic Biology* (2009).

[3] European Union, *Treaty of Lisbon; European Charter of Fundamental Rights*. Online version http://bookshop.europa.eu/is-bin/INTERSHOP.enfinity/WFS/EU-Bookshop-Site/en_GB/-/EUR/ViewPublication-Start?PublicationKey = QC3209190.

RECALLING the historic importance of the ending of the division of the European continent and the need to create firm bases for the construction of the future Europe,
CONFIRMING their attachment to the principles of liberty, democracy and respect for human rights and fundamental freedoms and of the rule of law,
CONFIRMING their attachment to fundamental social rights as defined in the European Social Charter signed at Turin on 18 October 1961 and in the 1989 Community Charter of the Fundamental Social Rights of Workers...

Article 1 of the Treaty deals with the establishment of the European Union. Article 2 then states:

The Union is founded on the values of respect for human dignity, freedom, democracy, equality, the rule of law and respect for human rights, including the rights of persons belonging to minorities.
These values are common to the Member States in a society in which pluralism, non-discrimination, tolerance, justice, solidarity, and equality between women and men prevail.

Article 3 continues on the place of peace and the well-being of peoples.

(ex Article 2 TEU)
1. The Union's aim is to promote peace, its values, and the well-being of its peoples.

In the next part of this chapter, I will reflect a little further on what these normative pillars of the European Union's ethics framework mean for an ethics of new technologies.

A Social–Ethical Approach to Ethics of New Technologies

In the following, I will introduce an alternative methodology for how to analyse ethical dimensions in new technologies. It tries to embrace evaluative as well as normative questions, and the moral perspective of individuals, as well as social values and/ or political regulations. It departs from the classical bioethical methodologies, summed up as deontological and teleological approaches that start with either the principle of autonomy, hence prioritising the individuals' goals, interests and responsibilities; or the social and/or political issues mainly addressed in theories of social goods and/or theories of justice. Both major bioethical approaches cannot grasp the complexity of the necessary ethical analysis that I will try to address.

Normative Principles: Human Rights

Formally speaking, ethics addresses first 'evaluative' implications of personal convictions and attitudes and individual and social ('teleological') visions of the good as well as the social norms that shape the interaction and integration among individuals and between societies. Indeed, social visions and norms shape and inform personal values and norm-systems long before individuals have developed their own moral identity enabling them to make their own choices,[4] while social conflicts result from the des-integration of individuals' interests and desires, or claims of recognition and respect. Second, ethics addresses the 'normative' implications of individual actions and social practices, namely rights claims and issues of political or social justice. Here, we make an important distinction: 'evaluative' issues are explicated, interpreted and then analysed with respect to consistency and relative to the good (or goods) argued for by the agents or moral communities (leaving room for plural approaches to the good(s). In contrast, 'normative' claims must be argued for from a universalistic perspective brought forward as categorical claims. Put briefly, reference to human rights – as is the case in the European and United Nations Policy papers – make only sense if (a) all human beings are covered by them and at least ideally could consent to them and (b) to claim a right means that the addressee of the claim is obliged to respect it. In claiming moral rights to be respected by others, one must have reasons insurmountable by other interests or desires.[5] From this rather abstract normative perspective, new technologies are considered in view of – and potentially as part of – the overall political struggle against the deprivation of health care, injustice of access, participation and distribution of health-related goods.

As an alternative to the technology-oriented ethical, legal, social aspect (ELSA) approach that I have referred to in Chapter 6 – partly because it enabled me to introduce the main goals, means, prospects and risks of a new technology – I propose to begin the ethical evaluation of a new technology with a social practices-oriented analyses, including contemporary research of social, cultural and religious studies, political philosophy, economics and ethical theory. This approach may be called 'social–ethical analysis of science and technology.'[6] Embracing this methodological framework, I presuppose that science and technology are first and foremost social practices that are certainly distinguishable, but neither independent of nor to be separated from other social practices. Like all social practices, science and technology should be as free as possible with respect to its norms, goals and

---

[4] For a thorough analysis of moral self-development and ethical reflection upon it in light of some contemporary ethical approaches. Cf. Haker, H. *Moralische Identität. Literarische Lebensgeschichten als Medium ethischer Reflexion. Mit einer Interpretation der 'Jahrestage' von Uwe Johnson* (Tübingen: Francke, 1999).

[5] For a thorough – if not uncontested – argument for human rights cf. Gewirth, A. *Reason and morality* (Chicago: University of Chicago Press, 1978). To refer to human rights as the normative basis of ethics still requires us to argue for their content, range and integration between several rights. In contemporary ethical discussion furthermore, the relationship between negative and positive rights is a highly debated issue, especially with respect to the corresponding obligations. This debate is beyond the scope of this chapter. However, since all relevant policy papers refer to human rights they can be assumed to be the normative reference point for the ethical analysis of nanomedicine.

[6] To my knowledge, it was Dietmar Mieth who first distinguished between these two approaches, labelling them 'technisch-induziert' und 'sozial-induziert'. Cf. Mieth, D. "Was wollen wir können? Ethik im Zeitalter der Biotechnik" (Freiburg i.Br: Herder, 2002).

means, but they should also be considered as important social measures that help to protect or foster the rights of members of society.[7] Taking serious the normative task of ethics, namely to justify, advocate and prioritise rights and duties, I work on the assumption that science and technology play an important role in all societies adhering to the protection and promotion of human rights, the self-fulfilling and flourishing of individuals, social justice and well-being. As particular social practices that offer the 'tools' to achieve the goals of a 'better life' for individuals and societies, sciences and technologies are praised and accepted – and are praiseworthy and acceptable.

The social–ethical analysis of science and new technologies demands that we reverse the perspective: it does not ask what societies may or may not do with the new developments, how they can adapt to the applications or how they will need to change, but rather asks which societal goals (in fact some of these goals are obligations) are the most urgent from the perspective of human rights claims, and which social practices are best equipped to bring about changes. As an overall practical framework for the implementation of human rights policies, we may take the Millennium Goals as an example of political strategies prioritising international and global policies. This is a strategy that the European Union has strongly endorsed. The Millennium Goals address the most urgent global problems in accordance with the human rights declarations that (ideally) guide the United Nations' actions; hence, the emphasis on global poverty, health care and standards of life necessary to live a minimally 'decent' life. Science and technology play an important role in this global struggle that is then broadened to other concerns, e.g. the environmental crisis or crisis of energy supply. Taken from the point of view of these priorities of political and social actions – derived from an ethical reflection of human rights claims – new technologies are to play a specific role in the struggle against hunger, infancy mortality and/or malnutrition, in the provision of basic health care, or in the struggle against lack of general means to self-sustainability.[8]

Emerging technologies are welcomed and accepted or praised, and as a result are funded with public money, if and insofar as they can reasonably argue that they, first, serve the needs and desires of individuals and society and, second, that the requirement to respond to these needs and desires falls into the range of social and political action. This role – the sciences for society – is to be balanced with autonomy within society that is, for example, the basis for the right to 'freedom of research'; research legitimately receives funding for projects whose results cannot be predicted in detail but are considered valuable and realistic according to the sta-

---

[7] While human rights are considered commonly in terms of political or freedom rights, technologies play an important role particularly with respect to social and economic rights. These rights are to be considered as *basic* rights, because they entail a right to life, to (basic) well-being and to the (basic) means to lead a 'decent' life.

[8] Cf. for the newest data on progress of the Millennium Goals: http://www.un.org/millenniumgoals/pdf/ MDG%20Report%202010%20En%20r15%20-low%20res%2020100615%20-.pdf.

tus quo knowledge.[9] Interestingly, the European Union operates on the Principle of Precaution, while the US Bioethics Commission recommended a far weaker (and legally not binding) principle of responsible stewardship.[10]

The ethical reflection I argue for is by no means an easy enterprise: ethicists have to learn the language of the new technologies including the physical, chemical and biological dimensions. In this process, we select from the outset what might turn out to be relevant and what we assume to be irrelevant for ethical reflection, and among other things, these selections need to be informed and corrected by scientists. As a corollary to that, the social practices-oriented approach (reasoning about social goals, biomedical means to reduce deprivation in basic health care and social and/or political injustice related to health care) can also only be realized in inter-disciplinary research, including technology assessment, ethical analysis and public discourse.

It is crucial to accept that ethicists are dependent on information, education, communication and collaboration with scientists from the sciences and humanities. Ethics as a scientific (or academic) discipline certainly is in a prominent position as moderator of normative claims between different agents or stakeholders – such a moderation and reasoning is necessary within the social and political discourses insofar as social integration and governance of practices is an important dimension in modern societies. By nature, ethics will not be neutral in this reasoning process; in contrast to systems theory, ethics presupposes agency and agents making choices and taking (or denying) responsibility for their actions. Even in cases where agents deny responsibility, they are legally liable and, furthermore, society holds them morally accountable. Ethical reflection does not only take place within the scientific community but is part of everyday reflection, insofar as people make deliberate choices about the way they want to live or how to deal with social and moral norms they are confronted with. Scientific ethical reflection in contrast is pushing this reflection a step further: its task is to interpret (articulate and analyse) values and norms at work in different and pluralistic settings and to confront them with moral principles considered to be essential for human life and human flourishing.[11] Ethicists argue about which normative claims entailed in the different value systems can be upheld reasonably in secularised societies.[12] Thus, professional

---

[9] Hence, it is obvious that visions and prospective technology assessment studies of nanotechnology or synthetic biology, as produced by the institutes of technology assessment, play an important part in this balancing process, and thorough evaluation of the prospects is crucial. One important instrument for this assessment that is used in the European Union is the Precautionary Principle that operates in the case of inconclusive or incomplete data concerning risks of particular technologies. Cf. http://eur-lex. europa.eu/smartapi/cgi/sga_doc?smartapi!celexplus!prod!
CELEXnumdoc&lg = en&numdoc = 52000DC0001.

[10] Presidential Commission for the Study of Bioethical Issues, *New Directions: The Ethics of Synthetic Biology and Emerging Technologies* (2010).

[11] Taylor, C. *Sources of the Self: the making of the modern identity* (Cambridge: Harvard University Press, 1989).

[12] Cf. Gewirth, A. *Reason and morality* (Chicago: University of Chicago Press, Chicago, 1978), Habermas, J. *Faktizität und Geltung. Beiträge zur Diskurstheorie des Rechts und des demokratischen Rechtsstaats* (Frankfurt a.M. Suhrkamp: 1992) and Gewirth, *The Community of Rights*.

ethicists are needed for this task, but they do not (and should not) be considered as 'experts' in morality as such, and they do not (and should not) make policy-oriented decisions themselves. On the contrary, these must be left to public debate and democratic procedures and an approach that tries to take into considerations these different levels of ethical reasoning.[13]

Ethics in the Humanities

The normative framework that I have referred to is neither ahistorical nor decontextualised. An ethics in the sciences that aims at integrating the humanities, mostly historical, social and cultural studies, needs to reflect upon the location from where its analyses start. Ethicists are moral agents, and as such, they enter their studies with convictions, interests and goals that need to be justified in the same way as the convictions, interests and goals of researchers or any other agents. However, the role of ethics is 'reflective': it reflects upon the basic structures of moral reasoning, critically checks arguments and judgements according to consistency, coherence and adequacy, and aims to justify moral claims in view of normative theories. Democratic societies consider themselves as 'open societies', based upon tolerance towards pluralistic value traditions. The role of the state is complex, and it is far from clear how ethical communication is best organised.[14] To explore the views of citizens, the European Union, for example, regularly issues polls such as the Eurobarometer asking about the opinions on new technologies. These, however, cannot overcome the lack of information about the new technologies that is almost always the finding of such polls. Many societies therefore promote public discourse, consultation and hearings, and media take up the task to mediate between science and society. Again, ethics plays an important, albeit not central, role in this communication process. It must listen to as many considerations as possible to gain an understanding of the different values or concerns that are being raised. Cultural studies as well as social analyses are needed for this task, and ideally will be integrated into the ethical analysis that addresses the ethical dimensions. In the reversed methodology that I propose, ethics starts its examination not only with the normative framework expressed in the different ethical frameworks, such as the United Nations Human Rights Declaration or the European Charter of Human Rights, but also with the historical, cultural and social analysis of how these reference points are actually embedded and articulated in the given contexts. Obviously, the gap between the normative framework and the 'lived morality' of modern societies will be apparent, but it is exactly the task of ethics to articulate this accurately and work towards greater consistency between normativity and facticity.

---

[13] Haker, H. *Ethik der genetischen Frühdiagnostik. Sozialethische Reflexionen zur Verantwortung am menschlichen Lebensbeginn* (Paderborn: Mentis, 2002).

[14] I cannot enter the long discussion on the best ways to mediate between pluralistic value traditions and the state in this paper, as, for example, addressed in the 'liberalism' versus 'communitarianism' debate, but certainly it is necessary to account for the presuppositions of different ethics approaches that are linked to this debate. Cf. Honneth, A., Ed.. *Kommunitarismus. Eine Debatte über die moralischen Grundlagen moderner Gesellschaften.* (Frankfurt am Main, 1993).

The EGE Opinion on Synthetic Biology

The political role of the EGE is to interpret the ethical frameworks in light of the new technologies. In addition to the general moral principles of rights and dignity, safety, sustainability, justice, precaution, freedom of research or proportionality, also need to be taken into account.

Following up on their opinion on the ethics of nanomedicine, in 2009, the EGE issued its Opinion on Synthetic Biology.[15] The report introduces the scientific findings and addresses the main areas of application; health, energy, environment and agriculture. The military sector, though considered extremely important, is not thoroughly examined because information is very difficult to obtain. The EGE also addresses this area, however, in the recommendations. In its Opinion, the EGE proposes a number of specific recommendations on synthetic biology that are connected to the recommendations on nanomedicine:

- *Safety*: The EGE advocates that any use of synthetic biology products should be conditional on meeting safety requirements identified in the Opinion. Echoing the Nanomedicine Opinion, the EGE recommends among other things a Code of Conduct for research in synthetic biology.
- *Environmental applications*: Before an organism, fabricated or modified via synthetic biology, is released into the environment, ecological long-term impact assessment must be carried out. The results of the study should be evaluated taking into account the precautionary principle and EU legislation.[16]
- *Energy and sustainable chemical industry*: The Group proposes that the use of synthetic biology for alternative energy supply in EU Member States should be complementary to the EU renewable energy plan. Advocating for the protection of consumers' rights, the EGE stresses that labelling of specific synthetic biology products, such as cosmetics and textiles, should be explored.
- *Biomedicine and biopharmaceutical applications*: In addition to the application of scientific and legal frameworks, specific ethical considerations that are addressed in the Opinion text have to be addressed by the competent authorities (such as EMEA) when drugs and medical products will result from synthetic biology protocols.
- *Biosecurity, prevention of bioterrorism and dual use*: New tools may be derived from synthetic biology for the military sector such as biomaterials or bioweapons. Ethical analysis must assess the goal of security in relation to transparency. In addition, the EGE recommends control mechanisms such as licensing and registering of tools to prevent terrorist uses of synthetic biology. The Group also recommends that the Convention on the Prohibition of the Development, Production and Stockpiling of Bacteriological (Biological) and Toxin Weapons and on Their Destruction should incorporate provisions on the limitation or prohibition of research in synthetic biology.

---

[15] The following paragraph uses the press release that the EGE issues as a short summary of its Opinions. Cf. http://ec.europa.eu/bepa/european-group-ethics/docs/press_release_opinion_25_en.pdf. For the full text cf. European Group on Ethics in Science and New Technologies. *Opinion 25: Ethics of Synthetic Biology* (2009).

[16] This point diverges radically from the US Report on Synthetic biology which uses the principle of 'responsible stewardship' instead of the Precautionary Principle (which has a legal status in the EU).

- *Governance*: The EGE urges the EC to propose and put in place a robust framework for synthetic biology identifying the relevant stakeholders and indicating their responsibilities. The EGE proposes that the EU takes up the question of governance of synthetic biology in relevant global forums.
- *Patenting and common heritage*: The EGE proposes that debates on the most appropriate ways to ensure the public access to the results of synthetic biology is launched. The EGE stresses that general ethical issues raised by patent applications have to be addressed properly in the patent allocation system.
- *Trade and global justice*: The EGE recommends that the ethical issues of synthetic biology should be addressed at the international level, including the World Trade Organisation. This should be taken into account in the Doha round negotiations. The EGE urges that EU Biosafety standards for synthetic biology products are adopted as minimal standards for EU import–export of synthetic biology products.
- *Science and society dialogue*: The Group asks the EU and EU Member States to take actions to promote public debates and engagement amongst the stakeholders to identify main societal concerns in the different areas covered by synthetic biology.
- *Research*: The Group invites the Commission to support basic research in the fields of biology, chemistry, energy, materials science and engineering, as well as applied and inter-disciplinary research, as identified in this Opinion. However, as synthetic biology could lead, in the future, to a paradigm shift in understanding concepts of life, the EGE recommends that an open inter-cultural forum is initiated to address the issues and to include philosophical and religious input.

These are some examples of how ethics committees can become part of broader political governance that must ensure that research and development of new technologies are conducted responsibly. And yet, this political and public role for ethics must not replace the thorough ethical analysis that needs a different methodology.

A Framework of Ethical Reasoning

Over the last few decades, the life sciences, neurosciences, information technology, and for the last few years, the nanosciences and synthetic biology have raised major concerns about the concept of 'nature'. As vague as this term is, philosophers and ethicists have asked about the 'future of human nature' (Habermas); the concept of personal identity; or the concept of reason when it is reduced to 'instrumental-reason' only. Another concern raises the question of the scope of responsibility and accountability when we know so little about the impact and risks accompanying these technologies. Furthermore, it has been argued that new technologies broaden the technology gap rather than narrow it, with the effect that the global health crisis is not attended to: the costs, especially for health care, may well rise because of patent laws and the interests of pharmaceutical companies who invest a lot of money to develop drugs or medical products based upon nanoproducts or synthetic biology. It has been argued, on the other hand, that costs will in fact go down because of more efficient diagnostic or therapeutic applications. Social ethics needs to take up these concerns but will raise further questions, concerning the underlying interests, the values that are promoted with particular research agendas, or the relation of new technologies and the challenge of global justice. It will ask whether new technologies embrace the finitude of human existence or whether they rather increase our vulnerability, whether they promote (implicitly or explicitly) what has been called the *Homo faber* or even *Homo creator*, and what this means for our self-understanding.

To structure the social and ethical discourse on new technologies, I suggest a basic framework that allows us to distinguish between the different dimensions of ethical reflection. I use both personal/individual ethics – to address those dimensions that focus on the actions, convictions and values, and rights and respective obligations of individual agents – and institutional/social ethics – to address those dimensions that focus on social settings and social values enabling and constraining human relationships, cultural and social norms, social and political structures and constraints for individuals' actions, and political, professional and/ or civil society institutions that enable collective actions and social practices, and issues of social and political justice. This describes the first axis in Table 14.1. In the second axes, I distinguish between evaluative/teleological and normative/ deontological dimensions.

This general framework, that entails values as well as rights and obligations, can then be applied to generate the ethical questions concerning new technologies (Table 14.2).

Although this framework is basic for any kind of ethical reasoning, it allows us to distinguish between different fields within new technologies and the different dimensions of ethical reasoning. Personal ethics – addressing teleological dimensions, for example – still must reflect upon, articulate, and interpret personal choices and life-planning, the competence and education that is needed to enable individuals to make reasonable choices (reasonable meaning in this case: making sense in view of their own desires, interests and moral convictions); it must analyse requirements of psychological and/or pastoral care and counselling, and find ways to show how the individual can handle biomedical information, such as considering the risks of nanomedical interventions. As we have seen, social–ethical, teleological issues concern social imagination and social visions, and also norms of social

Table 14.1 The General Framework of Ethical Reasoning

Status of Ethical Reflection	Personal/Individual Ethics	Institutional/Social Ethics
Teleological considerations with diverse and pluralistic answers	*Individual values*: Self-fulfilment, well-being, autonomy and freedom	*Social values*: Mutual recognition of individuals and groups, solidarity, common good
Deontological considerations with universalistic normative claims	*Individual rights*: Human rights based on the respect for the dignity of others, resulting in the obligation to respect the other and support his/her flourishing	*Political and social justice*: Distribution based on fairness and equality, compensation by redistribution, corrections of structural injustice

Table 14.2 Framework for Ethical Reflections of New Technologies

Status of Ethical Reflection	Personal/Individual Ethics (Exemplary Questions)	Institutional/Social Ethics
Teleological (goal-based) considerations with diverse and pluralistic answers	*Individual values* Dealing with heteronomy and autonomy in medical decision-making (control versus contingency and vulnerability) Personal Responsibility for one's life and health	*Social values* Social values and social norms of health, well-being and being a 'good enough' member of society Social visions of perfection and/or acknowledgement of 'imperfection'
	Choices with respect to quality of life, based on desires, interests and value convictions Priority setting of health goods over against other goods, assessment of risks, desire and interest to know or not to know Relational autonomy: Care for oneself in relation to and with others	Social concepts of life and death, of health and disease Solidarity among communities, solidarity among strangers Social, economic and health care goals and perspectives for developed and developing countries
Deontological (duty-based) considerations with normative claims	*Individual Rights* Respect of human rights as far as they are concerned with medical interventions (negative obligations) Respect of the decisions of others Respect of intellectual property rights and freedom of research Obligation to assist and support the well-being of others and to empower them to become agents or maintain agency, who can act according to their own interests (positive obligations, within limits of rights' claims)	*Political and social justice* Governance and legislation on human experiments, on research and application based on justice Just distribution of health care goods Fairness and equality in access to participate in all relevant medical practices Compensation and corrections of past and present structural injustice (e.g. special funding for infectious diseases to compensate for structural shortcomings of the past)

interaction, practices of solidarity or group identities. On the one hand, personal/ individual ethics – addressing the normative question of human rights, obligations, respect for the freedom of others – will need to be worked out with respect to some of the traditional bioethical concerns: privacy and data protection, protection against harm among others. Especially with respect to global health care, positive rights are open for debate, determining how much assistance is needed by exactly whom, to enable individuals to 'lead decent lives'. Additionally, social ethics addressing the normative question of justice is linked to policies and international strategies of global health care. It is on this level that the Millennium Goals of the United Nations need to be integrated in the reflection upon nanomedicine, and we need to integrate political and economic theories in the overall reflection. The task of ethics in this multi-disciplinary reflective enterprise is to address and analyse the personal values and social norms underlying different claims, to address their inter-relation, and to work on the normative claims that enable us to identify and priori-tise rights and obligations. With regard to individual decision-making, the task of ethics is to address the ethical dimension of the choices within the limits of moral pluralism and diversity, and to help all actors, scientists, legislators, ethicists and patients, in making responsible decisions.

As this framework shows ethical analysis cannot be realized as an appendix to technology assessment or scientific developments, but requires us to reverse the perspective to complement the technology-oriented ethical analysis with a social practice-oriented analysis. It was the aim of this chapter to argue for this comple-mentary method that is closer to ethics' own competence, and desperately needed to set the right priorities in and for science and new technologies.

Bibliography

Cahill L, Haker H. "Natural law. A Controversy". *Concilium* 2010;46:3.

European Group on Ethics in Science and New Technologies. *Opinion 25: Ethics of Synthetic Biology*; 2009. Online version: <http://ec.europa.eu/bepa/european-group-ethics/docs/opinion25_en.pdf/>

European Union. *Treaty of Lisbon; European Charter of Fundamental Rights*. Online ver-sion: <http://bookshop.europa.eu/is-bin/INTERSHOP.enfinity/WFS/EU-Bookshop-Site/en_GB/-/EUR/ViewPublication-Start?PublicationKey = QC3209190/>

Gewirth A. *Reason and Morality*. Chicago: University of Chicago Press; 1978.

Gewirth A. *The Community of Rights*. Chicago: University of Chicago Press; 1996.

Habermas J. *Faktizität und Geltung. Beiträge zur Diskurstheorie des Rechts und des demok-ratischen Rechtsstaats*. Frankfurt am Main: Suhrkamp; 1992.

Haker H. *"Moralische Identität. Literarische Lebensgeschichten als Medium ethischer Reflexion. Mit einer Interpretation der 'Jahrestage' von Uwe Johnson"*. Tübingen: Francke; 1999.

Haker H. *Ethik der genetischen Frühdiagnostik. Sozialethische Reflexionen zur Verantwortung am menschlichen Lebensbeginn*. Paderborn: Mentis; 2002.

Honneth A, editor. *Kommunitarismus. Eine Debatte über die moralischen Grundlagen mod-erner Gesellschaften*. Frankfurt am Main: Main; 1993.

Keasling J. "A Life of Its Own". *The New Yorker* 2009;: Cf. online: <http://www.newyorker.com/reporting/2009/09/28/090928fa_fact_specter.3/>.

Mieth D. *Was wollen wir können? Ethik im Zeitalter der Biotechnik.* Freiburg im Breisgau: Herder; 2002.

Presidential Commission for the Study of Bioethical Issues. *New Directions: The Ethics of Synthetic Biology and Emerging Technologies*; 2010. Online version: <http://www.bioethics.gov/documents/synthetic-biology/PCSBI-Synthetic-Biology-Report-12.16.10.pdf/>

Taylor C. *Sources of the Self: The Making of the Modern Identity.* Cambridge: Harvard University Press; 1989.

15 Lessons from Teaching Research Ethics Across the Disciplines

Amy Daughton

Director of Studies, Margaret Beaufort Institute of Theology,
Cambridge, UK

Abstract

Ethics as a subject for post-graduate researchers is both a discipline and a practice. What this means is that any researcher must develop a framework of thinking which can then be applied for the practical ethical challenges of her research, and crucially, can be communicated to her supervisors, peers and research participants. This necessarily includes those structures that provide ethical oversight on research, which take different forms in different institutional contexts.

As a teacher of ethics then, regardless of one's own location amongst ethical traditions of ethics, one has three clear responsibilities: enabling researchers to relate their practice to ethical concepts, supporting them as they develop their ethical argumentation in response and clarifying and refining the language they use to discuss ethical concepts and practice. My purpose in this chapter is to emphasise the necessary dialogical character of these tasks.

Key Words

Pedagogy, discussion, vulnerability, practical wisdom, translation

Introduction

Ethics as a subject for post-graduate researchers is both a discipline and a practice. What this means is that any researcher must develop a framework of thinking which can then be applied for the practical ethical challenges of her research, and crucially, can be communicated to her supervisors, peers and research participants. This necessarily includes those structures that provide ethical oversight on research, which take different forms in different institutional contexts.

As a teacher of ethics then, regardless of one's own location amongst ethical traditions, one has three clear responsibilities: enabling researchers to relate their

Ethics for Graduate Researchers. DOI: http://dx.doi.org/10.1016/B978-0-12-416049-1.00015-5

practice to ethical concepts, supporting them as they develop their ethical argumentation in response and clarifying and refining the language they use to discuss ethical concepts and practice. My purpose in this chapter is to emphasise the necessary dialogical character of these tasks.

By outlining these goals for teaching ethics, I will show that such work should not be focused on disseminating a series of isolated models, but rather on the range of ways of thinking available for discussion and critique. This view is partly shaped by my own research experience with the ethics of French philosopher Paul Ricoeur. What Ricoeur's ethics will help me to emphasise is the increased precision that can develop in discursive contexts. Ricoeur's own methodology reflects this, standing firmly in the European continental tradition yet also engaging closely with the Anglo-American analytical tradition. Ricoeur therefore provides a framework for thinking about the value of dialogue in ethics teaching across discipline and ethical perspective.

My own experience with peer-to-peer teaching of ethics to post-graduate researchers has also shaped this viewpoint and has ultimately borne out the emphasis I place on the value of dialogue in pedagogical approaches to ethics. Therefore, before I present the three aspects of ethics teaching that I list above and seek to argue for a deliberately discursive approach, I will outline that teaching experience.

Teaching Context

During my time as a post-graduate researcher and fellow at Trinity College Dublin (TCD), I was involved in two major projects aimed at communicating ethics and ethical research skills to post-graduate students. The first of these was as a support and co-teacher in a national fourth level generic skills module for graduate researchers. This project was launched in 2008–2009. The second was through the Trinity Long Room Hub (TLRH) at TCD, an inter-disciplinary centre directed towards capacity building for research in the arts, humanities and social sciences. Here, I designed and disseminated a project on ethics discussion as the TLRH Postgraduate Fellow in 2009. I will detail the teaching involved in each project in turn.

The generic skills programme was titled 'Research Ethics' and was designed and facilitated by the School of Religions, Theology and Ecumenics (TCD) in collaboration with University College Cork and the National University of Ireland-Galway (NUI-G). The module was aimed at early-stage graduate researchers from across all disciplines at the three institutions and was conducted in two distinct year groups from 2008 to 2009.

In the first year, the teaching of the component was through the gathered expertise of ethics scholars and practitioners from across Europe. This volume contains the rich and varied insights of many of those experts.

In the second year of the project, I co-taught alongside Dr. Cathriona Russell, working from the themes and ideas of the generic skills programme. We were able to take further advantage of European expertise through individual lectures hosted at TCD by Sigrid Graumann and Hille Haker. The teaching of this module was undertaken under two streams: 'Humanities and Social Sciences', which was my responsibility; and 'Natural and Health Sciences', which was the responsibility of Dr. Russell. Both streams were taught together. The thinking behind this structure was to identify for participants the appropriate ethics expertise, but to reject any isolation of discipline and thereby to enrich the resulting class discussion. My teaching covered theoretical and practical concerns, incorporating, e.g. Bosk,[1] and philosophical overviews of related challenges from Ricoeur[2] and Nora.[3]

A part of this teaching process that is worth noting was the emphasis placed on supporting students in the practical ethical challenges they encountered in their research. Students were called on to outline their research projects in terms of the potential ethical dilemmas and pitfalls they may encounter. For example, research involving children needs to take account of how to best communicate with younger participants, how to avoid leading any discussion and how to perform the research in safe, comfortable and supervised environments so as to best protect both child and researcher. Another example might include how to manage participant incentives, and reporting back to participants, to protect researchers from too many demands on their resources.

Final evaluations of these outlines were considered at the conclusion of the course, partly conducted as an open class-based discussion, and partly as direct commentary from myself and Dr. Russell as stream leaders. This allowed a concrete outcome for participants, and allowed teachers to both gauge the success of the teaching and have a direct impact on the ethical conduct of the future research of these participants. This year's group represented the conclusion of the work on the Research Ethics component of the fourth level generic skills project.

The second major teaching project derived from this initial experience. Feedback from the first year of the generic skills project had indicated that there was a student-led desire for a continuing discussion space – something that was specifically requested by a number of participants from TCD. In this collection of student responses, ethics was understood to be a key additional resource for understanding one's own research and was aided by being facilitated and discursive.

It is at this point that I introduce the Trinity Long Room Hub that became the context in which I was able to meet this desire for ongoing ethics discourse. The overall mission of the Hub is to ensure the long-term sustainability and vibrancy of the arts, humanities and social sciences. In the summer of 2009, the Trinity Long Room Hub was focused on developing its ability to meet the needs of early-stage researchers. My ethics teaching project was designed to contribute to these goals.

The project I designed, and the Hub hosted, focused on developing a structured opportunity for post-graduate and early-stage researchers to develop their knowledge of ethical traditions in a discursive context. Over 2 years, I led two courses of

---

[1] C. Bosk and V. de Vries, "Bureaucracies of Mass Deception: Institutional Review Boards and the Ethics of Ethnography Research," *AAPSS*, 595 (2004), 249–63.

[2] P. Ricoeur, "Approaching the Human Person" (D. Kidd, trans.) *Ethical Perspectives*, 1 (1999), 45–54.

[3] P. Nora, "Between Memory and History: Les Lieux de Mémoire," *Representations: Memory and Counter-Memory*, 26 (1989), 7–24.

discussion-based seminars, focused on responding to texts from different ethical traditions. Participants were post-graduate volunteers from throughout the Arts, Humanities and Social Sciences Faculty (AHSS). They were invited to participate through Faculty lists. Each participant was requested to confirm their attendance for each seminar, allowing continuity between each discussion session. This created a genuinely inter-disciplinary group.

Key to the long-term value of this was facilitating discussion on the connections between specific ethical challenges in each researcher's work and some wider themes. To this end, I identified four central themes that would allow the contextualising of the participants' work within broad contemporary ethical discussions: narrative, identity, memory, community.[4] The texts chosen for each seminar fell within one or more of these themes. It is important to note that these texts were situated within different ethical traditions, allowing opportunity for critique between traditions of thought in the light of concrete research projects.[5] My primary teaching role in this was thus one of comparison and contextualisation. In this way, over 3 years, I have taken a variety of roles in ethics teaching and in multiple teaching contexts. As I now turn to consider the responsibilities that I identified for the teacher of ethics at the beginning of this chapter, the insights gained from these processes direct my thinking.

As noted earlier, there are three main pedagogical tasks: linking ethics to practice, ethical argumentation and communication. I will outline these using emphases from Ricoeur's ethical theory, paralleled by my teaching experience with AHSS students. I will focus on the significance placed on practical wisdom, the emphasis on seeking the best argument and the need to communicate the insights of ethics to multiple audiences. Ultimately, I intend to advocate a discursive, inter-disciplinary approach to ethics teaching, balanced and facilitated by ethical expertise.

Practical Wisdom

I will look first at practical wisdom in its significance for Ricoeur's ethical theory and its role in working out concrete responses to complex ethical dilemmas. I will go on to note the value of the inter-disciplinary context for developing this kind of practically focused expertise.

Ricoeur's own ethical theory is constructed in stages. He characterises the entire enterprise of ethical theory in terms of the ethical aim, the moral norm and the practical wisdom. To clarify, Ricoeur's ethical aim is expressed as 'aiming at the

---

[4] The centrality of these themes for researchers within the Arts, Humanities and Social Sciences Faculty was underscored by their wider use in TLRH projects. These four titles were used to organise the digital presentation of post-graduate research on the internal TARA system.

[5] A good example would include a direct comparison between the views of Charles Taylor and Jürgen Habermas on the concept of multiculturalism: C. Taylor, "Politics of Recognition," in A. Gutmann, (ed.) *Multiculturalism: Examining the Politics of Recognition* (Princeton University Press, 1992), pp. 37–73, and the response is J. Habermas, "Address: Multiculturalism and the Liberal State," *Stanford Law Review*, 47, (1995), 848–53.

"good life" with and for others, in just institutions'.[6] Ricoeur deliberately acknowledges the multiplicity of views on what the 'good life', or living well can be taken to mean. The culturally subsistent concept of living well is held in the light of the universal duty to the person: in reference to the other, inter-personal ethics, and to the institution, the ethical relationship with the anonymous other.

So Ricoeur's ethical aim cannot be taken in isolation.[7] He constructs a constant movement between an understanding of the goals of living well, and the moral obligation to the other, thus testing the ethical aim in terms of the moral norm. He shows how the two approaches can be systematically combined and can be interpreted as bridgeable even on their own terms: virtue and good will. In this way, Ricoeur opens his ethics into the moral test, while acknowledging the culturally significant bases for decision-making.

This dialogue is made constructive by Ricoeur's addition of a further sphere of thinking about ethical action: the sphere of practical wisdom. He views practical wisdom as the mediation of the teleological and the deontological that constantly requires negotiation. The significance of this aspect of Ricoeur's ethical theory should not be under-estimated. Ricoeur himself laments that 'my chapter devoted to practical wisdom still looks like an appendix, and it should become the crucial chapter'.[8] Practical wisdom provides the decisive concrete insight to develop a creative path through the ongoing tensions.

For example, Deneulin, working primarily in development theory, has argued that practical wisdom 'is to have the last word in decision making'[9] because it is at this point that the 'necessary thickening'[10] of ethics is developed. Deneulin provides a useful example of this in the dialogue she constructs between Ricoeur and Amartya Sen on questions of international development. Ricoeur's own work on medical ethics, juridical issues and the ethics of memory also provides examples of this in its characteristically dialogical nature. He deliberately works by detours through significant texts from other thinkers. Essentially, both Ricoeur and his commentator Deneulin see practical wisdom as the crucial sphere for bringing the ethical aim and the test of the moral norm to a specific concrete decision.

In my view, the significance placed on practical wisdom within Ricoeur's wider ethical theory reinforces the dialogical nature of ethics teaching. It is an 'ethics of argumentation' that he proposes, employing Jürgen Habermas's term. This critical process is made necessary by multiple grounds of ethical argument, and also made richer by its encounter with that plurality. Ricoeur considered part of the solution

---

[6] P. Ricoeur, *Oneself as Another* (Chicago University Press, 1996), p. 172.
[7] Indeed, I consider the most significant characteristic of Ricoeur's ethical theory to be his attempt to marry traditionally opposed approaches to ethical questions – in this case Aristotle's virtue oriented life, and Kant's emphasis on moral duty.
[8] P. Ricoeur, "Ethics and Human Capability – A Response," in J. Wall, W. Schweiker, W. David Hall, (Eds.) *Paul Ricoeur and Contemporary Moral Thought* (London: Routledge, 2002), pp. 279–98. p. 288.
[9] S. Deneulin, "Necessary Thickening," in S. Deneulin, M. Nabel, and N. Sagovsky, (eds.) *Transforming Unjust Structures – The Capability Approach*, (Dordrecht: Springer, 2006) pp. 27–45. p. 40.
[10] Deneulin, 2006, p. 27.

of practical wisdom to be rooted in the enriching possibilities of the encounter with the other. For research ethics, the conclusion to be drawn from this theoretical structuring of ethical discourse is that the researcher must contribute to establishing ethical practice.

This is the challenge for the AHSS researcher, who must make concrete decisions for his/her own protection and for the protection of the research participants. It is through this expertise that any given ethical theory must be applied.

For this to be done well, the practical insights of the researcher are essential. In the context of the US debate on Institutional Review Boards, the insights of Bosk and de Vries emphasise that it is often *only* in the daily details of research that the ethics of a particular research project can be worked out. They argue that for some humanities and social sciences researchers, establishing an ethical framework in advance is a difficult process. Ethnographers, for example, 'cannot specify risks because we do not know what we will find, what interpretive frameworks we will develop for reporting what we do observe, and how the world around us will change to make those findings seem more or less significant'.[11] The way that the research itself is conducted must be deliberately set outside such frameworks so that it can be responsive to what is being found during the research. 'We cannot state our procedures any more formally than we will hang around here in this particular neighborhood and try to figure out what is going on among these people'.[12]

For example, during my co-teaching of the fourth level skills module, one researcher's project was intended to begin to map the impact of HIV/AIDS on Rwandan children born from rape during the 1994 genocide. Class discussion on this project emphasised the unpredictability of identifying and responding to vulnerabilities in both individuals and the wider community. What this broader point of the protection of vulnerable persons may mean in practice is necessarily led by the on-project conversations between researcher and participant. It will be the researcher's role to determine what constitutes the protection of the participant in any given conversation, in the context of the research goals, and to choose their questions accordingly.[13]

This means that the expertise of researchers in their disciplines, and their research practice is highly valued. Still, while the researcher is called to make the ultimate decision, this does not remove responsibility from the ethicist. What is required of ethics teaching is therefore twofold: first, there is the need to recognise the importance of inter-disciplinary discussion for the development of practical wisdom. Second, given this discursive approach, the role of the ethicist is

---

[11] Bosk and de Vries, 2006, p. 53.
[12] Bosk and de Vries, 2006, p. 253.
[13] This indicates child-centred research in the immediate information-gathering stage; a strong sensitivity to the potentially traumatic nature of any family discussion; and a view towards the future outcomes of research benefiting the participating community. The researcher must also be protected from undertaking work that requires too much of them: for example, the potentially therapeutic aspects to discussion. Such research may therefore be best done by working through NGOs and other organisations with the appropriate resources, and can add further practical wisdom of those experienced in the sector and the region.

understood as one that involves providing the tools which a researcher can take into the research context for those moments that demand practical wisdom. I will briefly discuss these points.

First, ethics teaching should provide opportunities for inter-disciplinary discussion, thereby creating a space for developing that judgement for situations that call for practical decision-making. 'It is through public debate, friendly discussion, and shared convictions that moral judgement in situation is formed.[14] This is Deneulin's necessary thickening of the ethical aim with the moral norm, and ultimately with practical wisdom. An inter-disciplinary context allows for multiple viewpoints from different angles and practical contexts. In this way, the necessary thickening can be developed with a wider and deeper critique.

This is the significance of practical wisdom which seeks to articulate 'convictions which have their origins in the aims of real life'.[15] What Ricoeur's emphasis on the word conviction reveals for my purposes in this chapter is the significance of the particular circumstance in which an ethical challenge has arisen. 'The last word belongs to the convictions which receive the stamp of a specific culture and historical context'.[16] In this sense, again, it is the researcher's own discipline and research context that must be the final word in how to respond ethically to the research situation. In this way, it becomes clear that teaching ethics must be aimed at providing the researcher with an appropriate range of tools to then respond practically.

This brings me to my second requirement for ethics teaching. Assuming a pedagogical context that is discursive and inter-disciplinary, the work for an ethics teacher lies in enabling that discussion to proceed as precisely and rigorously as possible. What is key for this is how to develop the researcher's best argument.

Developing the Best Arguments

It is under this heading of seeking the best argument that I will further clarify the pedagogical approach to developing practical wisdom. Given the context of an 'ethics of argumentation', where better arguments are pursued through inter-disciplinary discussion, there is a responsibility to produce the best argument one can. I noted earlier the source of the 'ethics of argumentation' in Habermas. In discussing this, Ricoeur asks the following question: 'what does an "ethics of argumentation" mean? It is to be ready to give the best argument and to allow the other one to give their best argument'.[17] The discussion itself is to be valued as a way of publically testing one's own argumentation. The aim is not resolution, but to fully explore the ethical dilemma and for 'reasonable disagreement' to be fully heard. A

[14] Ricoeur, 1996, pp. 290–1.
[15] J. Greisch, "From Testimony to Attestation," in R. Kearney (ed.), *Paul Ricoeur: The Hermeneutics of Action* (London: Sage, 1996), pp. 81–98. p. 94.
[16] Greisch, 1996, p. 95.
[17] P. Ricoeur and Y. Raynova, "All that gives us to think: Conversations with Paul Ricoeur," in A. Wiercinski (ed.) *Between Suspicion and Sympathy* (Toronto: The Hermeneutic Press, 2003), pp. 679–96. p. 694.

good example of the working out of this is the practice of the European Group on Ethics in Science and New Technologies (EGE), which advises the European Commission. This group will provide an agreed recommendation, but includes in its written reports the justifications for multiple perspectives on the argument.[18]

Indeed, this is the 'most I can ask of others', suggests Ricoeur, when there is disagreement, 'not to subscribe to what I believe to be true, but to present their best arguments'.[19] As a model for how to go about a debate on ethics, this acknowledges both the limits of the best argument and its valuable dialogical context. It is necessary to accept 'the fact that there are unresolvable differences... by recognizing the reasonableness of the parties present, giving dignity and respect to opposing viewpoints and acknowledging the plausability of arguments invoked on both sides'.[20]

Ultimately, this continued discursive approach is not possible within a set research project and the AHSS researcher will have to make concrete decisions. Here is where the pedagogical roles of the philosopher appear for Ricoeur. 'Concisely, the task of philosophy would be firstly, to protect our inheritance, secondly, to enter into discussion with scientists,[21] and thirdly, to enact what I call practical wisdom'.[22] I have already noted this emphasis on developing practical wisdom in the classroom, but Ricoeur adds a further requirement: 'the task of the mediation between everyday problems, but only on condition of having addressed the other two tasks'.[23] It is these tasks that I now examine.

In terms of translating to the classroom, the 'protection of our inheritance' means for Ricoeur that 'we should see to it that people still read Plato, Aristotle, Kant, etc.'.[24] What is required pedagogically then is the systematic input an ethics teacher can give, introducing research ethical vocabulary, concepts and traditions of thought. These constitute the tools that the researcher can use to respond to their particular research context.

The positive impact that such systematic introductions have on discursive teaching is borne out by my own classroom experience. The value of this for the teaching context is emphasised by my experience with the TLRH teaching project. The first tranche − in response to the feedback from the fourth level generic skills − focused primarily on peer-to-peer discussion. However, feedback on this first round indicated the need to have a stronger guide in terms of technical language and frameworks of thought. This prompted me to add formal teaching sections as routes into discussions for the second tranche of the project.

---

[18] See http://ec.europa.eu/bepa/european-group-ethics/publications/opinions/index_en.htm−last accessed 24 May 2012.

[19] P. Ricoeur, *Critique and Conviction. Conversations with François Azouvi and Marc de Launay* (K. Blamey, trans.), (Oxford: Polity Press, 1998), p. 129.

[20] Ricoeur, 1998, p. 129.

[21] Later in the discussion, Ricoeur notes that his meaning of scientists includes such disciplines as historical studies and sociology, as well as bio- and chemical sciences.

[22] Ricoeur and Raynova, 2003, p. 693.

[23] Ricoeur and Raynova, 2003, p. 693.

[24] Ricoeur and Raynova, 2003, p. 693.

This theory-based discussion then led to the concrete specifics of the research projects of the group. The teaching input here becomes about guiding research students into articulating these theoretical frameworks in practical expressions.

At this stage, in Ricoeur's terms, the goal is to require correct arguments in the discussion.[25] Partly this is a question of continuing to demand precision in language. 'All these words have complex usage; and, as always, one of the tasks of philosophical reflection is to clarify concepts... distinguish the uses of terms'.[26] Pedagogically this can be easily pursued by an ongoing process of questioning[27] : 'If you use the word freedom, what do you mean by that word?'.[28] This allows the student to further contextualise his/her argument, refining its impact. The need to make these ways of thinking practical for the research project provides the researchers with experience of judging what is reasonable, in dialogue with critical input from the teacher and the practical wisdom of her peers.

In this way, the researcher is guided to develop their best argument in the context of multiple bases for ethical thinking.

It is worth noting here the responsibility present for the teacher in this approach. The goal of enabling the researcher to develop his/her best argument also means responding to the vulnerability of students. If one accepts that there is in obligation to bring one's best argument to articulation and that such articulation is best refined in discussion, there is a clear responsibility on the part of the teacher, guiding that discussion, to manage circumstances where there is an inability to speak. There is an ethical task within the classroom to ensure vulnerable students are enabled to contribute to this discussion. In practice, this is a question of directing discussions to ensure that all opinions are heard – a task not limited to ethics teaching.

This can include circumstances where there is a straightforward question of facilitation. Some practical examples from different teaching contexts of mine include: accounting for dyslexia in handout formats: large print, coloured paper, coloured ink; giving out readings in time for alteration and ensuring hearing aid loops are switched on; varying discussion formats to allow different kinds of contributions: small groups, response to readings, written exercises.

However, there can be an inability to participate in a class discussion that has more to do with what Ricoeur calls 'fragility'. Anderson has written on the concrete incapacity of feeling unable to speak.[29] Ricoeur too, frames this question in terms of what an individual can do to prevent or respond to inequalities that impact

---

[25] Ricoeur and Raynova, 2003, p. 694.

[26] Ricoeur, 1998, p. 133.

[27] As I will note below, this ongoing process of refinement will be best conducted in different ways for different students. It is important that the pursuit of a precise definition not be seen by the student as a rejection of the argument, but a shared constructive discussion for improvement. I am about to discuss the pedagogy of this below.

[28] Ricoeur and Raynova, 2003, p. 694.

[29] P. S. Anderson, "Loss of Confidence: Dissymmetry, doubt, deprivation in the power to act and (the power) to suffer," in J. Carter, J. Carlisle, and D. Whistler, (eds.) Moral Powers, Fragile Beliefs: Essays in Moral and Religious Philosophy, (London: Continuum, 2011) pp. 83–108.

on concrete abilities. For a teacher, facilitating the varying capabilities in the classroom is a crucial responsibility.

Ricoeur has written on the significance of this responsibility in the face of vulnerability in the juridical context. While not juridical, ethics teaching takes place in an institutional context that carries responsibility for its participants. In the same way it is 'vulnerability that makes autonomy remain a condition of possibility that juridical practice turns into a task',[30] so too does it for teachers. The reason for this is that '[p]eople do not simply lack power, they are deprived of it'.[31] In response, the real capacities of each person are to be emphasised in the face of possible fragility or inability. The crucial counterpart that Ricoeur forms in response to fragility is therefore a 'pedagogy of responsibility'.[32]

In terms of practical teaching choices, this is often a question of responding to the particular group of students, but ultimately the goal of seeking the best argument is a good one for shaping pedagogy on this point. The aim of drawing out the best argument in dialogue means being alive to the dangers of a didactic approach. To this end, the teacher should be seeking to draw out more precise definitions, and to further the implications of arguments, rather than applying his/her own ethical position. In terms of drawing out students less able to contribute to this discussion, it is valuable to consider different discursive opportunities, such as responding to previously written work. In this way, quieter students can be drawn into the conversation by explicitly drawing in these contributions. Moreover, emphasising the constructive role of that discussion can be done by building on students' work. The goal is to help reframe students' work, or identify important steps in an argument that should be more fully articulate, supplying criticism to build up the argument more strongly, rather than rejecting it.

Most significant is the role that student evaluation can take. The constructive nature of the discourse is underlined for the student by the attitude of the teacher to the input of students on the teacher's own thinking. For example, a useful way of framing the teaching course is to explicitly note the ongoing opportunities for input regarding what would be most valuable for the students. This can be done in terms of soliciting reading ideas, by listing initial student responses to a text and using these to structure the subsequent conversation, noting the current structure of the course in relation to previous students' course evaluations. Indeed, these course evaluation forms should be highlighted at the very beginning of the course in terms of their genuine contribution to the shape of the class. I have already noted the way student evaluation prompted the existence of the TLRH project and helped shape it for future tranches. Acknowledging this explicitly emphasises the value placed on student contribution, further enabling the student in terms of their capability of speaking and evaluating.

This is an embodiment by the teacher of valuing the viewpoint of the other, thus shaping a deliberately discursive and inclusive space. Teaching then becomes one

---

[30] P. Ricoeur, *Reflections on the Just,* D. Pellauer, (trans.), (University of Chicago Press, 2007). 72.

[31] Ricoeur, 2007, p. 77.

[32] Ricoeur, 2007, p. 77.

of the 'practices applicable to the paradox of autonomy and fragility'.[33] A further useful description comes from Maureen Junker-Kenny's overview of approaches to Habermas's analysis to this question. She points to a phase of Hermann Nohl's, the 'pedagogical paradox',[34] to describe the difficulty in assuming the autonomy of the student to properly create it. However, '[t]he pedagogical paradox is oriented towards the future and can be resolved by an adequate structuring of the interaction which respects the emerging identity'[35] of the dialogue partner. As a teacher then deliberately making one's own thinking available for critique displays for the student the productive nature of that critique. Autonomy is claimed by appropriating, or further debating a critique, in the face of the fragility that could occur in a power-based confrontation. Again, the teacher develops the conditions in which the student is ultimately enabled to pursue his/her best arguments in dialogue, in the light of the practical wisdom and ethical expertise in the classroom.

There are two valuable outcomes to this. The first is the development of the student's best argument and the development of one's own in that engagement. This has already been emphasised by Ricoeur's focus on ethics as an inter-disciplinary responsibility, where the ethicist learns from the scientist. The second is in the model of discussion it can perpetuate for ethical research itself.

To expand on this point, the researcher is also called upon to account for the necessarily fragile relationship between herself and her research participants. Developing a sensibility towards incapacities for speech within the experience of ethics teaching can promote that within research.[36]

Again, '[p]eople do not simply lack power, they are deprived of it'.[37] The researcher (and the Ethics Board that supports her) must therefore be alive to the possibility of creating such incapacity in others in the research process, or indeed of failing to identify it. General examples might include preventing a narrative being told by the participant by asking leading questions, or by structuring the discussion too rigidly.

The researcher must therefore respond to the needs of the participant. The teacher of ethics can provide a model for this by, in Ricoeur's terms, being ready '[t]o learn how to tell the same story in another way, how to allow our story to be told be others, how to submit the narrative of a life to an historian's critique'.[38] The availability to the viewpoint of the other is thus at the heart of the significant pedagogical experiences Ricoeur highlights.

---

[33] Ricoeur, 2007, p. 80.

[34] For another working out of this tension see I. Kant, *On Education*, A. Churton, (trans.), (Mineola, NY: Courier Dover Publications, 2003).

[35] M. Junker-Kenny, *Habermas and Theology*, (New York: Continuum, 2011), p. 26.

[36] In relation to this, significant responsibility for oversight is also placed on Research Ethics Boards in their various forms, which provide the institutional protocol for recognising and managing necessarily fragile relationships. This third party viewpoint is crucial for clarifying the inter-personal relationships that often form the basis for AHSS research.

[37] Ricoeur, 2007, p. 80.

[38] Ricoeur, 2007, p. 80.

An example from the TLRH teaching project is of an early-career researcher in the Department of Business and his experience recording narratives of voluntary activity. When transcribing testimony, there is a possibility of writing the story in a way that does not authentically reflect the experience the participant meant to express. At the same time, the researcher may see points of interest not visible to the participant. Owing to this, the researcher seeking to record narratives built additional follow-up with his research participants into the project. This ensured a clear and agreed narrative representation that could be used with consent, but more broadly also allowed the participants to both feel in control of their own stories[39] and allow them the opportunity to reflect on their experiences in dialogue. Most crucially, it avoids the researcher directing the narrative too strongly.

Recognising the fragility, and the concrete needs of the participant, through the discursive model of ethics teaching and the practical wisdom exchanged there, leads me to my final point: the need to translate.

Translation

I noted in my introduction the need to be able to communicate well, one's ethical standpoint. I turn again to Ricoeur, who suggests translation as a lens for understanding dialogue that is ostensibly within a language but is across discipline.[40] Here, 'translation' describes both the classroom discussion and the conducting of research itself. I will deal with each context in turn.

First, as I have already noted, ethical reflection can be inter-disciplinary. Acknowledging this within the classroom is valuable. For example, Ricoeur points to philosophically significant *Grundwörter*, which 'are themselves summaries of long textuality where whole contexts are mirrored... [and i]ntertextuality which is sometimes equivalent to revival, transformation, refutation of earlier uses'.[41] This is all the more significant in the context of inter-disciplinary development of ethical thinking where dialogue has directly contributed to the research ethics of a given project. As I noted earlier, the clarification of the meaning of words is crucial for this. Again, this is matched by the ethical expertise of the teacher, philosopher, providing direct and systematic input from the intellectual history, and renewed by the researcher's self-critical articulation of ethical thinking itself.

The best example from my experience of teaching comes from the fourth level generic skills course, co-taught by Dr. Russell and myself. One student's research focus was online research using virtual environments such as Second Life. It would be difficult for an ethicist to make an absolute judgement on relevant ethical safeguards without being in conversation with the researcher, who has a more complete picture of the technological implications and limitations. The value of this conversation is further shown as the researcher was subsequently able to contribute to the growing ethical awareness in Internet-based research by publishing on the ethical

---

[39] This is particularly important for testimonies given in relation to ongoing circumstances or trauma.
[40] P. Ricoeur, *On Translation*, E. Brennan, (trans.). (London: Routledge, 2005).
[41] Ricoeur, 2005, p. 6.

implications of her research project.[42] This is an instance of ethical expertise being drawn into a different context through the translation of an ethical framework into practical research concerns, in this case computer science.

It is also crucial that the researcher be able to properly communicate to participants. This is partly a question of being able to explain the measures taken to protect both participant and researcher and the reasons for these, and also in pitching the research questions in such a way that the answers are not directed, that the questions themselves are understood,[43] and that the discussion goes on in such a way that the participant is enabled to answer as emphasised earlier. Including unnecessary technical language is no help to any of these goals and ultimately the specialist vocabulary of research ethics could benefit from a translative approach. This may appear a basic point, but the way in which communication from one's academic discipline to another context is improved is by continuing to seek a better translation. The practical experience and the discursive context outlined earlier remains critical, as an opportunity for constructive criticism.

An obvious example is found in any research project focused on inter-linguistic and inter-cultural relationships. Through the TLRH group, one such example emerged, namely a study on the decline and renewal of the French dialect Occitan, in which the researcher was confronted with the issue of how a non-Occitan speaker could evaluate the renewal of a language from the outside. This was an ongoing challenge for the researcher in question and was eventually addressed through the researcher engaging in as strong a dialogue as possible with research participants who were first-language Occitan speakers. It is an instance where practical wisdom developed within the research context will be key. This underlines my points regarding the enriching of research frameworks by involving the thinking of the other. Understanding this in terms of translation emphasises the genuine contribution to be experienced within the research context and within the interdisciplinary discourse I advocate for ethics teaching.

Conclusion

In this way, the steps of teaching ethics to a researcher are threefold: systematic input from the ethics teacher, enabling a broader discursive context of the classroom discussion and its input from practitioners, and the subsequent adaptation to the practical experience of the research context. The goal is to enable the researcher to develop his/her ethical expertise with a view to articulating his/her ethical basis

---

[42] C. Girwan, and T. Savage, "Ethical considerations for education research in a virtual world," in *Interactive Learning Environments* (in press, 2012).

[43] This impacts on questions of consent: there is a clear moral obligation to ensure full consent from the participant and this can only be achieved if the participant fully understands all the implications of the project. A good example from the first tranche of the fourth level generic skills module, which incorporated the expertise of Professor Sheila Greene, who specialises in research with children. See S. Green and D. Hogan, *Researching Children's Experience: Methods and Approaches*, (London: Sage, 2005).

and improving his/her ethical argumentation. Ultimately, what my experience of teaching ethics has emphasised is that, without a context of dialogue, ethics teaching does not go forward in a way that is useful to the researcher, or that is productive for the ongoing development of ethical responses to practical situations.

The ultimate pedagogical responsibility in ethics teaching is to enable the researcher to engage with an ongoing critical and constructive dialogue. This will be key for the classroom itself, for a dialogue with any given ethics oversight committee, and for the research context. In this way, it is essential to emphasise: the translative aspects of communication on ethics; the pedagaogical experience of constructive and inclusive classroom discussion; and the insights of practitioners within and outside the peer group.

Throughout my teaching, my practical enabling of the researcher has been improved by modelling an explicit pedagogy around valuing the input of the other. This involves a translative awareness of multiple disciplines and contexts, the critically dialogical nature of reasonable disagreement and the development of the best argument, and the need for ongoing discussions between ethical experts and practitioners. Ultimately the fact that this has been a process of improvement emphasises the pedagogical point I have made throughout this chapter, that the best teaching context for ethics, with AHSS researchers and beyond, is one of respectful dialogue: improving technical knowledge and the quality of arguments, and ultimately providing a model for a respectful and inclusive approach to ethical dilemmas in the future.

16 Conclusion

Linda Hogan

University of Dublin, Trinity College, Dublin, Ireland

Abstract

This essay reprises the major themes of the collection, arguing that the credibility of all research depends on our having confidence that it is being conducted with integrity.

Key Words

Inter-institutional collaboration, globalisation, common good

This e-book began life as a collaboration between a number of Irish universities under an initiative of the Irish government's Strategic Investment Fund, launched in 2006. The fund was directed towards support for innovation in higher education institutions, and focused particularly on developing new approaches to excellence within higher education and research.[1] Within this context, there was an explicit focus on the provision of graduate education, and specifically on training through the development of tailored generic skills modules. The focus on generic skills at graduate level has been tremendously successful, it has improved both the quality of research projects and has been an important feature in the future employability of graduates. Moreover, a second feature of the Strategic Investment Fund has been its concern for the benefits that accrue to students and academics alike through inter-institutional collaboration. The 'Research Ethics for Graduate Researchers' programme actively pursued this inter-institutional model, in both the development and the delivery of its graduate training programme.

It is now well understood that graduate researchers must be facilitated in the development of transferrable skills alongside discipline-specific knowledge and understanding. Moreover, the transferrable skills upon which graduate researchers now need to draw are manifold. This collection is focused on the skills and competencies in research ethics and proceeds from the conviction that all graduates should be both encouraged and required to develop such competencies, and that this ought to form an integral part of their graduate education. The teaching programme from which this collection derives was delivered a number of times

---

[1] Higher Education Authority, *Strategic Investment Fund*, Call for Proposals, July 2006.

Ethics for Graduate Researchers. DOI: http://dx.doi.org/10.1016/B978-0-12-416049-1.00016-7

between 2007 and 2009, and involved graduate researchers from across many disciplinary fields and from a number of different universities in Ireland, namely Trinity College Dublin (the host institution), University College Cork and the National University of Ireland, Galway. It had the explicit support of the respective Deans of Graduate Studies, who recognised the merits of encouraging early researchers to interrogate the objectives and progress of their research projects, not only in terms of the contribution to knowledge in their respective disciplines, but also in terms of the ethical dimensions of the research. The aim of the programme has been to ensure that the graduate researcher him/herself develops the skills of ethical reflection and argumentation so that he/she can think critically, and to articulate to his/ her peers the core values that are expressed and developed in the research process. Notwithstanding this concern with developing the skills of the individual graduate researcher, however, a strong theme of this programme has been the recognition that ethical reflection occurs in a social and scientific context and is inevitably shaped by the values, norms and principles that are embedded in such contexts.

Philosophers regularly remind us that human beings are 'ethical animals', that we constantly 'grade and evaluate, and compare and admire, and claim and justify' ... and that 'events endlessly adjust our sense of responsibility, our guilt and our shame, and our sense of our own worth and that of others'.[2] In the context of research ethics, this process of evaluation and assessment functions within a framework for ethical reasoning that has a number of important dimensions. Philosophers characterise these dimensions differently, although they broadly agree that ethical analysis inevitably involves a consideration of operative values at both the individual and the societal levels. In the research context, ethical reflection begins with the decision-maker, i.e. the individual who makes a choice. Each individual functions within a particular moral framework, although it may be more or less explicit. This moral framework is the basis on which a person can say what his or her core values are; why they are important; how he or she would go about choosing among competing moral values; and what he or she regards as the relative importance of one value, e.g. truthfulness, over and against another value or honouring one's professional commitments. The second relates to the systems and the social arrangements within which we make our decisions. The culture within which we function has a major impact on how we operate as individual agents, and in the research context, it can exert pressures, particularly on early and graduate researchers, to operate within its norms. A particular feature of the 'Research Ethics for Graduate Researchers' programme therefore has been its focus on personal moral responsibility, and its desire to equip graduate researchers to think through complex issues in a thoughtful and honest manner.

The collection began by suggesting that ethics must be seen as a core competency in research education, and argues that there can be no substitute for a process whereby the graduate researcher him/herself engages with, interrogates, and attempts to resolve the ethical issues that he/she encounters in the course of his/her research. In particular, it highlights the dangers associated with models of research ethics in which issues of compliance figure prominently and insists that ethics

---

[2] Blackburn, Simon, *Ethics, A Very Short Introduction*, (Oxford: Oxford University Press, 2000) 16.

cannot be subordinated to compliance, but rather must be understood to be integral to the practices of good research. In Section 1, the chapters focused on a number of different dimensions of this core competency. Maureen Junker-Kenny's essay discusses one of the fundamental dimensions of ethical reflection, namely the fact that it is grounded in the shared human capacity to generate value judgements based on our ability to be self-reflective. From this fundamental starting point, she goes on to assess the many different traditions of argumentation that are embedded in ethical discourse, drawing attention to the implications of these different approaches for graduate researchers as they consider how to resolve the complex ethical issues that arise in their research programmes. This spotlight on competency in ethical reflection is developed further by Alan Kelly with his focus on the design and development of research methods. Kelly discusses a host of practical considerations that have an impact on the ethical conduct of research, insisting that honesty is a fundamental value that cannot be compromised or undermined in any aspect of research. Kelly is very clear that inequalities of power in the research context can and do have a corrupting influence. He also highlights the pressures associated with results-driven research cultures which, he argues, can often undermine and challenge even the most responsible of researchers. Frank Gannon's discussion of the ethical integrity of the researcher also develops these precise issues, but focuses on the institutional context of the research laboratory. His conclusion reinforces the central theme of this first section, namely that individual researchers must be habituated in the norms of ethical research and, moreover, that the integrity of the research process depends on the maintenance of the highest of ethical standards throughout the process and in the institutional settings in which research is conducted.

In Section 2, the spotlight is on the existing parameters in which all research takes place, focusing particularly on the international documents that determine the conditions under which research occurs. There is a consideration of the processes whereby agreement on these conditions is reached, as well as discussions of occasions where there has been a failure to do so, as in the United Nations Declaration on Human Cloning in 2005 examined by Sigrid Graumann. Consideration is also given to discussions in which there have been compromise solutions between the different states in the European Union (EU) which leave the interpretations of guiding concepts and the decisions on which practices are to be permitted to national jurisdictions. The understanding underlying research governance in the EU is one in which there is a concern to formulate an ethical framework for research and to specify its limits, but to refrain from aiming for a uniform policy. In this way, the EU hands the task of democratic will formation back to civic debate in the member states. However, it is clear that a European public realm in which these national discourses can be encountered and compared, reassessed at home and brought back to contribute to a larger European consensus is only beginning to emerge.

The international conventions that formulate goals and limits of research differ in how legally binding they are. In contrast to Council of Europe Conventions and the Declaration of Helsinki (1964) with its subsequent revisions by the World Medical Association, United Nations conventions and declarations have the status of international law. Within the EU, however, principles such as the 'precautionary principle' have the status of a legal constraint. It marks one of the major differences in approach to new technologies in comparison with the United States, which refers to the human responsibility for 'stewardship' that does not carry any power to be legally asserted. In some chapters of this section, professional ethicists reflect on their work in the national and European ethics committees and on the advisory boards to which they, together with scientists and lawyers, contribute. As they work between different constituencies and with a range of different expectations, their role requires continuous self-reflection on how they realise their independence, on how they accomplish their task of representing different moral perspectives and traditions of thinking in a society, including religious ones, and on how they interpret the principles of the constitutions and the values articulated in European treaties. The process of relating these sources to new technologies under discussion is reflected in the articles of Dietmar Mieth and Hille Haker. While the goal in such committees is to achieve a balanced consensus, different methods have emerged for dealing with these ongoing differences. Just like countries have opted out of signing conventions, as has been the case with the 1997 Council of Europe Convention on Human Rights and Biomedicine, where Germany and the United Kingdom refused their signature for different reasons, so can individual members of an ethics committee signal differences in conclusions and points of view. They can also formulate a minority vote, which signals to civil society that further debate is needed. In a different context, when a procedure is adopted by the President's Council of the United States, there is a comparable process whereby the provisional character of these decisions can also be signalled. In this case, the Council not only documents the consensus that has been reached, but it also equally notes the sources from which the different members have come to their positions and argumentations they have employed and which may point to a way forward that acknowledges the 'work in progress' character of decisions on novel technologies.[3] In this way, they recognise that such decisions need to be open to revision and to re-assessment in the public sphere from which both ethicists and scientists have only been delegated.

The chapters in Section 3 showcase the experience and creativity with which professional researchers articulate ethical argumentation in practice in different domains; Desmond O'Neill in medicine, Sigrid Graumann regarding medical research, Deirdre Stritch in archaeology, Gladys Ganiel in social scientific action research and Elizabeth Nixon in psychology. The motivation and ability to reach across disciplines to integrate other perspectives requires a degree of commitment and even imaginative risk taking which are not without reward. A sound ethical 'proofing' of a research project in its inception and execution protects the researcher from the consequences of breaches of ethics codes, professional norms and international commitments, which is important as a first step. More importantly, it also directs research goals towards a better ultimate 'fit' and consequently wider applicability, as the outcomes will better cohere with social, ethical and

---

[3] The President's Council on Bioethics, *Human Cloning and Human Dignity* (July 2002). This report and others are available at www.bioethics.gov.

institutional mandates to respect the dignity and integrity of the human person, the societies in which they live, as well as the sustainability of the natural world.

The responsibility for sound ethical practice in research is there at all levels and stages of the process, with the individual researcher, their supervisors and teachers, and with the professional bodies that oversee standards nationally and internationally. These skills take time to develop and need to be fostered in supportive working and teaching environments with skilled facilitation, as Amy Daughton tells us in her lessons from the ethics classroom. If we are to learn anything from the experience of medical ethics curricula and teaching, as Desmond O'Neill reminds us, it is that initiatives in facilitating ethics training at graduate level need not just ethics teachers but the support of faculty at all levels, and most significantly, the fostering of a research culture that engages actively with the ethics literature within and between disciplines and values integration, inter-disciplinarity, ongoing interpretation and challenging critique. For many early-career researchers gaining skills in ethics, no more than statistics, or technology transfer, may appear an arduous sojourn on the path to professionalisation. This collection hopes to have provided resources for those first steps in what will be a lifetime of intellectually vibrant, productive and socially responsive work within and beyond the researchers' chosen discipline.

In Section 4, the focus is on emerging debates and future prospects, and this, inevitably, has many different dimensions. Of course, new developments in science and technology throw up new ethical dilemmas, and raise fundamental questions about how human beings understand themselves and their world. This is expertly discussed by Hille Haker. In addition, new methodologies and new modes of working also have a major impact on the emerging issues in research ethics, as Cathriona Russell and Amy Daughton illustrate. However, it is the changed social context in which research is now conducted that has the most critical role in determining the future shape of research, and therefore the most significant impact on the ethical issues embedded therein. In this regard, issues of social justice and the distribution of the benefits of research have come sharply into relief. In the globalised context in which scientific and technological research take place, the challenges associated with the market-driven, utilitarian culture in which it is often embedded are of legitimate concern for many citizens. Indeed, as the essays in this section illustrate, such challenges are ultimately about ensuring that the objectives, conduct and outcomes of research are pursued in service of the common good.

As they embark on their research careers, graduate researchers must be equipped to deal with the ethical issues that will inevitably arise in the course of their research. They must be educated in such a way that they will be capable of resisting many pressures associated with the contemporary context in which research is conducted and must be able to discern the limitations and blind spots of existing research norms and practices. Moreover, they must be able to articulate and defend their own ethical positions and to pursue their own research with integrity. The form of education and training that is advocated, therefore, is one that encourages graduate researchers to interrogate the norms of their disciplines, to acknowledge the complexities of the conflicts that they may encounter in their research, to be clear-sighted about the pressures under which they may come and to recognise that certain moral dilemmas may not always be amenable to clear-cut resolutions. Aristotle reminds us that ethics is not an exact science, and that one should not expect the same degree of certitude from morality as one might expect from other disciplines.[4] Research ethics training must enable graduate researchers to live with this complexity and uncertainty, while also ensuring that they have the requisite skills to conduct their research ethically. The credibility of all research ultimately depends on our having confidence that it has been conducted with integrity.

[4] Aristotle, *Nicomachean Ethics*, translated by Thomson, J., (Harmondsworth: Penguin, 1976), 1.3, 1−4, 1094b.

Printed in the United States
By Bookmasters